Clinical and Electrophysiologic Management of Syncope

Editors

ANTONIO RAVIELE
ANDREA NATALE

CARDIOLOGY CLINICS

www.cardiology.theclinics.com

Consulting Editors
ROSARIO FREEMAN
JORDAN M. PRUTKIN
DAVID M. SHAVELLE
AUDREY H. WU

August 2015 • Volume 33 • Number 3

ELSEVIER

1600 John F. Kennedy Boulevard • Suite 1800 • Philadelphia, Pennsylvania, 19103-2899

http://www.theclinics.com

CARDIOLOGY CLINICS Volume 33, Number 3
August 2015 ISSN 0733-8651, ISBN-13: 978-0-323-39328-7

Editor: Adrianne Brigido
Developmental Editor: Susan Showalter

Cardiology Clinics (ISSN 0733-8651) is published quarterly by Elsevier Inc., 360 Park Avenue South, New York, NY 10010-1710. Months of issue are February, May, August, and November. Business and Editorial Offices: 1600 John F. Kennedy Blvd., Ste. 1800, Philadelphia, PA 19103-2899. Customer Service Office: 3251 Riverport Lane, Maryland Heights, MO 63043. Periodicals post-age paid at New York, NY and additional mailing offices. Subscription prices are $320.00 per year for US individuals, $530.00 per year for US institutions, $155.00 per year for US students and residents, $390.00 per year for Canadian individuals, $665.00 per year for Canadian institutions, $455.00 per year for international individuals, $665.00 per year for international institutions and $220.00 per year for Canadian and international students/residents. To receive student/resident rate, orders must be accompanied by name of affiliated institution, data of term, and the *signature* of program/residency coordinator on institution letterhead. Orders will be billed at individual rate until proof of status is received. Foreign air speed delivery is included in all *Clinics* subscription prices. All prices are subject to change without notice. **POSTMASTER:** Send address changes to *Cardiology Clinics*, Elsevier Health Sciences Division, Subscription Customer Service, 3251 Riverport Lane, Maryland Heights, MO 63043. **Customer Service: 1-800-654-2452 (U.S. and Canada); 314-447-8871 (outside U.S. and Canada). Fax: 314-447-8029. E-mail: journalscustomerservice-usa@ elsevier.com (for print support); journalsonlinesupport-usa@elsevier.com (for online support).**

Reprints. For copies of 100 or more, of articles in this publication, please contact the Commercial Reprints Department, Elsevier Inc., 360 Park Avenue South, New York, NY 10010-1710. Tel.: 212-633-3874; Fax: 212-633-3820; E-mail: reprints@elsevier.com.

Cardiology Clinics is also published in Spanish by McGraw-Hill Interamericana Editores S. A., P.O. Box 5-237, 06500, Mexico D. F., Mexico; in Portuguese by Reichmann and Alfonso Editores Rio de Janeiro, Brazil; and in Greek by Dimitrios P. Lagos, 8 Pondon Street, GR115-28 Ilissia, Greece.

Cardiology Clinics is covered in *MEDLINE/PubMed (Index Medicus), Excerpta Medica, The Cumulative Index to Nursing and Allied Health Literature* (CINAHL).

Contributors

EDITORIAL BOARD

ROSARIO FREEMAN, MD, MS, FACC
Associate Professor of Medicine; Director, Coronary Care Unit; Director, Echocardiography Laboratory, University of Washington Medical Center, Seattle, Washington

JORDAN M. PRUTKIN, MD, MHS, FHRS
Assistant Professor of Medicine, Division of Cardiology/Electrophysiology, University of Washington Medical Center, Seattle, Washington

DAVID M. SHAVELLE, MD, FACC, FSCAI
Associate Professor, Keck School of Medicine; Director, General Cardiovascular Fellowship Program; Director, Cardiac Catheterization Laboratory, Los Angeles County + USC Medical Center; Division of Cardiovascular Medicine, University of Southern California, Los Angeles, California

AUDREY H. WU, MD
Assistant Professor, Internal Medicine, University of Michigan, Ann Arbor, Michigan

EDITORS

ANTONIO RAVIELE, MD, FESC, FHRS
ALFA - ALliance to Fight Atrial fibrillation, Mestre-Venice, Italy

ANDREA NATALE, MD, FACC, FHRS
Executive Medical Director, Texas Cardiac Arrhythmia Institute, St David's Medical Center, Austin, Texas; Consulting Professor, Division of Cardiology, Stanford University, Palo Alto, California; Adjunct Professor of Medicine, Heart and Vascular Center, Case Western Reserve University, Cleveland, Ohio; Director, Interventional Electrophysiology, Scripps Clinic, San Diego, California; Senior Clinical Director, EP Services, California Pacific Medical Center, San Francisco, California

AUTHORS

ARNON ADLER, MD
Sackler School of Medicine, Tel Aviv Medical Center, Tel Aviv University, Israel

MEHMET AKKAYA, MD
Cardiovascular Division, Department of Medicine, Cardiac Arrhythmia Center, University of Minnesota Medical School, Minneapolis, Minnesota

PAOLO ALBONI
Syncope Unit, Section of Cardiology, Department of Medicine, Ospedale Privato Quisisana, Ferrara, Italy

ANGELO BARTOLETTI, MD
Cardiology Division, Syncope Centre, San Giovanni di Dio Hospital, Florence, Italy

CRISTINA BASSO, MD, PhD
Cardiovascular Pathology, Department
of Cardiac, Thoracic and Vascular
Sciences, University of Padova, Padova,
Italy

**DAVID G. BENDITT, MD, FACC, FRCPC,
FHRS**
Professor of Medicine, Cardiovascular
Division, Department of Medicine; Co-Director,
Cardiac Arrhythmia Center, University of
Minnesota Medical Center, University of
Minnesota Medical School, Minneapolis,
Minnesota

JEAN-JACQUES BLANC, MD
Professor of Cardiology, Department of Clinical
Research, Université de Bretagne Occidentale,
Brest, France

MICHELE BRIGNOLE, MD, FESC
Department of Cardiology, Arrhythmologic
Center, Lavagna, Italy

LISA BYRNE, RGN, Postgrad Dip Crit Care
School of Medicine, Trinity College Dublin,
Health Sciences Institute, St James's Hospital,
Dublin, Ireland

HUGH CALKINS, MD
Division of Cardiology, The Johns Hopkins
Hospital, Johns Hopkins University, Baltimore,
Maryland

PAOLA COPPOLA
Syncope Unit, Section of Cardiology,
Department of Medicine, Ospedale Privato
Quisisana, Ferrara, Italy

DOMENICO CORRADO, MD, PhD
Professor of Cardiovascular Medicine,
Arrhythmogenic Inherited Cardiomyopathy
Unit, Department of Cardiac, Thoracic and
Vascular Sciences, University of Padova
Medical School, Padova, Italy

JEAN-CLAUDE DEHARO, MD, FESC
Department of Cardiology, Timone University
Hospital, Marseille, France

OANA DICKINSON, MD
Cardiovascular Division, Department of
Medicine, Cardiac Arrhythmia Center,
University of Minnesota Medical School,
Minneapolis, Minnesota

FRANCO GIADA, MD
Cardiovascular Rehabilitation and Sports
Medicine Service, Cardiovascular Department,
PF Calvi Hospital, Noale, Venice, Italy

REGIS GUIEU, MD
Laboratory of Biochemistry and Molecular
Biology, Timone University Hospital,
Unité Mixte de Recherche Ministere de la
Defense, Aix Marseille Université, Marseille,
France

JUAN C. GUZMAN, MD, MSc, FRCPC
Syncope and Autonomic Disorder Unit,
Cardiology Division; Assistant Professor,
Department of Medicine, McMaster University,
Hamilton, Ontario, Canada

KHALIL KANJWAL, MD
Clinical Cardiac Electrophysiology Fellow,
Section of Cardiac Electrophysiology,
Johns Hopkins University, Baltimore,
Maryland

**ROSE ANNE KENNY, MD, FRCPI, FRCP,
FRCPE, FTCD**
School of Medicine, Trinity College Dublin,
Health Sciences Institute, St James's Hospital,
Dublin, Ireland

IAIN G. MATTHEWS, MBChB, MRCP
British Heart Foundation Fellow, Institute for
Ageing and Health, Newcastle University,
Newcastle upon Tyne, United Kingdom

SUNEET MITTAL, MD, FACC, FHRS
Director, Electrophysiology, Arrhythmia
Institute, Valley Health System, Ridgewood,
New Jersey and New York, New York

**CARLOS A. MORILLO, MD, FRCPC, FACC,
FESC, FHRS**
Director, Syncope and Autonomic Disorder
Unit, Cardiology Division; Professor,
Department of Medicine, McMaster University,
Hamilton, Ontario, Canada

ANGEL MOYA, MD, PhD
Cardiology Service, Unitat Arítmies, Hospital
Universitari Vall d'Hebrón, Universitat
Autónoma de Barcelona, Barcelona, Spain

BRIAN OLSHANSKY, MD
Professor Emeritus, University of Iowa
Hospitals, Iowa City, Iowa

STEVE W. PARRY, MBBS, MRCP, PhD
Senior Lecturer and Consultant Physician, Institute for Ageing and Health, Newcastle University; Falls and Syncope Service, Royal Victoria Infirmary, Newcastle upon Tyne, United Kingdom

MARK PREMINGER, MD
Arrhythmia Institute, Valley Health System, Ridgewood, New Jersey and New York, New York

VENKATA KRISHNA PUPPALA, MD, MPH
Hospitalist, St Joseph Hospital, Healtheast Care System, St Paul; Cardiac Arrhythmia Center, University of Minnesota Medical School, Minneapolis, Minnesota

CIARA RICE, RGN, BNS, Grad Dip Crit Care
School of Medicine, Trinity College Dublin, Health Sciences Institute, St James's Hospital, Dublin, Ireland

ROBERT SHELDON, MD, PhD
Professor of Cardiac Sciences, Medicine, and Medical Genetics, Libin Cardiovascular Institute of Alberta, University of Calgary, Calgary, Alberta, Canada

NICOLA STUCCI, MD
Syncope Unit, Section of Cardiology, Department of Medicine, Ospedale Privato Quisisana, Ferrara, Italy

RENEE M. SULLIVAN, MD
Assistant Professor of Medicine, University of Missouri, Columbia, Missouri

RICHARD SUTTON, DSc
Professor Emeritus of Clinical Cardiology, Imperial College, London, United Kingdom

GAETANO THIENE, MD
Cardiovascular Pathology, Department of Cardiac, Thoracic and Vascular Sciences, University of Padova, Padova, Italy

ISABEL A.E. TRESHAM, MBBS, MRCP
Consultant Geriatrician, Falls and Syncope Service, Royal Victoria Infirmary, Newcastle upon Tyne, United Kingdom

GIULIA VETTOR, MD
Department of Cardiac, Thoracic and Vascular Sciences, University of Padova Medical School, Padova, Italy

SAMI VISKIN, MD
Sackler School of Medicine, Tel Aviv Medical Center, Tel Aviv University, Israel

ALESSANDRO ZORZI, MD
Department of Cardiac, Thoracic and Vascular Sciences, University of Padova Medical School, Padova, Italy

Contents

> With the advent of implantable loop recorders capable of prolonged electrocardiographic monitoring, and following studies demonstrating the benefit of implantable cardioverter-defibrillator therapy in subgroups of patients with structural heart disease and depressed left ventricular function, the role of invasive cardiac electrophysiologic (EP) studies in patients with unexplained syncope has been substantially reduced. Nonetheless, in select high-risk patients presenting with unexplained syncope, EP studies still play an important role in identifying a diagnosis in these patients and assessing long-term risk of mortality.

> Convulsive syncope is a common cause of misdiagnosis in patients who present with a transient loss of consciousness. This misdiagnosis contributes significantly to the numbers of patients with a questionable diagnosis of epilepsy, and to those with apparently drug-resistant epilepsy. The most important step to an accurate diagnosis is a fastidious history. Inducing syncope with tilt table testing and documenting heart rate changes during events with implantable loop recorders have proved to be useful. These suggest the need for closer and ongoing collaboration among neurologists and cardiologists to provide optimal care for patients with the diagnostic dilemma of syncope or epileptic seizures.

> Important goals in the initial evaluation of patients with transient loss of consciousness include determining whether the episode was syncope and choosing the venue for subsequent care. Patients who have high short-term risk of adverse outcomes need prompt hospitalization for diagnosis and/or treatment, whereas others may be safely referred for outpatient evaluation. This article summarizes the most important available risk assessment studies and points out key differences among the existing recommendations. Current risk stratification methods cannot replace critical assessment by an experienced physician, but they do provide much needed guidance and offer direction for future risk stratification consensus development.

> Most strategies for managing syncope in children reflect data from studies involving the adult population. In the future, there will be a great need for studies in children and adolescents suffering from recurrent syncope. To date, there has been no Food and Drug Administration–approved therapy for neurocardiogenic syncope (NCS), the most common cause of syncope in both adults and children. None of the clinical trials of pharmacotherapy in NCS has shown benefit over placebo. NCS should be considered a chronic condition, and the aim of the therapy should be to decrease recurrence of syncope rather than to completely eliminate it.

Iain G. Matthews, Isabel A.E. Tresham, and Steve W. Parry

Syncope in the older person carries a high morbidity, mortality, and health economic burden. While neurally mediated disorders and orthostatic hypotension account for the majority of syncopal episodes in this age group, about a third of causes are cardiac, predominantly arrhythmic. Clinicians need to be aware of the management of potential comorbid issues such as osteoporosis and cognitive impairment and if not in a position to act on them, ensure that appropriate specialist help is sought. Further work is needed to understand the pathophysiology and hence the management of syncope in the older patient, with ongoing studies helping to tease out some of the treatment controversies.

Giulia Vettor, Alessandro Zorzi, Cristina Basso, Gaetano Thiene, and Domenico Corrado

Clinical evaluation of syncope in the athlete remains a challenge. Although benign mechanisms predominate, syncope may be arrhythmic and precede sudden cardiac death (SCD). Exercise-induced syncope should be regarded as an important alarming symptom of an underlying cardiac disease predisposing to arrhythmic cardiac arrest. All athletes with syncope require a focused and detailed workup for underlying cardiac causes, either structural or electrical. A major aim is to identify athletes at risk and to protect them from SCD. Athletes with potentially life-threatening etiologies of syncope should be restricted from competitive sports.

Arnon Adler and Sami Viskin

Since the discovery of the first mutation causing long QT syndrome (LQTS) in 1995, the field of hereditary arrhythmogenic syndromes has expanded greatly. Today, these syndromes include LQTS, Brugada syndrome, catecholaminergic polymorphic ventricular tachycardia, and short QT syndrome. There is also evidence suggesting that the newly described malignant early repolarization syndrome also has a genetic cause.

Michele Brignole, Jean-Claude Deharo, and Regis Guieu

Syncope due to idiopathic AV block is characterized by: 1) ECG documentation (usually by means of prolonged ECG monitoring) of paroxysmal complete AV block with one or multiple consecutive pauses, without P-P cycle lengthening or PR interval prolongation, not triggered by atrial or ventricular premature beats nor by rate variations; 2) long history of recurrent syncope without prodromes; 3) absence of cardiac and ECG abnormalities; 4) absence of progression to persistent forms of AV block; 5) efficacy of cardiac pacing therapy. The patients affected by idiopathic AV block have low baseline adenosine plasma level (APL) values and show an increased susceptibility to exogenous adenosine. The APL value of patients with idiopathic AV block is much lower than that of patients affected by vasovagal syncope, who have high adenosine values.

CARDIOLOGY CLINICS

THE CLINICS ARE AVAILABLE ONLINE!
Access your subscription at:
www.theclinics.com

Syncope: Definition, Epidemiology, and Classification

Jean-Jacques Blanc, MD

KEYWORDS

- Syncope • Transient loss of consciousness • Epidemiology • Cerebral hypoperfusion

KEY POINTS

- During the last 2 decades, major progress has been made in syncope as a consequence of the acceptance of a clear definition of this symptom.
- The strategy for diagnosis of syncope includes the following criteria: transient loss of consciousness must be established; rapid onset and short duration of transient loss of consciousness must be established; recovery must be "complete and spontaneous"; and head trauma and epilepsy must be ruled out.
- Awareness of this diagnostic strategy will help to avoid useless, costly, and painful examinations.

INTRODUCTION

For decades, in fact since the origin of medicine, syncope has not drawn much attention. For neurologists it was just a manifestation of epilepsy, for cardiologists, a manifestation of paroxysmal atrioventricular (AV) block, and for most physicians, a benign and not very positive expression of "weakness" (swoon, blackout, fainting). Interest in syncope arose in the mid-1980s when Kapoor and colleagues[1,2] published some articles in which, for the first time, syncope was not considered through the scope of one specialty but as a self-determining symptom not directed by an immediate diagnosis or therapy. A second major input occurred almost at the same time when Kenny and colleagues[3] reported the effectiveness of head up tilt test to reproduce syncope in patients with previous spontaneous episodes of loss of consciousness. These preliminary reports stimulated publications of many new findings on the subject, mostly by cardiologists, and finally in the late 1990s, syncope was considered sufficiently important in the area of cardiology to justify guidelines and recommendations directed by the European Society of Cardiology (ESC). A task force was therefore nominated and proposed the first ever published comprehensive document on syncope in 2001.[4] A complete revision of this first issue was published in 2009.[5] The present review of the definition, epidemiology, and classification of syncope makes ample reference to this latter document.

DEFINITION

One of the major contributions of the 2001 document and the subsequent 2009 version of the ESC guidelines is certain to have generated a precise and widely accepted definition of syncope.[4,5] Before that time, there was no widely accepted definition of syncope, which certainly helped explain the lack of interest in syncope observed for many years: everyone had their own definition, giving rise to conflicting and nonreproducible results and diagnosis.

In the 2009 version of the ESC guidelines,[5] syncope is defined as "a transient loss of consciousness (TLOC) due to transient global cerebral hypoperfusion characterized by rapid onset, short duration, and spontaneous complete recovery."

To satisfy this definition and to be classified as having syncope, a patient suspected of having this symptom must meet the following criteria: TLOC

This article originally appeared in Cardiac Electrophysiology Clinics, Volume 5, Issue 4, December 2013.
Disclosure: The author has nothing to disclose.
Department of Clinical Research, Université de Bretagne Occidentale, 2 rue de kerglas, Brest 29200, France
E-mail address: jjacques@jjgblanc.fr

Cardiol Clin 33 (2015) 341–345
http://dx.doi.org/10.1016/j.ccl.2015.04.001

cardiology.theclinics.com

must be established; rapid onset and short duration of TLOC must be established; recovery must be "complete and spontaneous"; and head trauma and epilepsy must be ruled out.

Transient Loss of Consciousness

The first mandatory step is to establish that the patient had a TLOC. This information is easily obtained by questioning patients and/or eyewitnesses. However, some studies have recently demonstrated that almost 50% of patients during head up tilt test, whatever their age but predominantly older patients, denied any TLOC, although the loss of consciousness was confirmed by nurses and/or doctors.[6] In patients in whom TLOC remains uncertain, occurrence of loss of postural tone is a strong argument to consider that TLOC has really occurred.

In the absence of TLOC, syncope can be definitively excluded and an alternative diagnosis should be sought, such as falls, dizziness, cataplexy, vertigo, psychogenic pseudo-TLOC, or transient ischemic attack (TIA) of carotid origin. The latter diagnosis is frequently and erroneously considered to be the cause of syncope, but as stated by Van Dijk "in clinical practice TIA is characterized by focal neurological signs without TLOC, whereas syncope is characterized by TLOC without focal neurological signs" (Van Dijk, personal communication, 2010). How many useless, time-consuming, and expensive computed tomographic scans or even magnetic resonance images would have been avoided if this sentence had been displayed in every emergency room?

Is TLOC Characterized by Rapid Onset and Short Duration?

Once the occurrence of TLOC has been established, the next step is to answer to the following question: "Was TLOC characterized by rapid onset and short duration"? The term "rapid onset" is not very accurate because it can mean a few seconds or a few minutes. This ambiguity is certainly a minor limitation of the definition, but "rapid" could infer that the delay between the beginning of symptoms and TLOC is between a few seconds to less than 1 minute. The same reproach can be directed at the term "short duration." In that case, however, the overlap between "short" or "long" does not seem significant and it could be assumed that the term "short" excludes TLOC lasting more than a few minutes. When a TLOC exceeds this delay, it is not syncope but coma, definite stroke, or intoxication (alcohol, drugs). A common error leading to underestimate the real cause is to consider that syncope could

be the consequence of hypoglycemia; however, hypoglycemia induces coma and not syncope.

Recovery

The third requirement before considering TLOC as a syncope is to establish that "recovery has been complete and spontaneous." This sentence has been added to exclude from the scope of syncope patients who had sudden death consecutive to malignant ventricular arrhythmias,[7] aborted as a result of resuscitation maneuvers and particularly external shocks. In that case the diagnostic strategy is totally different. However, that does mean, of course, that malignant ventricular arrhythmias when they are paroxysmal have to be excluded from the causes of syncope.

Rule Out Head Trauma and Epilepsy

Finally, even if the 3 preceding requirements have been satisfied, one is still missing to definitely consider a TLOC as syncope: "due to transient global cerebral hypoperfusion." This statement is certainly the most original contribution of the ESC definition but also the most crucial. The first 3 requisites included in the definition could also apply to 2 other conditions that are not syncope: TLOC due to head trauma and epilepsy. Without this addition, the 2 previous situations are considered syncope, which obviously could not be the case according to the experts selected in the task force of the ESC.[5]

For head trauma, TLOC is caused by cerebral concussion and not by global cerebral hypoperfusion. It is obviously diagnosed simply by questioning the patient. A rare situation could, however, be confusing: syncope could provoke head trauma as a consequence of loss of postural tone and fall. In this situation when patients are unable to describe which came first, trauma or TLOC, syncope should be consider the cause,[8] unless the alternative was proved.

Epilepsy is the result of cerebral neuronal discharge and not of global cerebral hypoperfusion. There are no simple methods to differentiate these 2 mechanisms: electroencephalography could be diagnostic when demonstrating clear abnormalities. However, it is not always indicative, particularly when the delay between the episode and the examination exceeds some days. Measurement of cerebral blood flow is only feasible in dedicated laboratories. Fortunately, syncope and epilepsy are sufficiently typical to be easily differentiated in most instances by questioning of the patient and/or witnesses.[9] If doubt persists, a multidisciplinary discussion is definitely indicated.

EPIDEMIOLOGY

Syncope is a common symptom[10] that affects at least half of human beings during their lifetime, although it is considered to be very uncommon among other vertebrates.[11,12] The first episode occurs generally in teenagers around the age of 15.[13,14] In Amsterdam, 39% of medical students reported syncope during their life, with a more frequent incidence among women.[14] In this age group vasovagal syncope is almost the exclusive cause of syncope.[15] There is a second peak after the age of 65. In the Framingham study the incidence of syncope shows a sharp rise after the age of 70 years, from 5.7 events per 1000 person-years in men aged 60 to 69, to 11.1 in men aged 70 to 79.[15,16] In this population, causes are more varied. For some, it is the re-emergence of vasovagal syncope, which first appears at a younger age; for others, it is the first manifestation of cardiac disorders.

Many studies report a remarkably constant frequency of syncope in European emergency departments, with an incidence of approximately 1% of all attendances.[17–23] However, it is noteworthy that only a minority of patients with syncope in the general population seek medical advice. In the Framingham offspring study, 44% of the participants (mean age 51 years) with an episode of loss of consciousness (not only syncope due to a different definition than used by the ESC) reported that they did not present in any clinical setting[16] and the proportion is much higher in the younger population.[13,15] Finally, in the Netherlands it seems that only approximately half of the patients with fainting visited their general practitioner, and less than 5% went to emergency departments.[15,24]

CLASSIFICATION

Syncope has multiple causes, which are generally cataloged under different subheadings, such as cardiac causes, orthostatic hypotension, and so forth. This presentation is still produced in all documents on syncope. However, it seems more appropriate to attempt to classify causes of syncope according to the underlying mechanism leading to TLOC. As mentioned in the definition section, syncope is the consequence of transient global cerebral hypoperfusion, but this hypoperfusion may be due to different mechanisms.

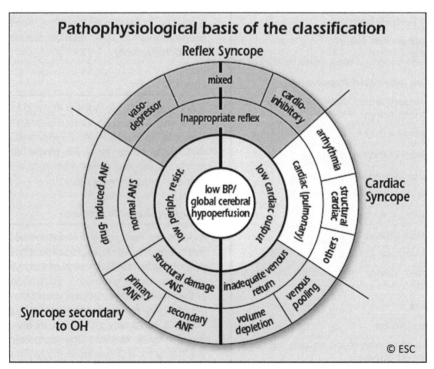

Fig. 1. Correlation between mechanisms of low global cerebral blood flow and main causes of syncope. ANF, autonomic nervous failure; ANS, autonomic nervous system; BP, blood pressure; low periph. resist., low peripheral resistance; OH, orthostatic hypotension. (*From* Moya A, Sutton R, Ammirati F, et al. The Task Force for the Diagnosis and Management of Syncope of the European Society of Cardiology (ESC). Guidelines for the diagnosis and management of syncope (version 2009). Eur Heart J 2009;30:2637; with permission. Copyright © ESC.)

Box 1
Classification of the main causes of syncope

Reflex syncope

Vasovagal:

  Mediated by emotion (pain, fear, instrumentation, blood)

Situational:

  Orthostatic position

  Cough, sneeze

  Gastrointestinal stimulation (swallow, defecation, postprandial)

  Micturition

  After intense exercise

  Miscellaneous (laugh, brass instrument playing, weight-lifting)

Carotid sinus syndrome

Atypical forms:

  Without evident triggers and/or atypical presentation

Syncope due to orthostatic hypotension

Primary autonomic failure

  Pure autonomic failure, multiple system atrophy, Parkinson disease with autonomic failure, Lewy body dementia

Secondary autonomic failure

  Diabetes, amyloidosis, uremia, spinal cord injuries

Drug-induced orthostatic hypotension

  Alcohol, vasodilators, diuretics, antidepressant, phenothiazines

Volume depletion

  Hemorrhage, vomiting, diarrhea

Cardiovascular syncope

Arrhythmias

  Bradycardia

    Sinus node disease

    Atrioventricular conduction system disease

    Implanted device malfunction or drug-induced

  Tachycardia

    Supraventricular

    Ventricular, whatever the underlying cause (drug, heart disease)

Structural heart disease

  Valvular disease, myocardial ischemia, tumors, hypertrophic cardiomyopathy, tamponade, prosthetic valve dysfunction

Miscellaneous

  Pulmonary embolism or hypertension, aortic dissection

Adapted from Moya A, Sutton R, Ammirati F, et al. The Task Force for the Diagnosis and Management of Syncope of the European Society of Cardiology (ESC). Guidelines for the diagnosis and management of syncope (version 2009). Eur Heart J 2009;30:2636; with permission.

PATHOPHYSIOLOGY

A decrease in global cerebral blood flow forms the basis of pathophysiology for syncope. An abrupt cessation of cerebral blood flow for less than 10 seconds in a supine subject has been shown to cause complete loss of consciousness. The best example is represented by paroxysmal AV block. However, even in the presence of normal cardiac electrical activity, experience from tilt testing has showed that a decrease in systolic blood pressure (BP) at or below 60 mm Hg is associated with syncope.[25] Systolic BP is the resultant of cardiac output (CO) and total peripheral vascular resistance; therefore, a decrease in one of these 2 components may provoke syncope. In fact, a combination of the 2 mechanisms is often present, even if their relative contributions may vary considerably.

Low CO

A decrease in CO important enough to induce syncope can be due to inappropriate reflex, as, for example, in carotid sinus syndrome, cardiac arrhythmias, paroxysmal AV block, severe tachycardia, or cardiac disease such as aortic stenosis or inadequate venous return.

Low Peripheral Resistance

A decrease in peripheral resistance can be due to inappropriate reflex, as, for example, in vasovagal syncope, structural damage of the autonomic nervous system (for example in Parkinson disease), or in the absence of structural damage of autonomic nervous system by drugs such as diuretics.

Fig. 1, originally published in the ESC guidelines,[5] nicely depicts the correlation between mechanisms of a decrease in cerebral blood flow and causes of syncope with low BP/global cerebral hypoperfusion at the center, adjacent to low or inadequate peripheral resistance and low CO.

Box 1 summarizes the main causes of syncope as usually reported in a catalog form.

SUMMARY

Major progress has been made during the last 2 decades on the different aspects of syncope. Most of the progress is the consequence of the acceptance of a clear definition of what is and what is not syncope. However, although this definition is widely accepted by physicians who are "specialists" in syncope, it still remains unknown or challenged by many other physicians. This lack of awareness leads to multiple useless, costly, and painful examinations. The next step is therefore to disseminate the knowledge of this definition and the strategy for diagnosis of syncope.

REFERENCES

1. Kapoor WN, Karpf M, Maher Y, et al. Syncope of unknown origin. The need for a more cost-effective approach to its diagnosis evaluation. JAMA 1982; 247:2687–91.
2. Kapoor WN, Karpf M, Wieand S, et al. A prospective evaluation and follow-up of patients with syncope. N Engl J Med 1983;309:197–204.
3. Kenny RA, Ingram A, Bayliss J, et al. Head-up tilt: a useful test for investigating unexplained syncope. Lancet 1986;1:1352–5.
4. Brignole M, Alboni P, Benditt D, et al. Guidelines on management (diagnosis and treatment) of syncope. Eur Heart J 2001;22:1256–306.
5. Moya A, Sutton R, Ammirati F, et al, The Task Force for the Diagnosis and Management of Syncope of the European Society of Cardiology (ESC). Guidelines for the diagnosis and management of syncope (version 2009). Eur Heart J 2009;30:2631–71.
6. O'Dwyer C, Bennett K, Langan Y, et al. Amnesia for loss of consciousness is common in vasovagal syncope. Europace 2011;13:1040–5.
7. Nair K, Umapathy K, Downar E, et al. Aborted sudden death from sustained ventricular fibrillation. Heart Rhythm 2008;8:1198–2005.
8. Bartoletti A, Fabiani P, Bagnoli L, et al. Physical injuries caused by a transient loss of consciousness: main clinical characteristics of patients and diagnostic contribution of carotid sinus massage. Eur Heart J 2008;29:618–24.
9. Sheldon R, Rose S, Ritchie D, et al. Historical criteria that distinguish syncope from seizures. J Am Coll Cardiol 2002;40:142–8.
10. Ganzeboom KS, Mairuhu G, Reitsma JB, et al. Lifetime cumulative incidence of syncope in the general population: a study of 549 Dutch subjects aged 35–60 years. J Cardiovasc Electrophysiol 2006;17: 1172–6.
11. Alboni P, Alboni M, Bertolelle G. The origin of vasovagal syncope: to protect the heart or to escape predation? Clin Auton Res 2008;18:170–8.
12. Van Dijk JG. Fainting in animals. Clin Auton Res 2003;13:247–55.
13. Serletis A, Rose S, Sheldon AG, et al. Vasovagal syncope in medical students and their first-degree relatives. Eur Heart J 2006;27:1965–70.
14. Ganzeboom KS, Colman N, Reitsma JB, et al. Prevalence and triggers of syncope in medical students. Am J Cardiol 2003;91:1006–8.
15. Colman N, Nahm K, Ganzeboom KS, et al. Epidemiology of reflex syncope. Clin Auton Res 2004; 14:i9–17.
16. Soteriades ES, Evans JC, Larson MG, et al. Incidence and prognosis of syncope. N Engl J Med 2002;347:878–85.
17. Ammirati F, Colivicchi F, Santini M. Diagnosing syncope in clinical practice. Implementation of a simplified diagnostic algorithm in a multicentre prospective trial—the OESIL 2 study (Osservatorio Epidemiologico della Sincope nel Lazio). Eur Heart J 2000;21:935–40.
18. Blanc JJ, L'Her C, Touiza A, et al. Prospective evaluation and outcome of patients admitted for syncope over a 1 year period. Eur Heart J 2002;23: 815–20.
19. Blanc JJ, L'Her C, Gosselin G, et al. Prospective evaluation of an educational programme for physicians involved in the management of syncope. Europace 2005;7:400–6.
20. Brignole M, Menozzi C, Bartoletti A, et al. A new management of syncope: prospective systematic guideline-based evaluation of patients referred urgently to general hospitals. Eur Heart J 2006;27: 76–82.
21. Crane SD. Risk stratification of patients with syncope in an accident and emergency department. Emerg Med J 2002;19:23–7.
22. Disertori M, Brignole M, Menozzi C, et al. Management of patients with syncope referred urgently to general hospitals. Europace 2003;5:283–91.
23. Sarasin FP, Louis-Simonet M, Carballo D, et al. Prospective evaluation of patients with syncope: a population-based study. Am J Med 2001;111: 177–84.
24. Olde Nordkamp LA, van Dijk N, Ganzeboom KS, et al. Syncope prevalence in the ED compared to that in the general practice and population: a strong selection process. Am J Emerg Med 2009; 27:271–9.
25. Stephenson J. Fits and faints. Oxford (England): Blackwell Scientific Publications; 1990. p. 41–57.

Initial Clinical Evaluation

Paolo Alboni*, Paola Coppola, Nicola Stucci, MD

KEYWORDS

- Cataplexy • Epilepsy • Fall • Psychogenic pseudosyncope • Syncope • Transient ischemic attack

KEY POINTS

- Syncope is a transient loss of consciousness (LOC) caused by global cerebral hypoperfusion; unfortunately, there are no signs or symptoms specific for this hypoperfusion.
- The initial evaluation of patients with transient LOC comprises a detailed medical history, physical examination, and 12-lead electrocardiogram.
- Because there are many causes of syncopal and nonsyncopal LOC, an adequate method of taking the clinical history, which is the cornerstone of diagnosing patients with transient LOC, should be used.
- The first question to answer is whether the patient has had a real LOC; events with similar features, such as falls, drop-attack, and so forth, should therefore be excluded.
- After a transient LOC has been diagnosed, one should try to exclude a nonsyncopal LOC. After syncope has been diagnosed, one should try to define the cause.

Syncope is a transient loss of consciousness (LOC) caused by transient cerebral hypoperfusion characterized by rapid onset, short duration, and spontaneous complete recovery.[1] There are several causes of syncope, which are reported in Moya and colleagues,[1] and are also discussed elsewhere in this issue. Unfortunately, there are no signs or symptoms specific of such hypoperfusion and there are other conditions that resemble syncope (ie, may produce or appear to produce transient LOC) but are not caused by a generalized reduction in cerebral blood flow. These conditions, which are reported in **Box 1**, must be considered in the differential diagnosis.

The initial diagnostic approach to patients with transient LOC comprises a detailed medical history (incorporating documentation of witness accounts); a through physical examination (including supine and standing blood pressure measurement); and 12-lead electrocardiogram. Other tests, including basic laboratory tests, are usually not indicated in the initial evaluation of patients with syncope.[1] The history and physical examination

are the core and the work-up for patients with transient LOC. They are able to define the cause of transient LOC in about 20% of patients, obviating the need for further evaluation and enabling treatment to be instituted; in 60% of patients they do not enable a definite diagnosis to be made, but suggest some causes and, therefore, specific examinations.[2] Because there are many causes of transient LOC, an adequate method of taking the clinical history should be used (**Fig. 1**). **Box 2** lists some of the most important questions that must be answered when the patient's history is taken.

WAS LOC COMPLETE?

The first question to answer is whether the patient has had a true LOC, which is characterized by loss of postural control and unresponsiveness to external stimuli, particularly acoustic. If there are witnesses, the question can generally be answered; if, however, the patient is alone, the diagnosis can be difficult, if not impossible. A state of altered consciousness and, above all, a fall

This article originally appeared in Cardiac Electrophysiology Clinics, Volume 5, Issue 4, December 2013.
Conflict of Interest: None declared.
Syncope Unit, Section of Cardiology, Department of Medicine, Ospedale Privato Quisisana, Viale Cavour 128, Ferrara 44121, Italy
* Corresponding author.
E-mail address: alboni.cardiologia@gmail.com

including a drop-attack must be considered in the differential diagnosis. Falls are more frequent in the elderly. Many falls can be attributed to an environmental cause, such as accidental collisions, slips, or trips. These extrinsic falls require a very different approach from falls associated with LOC. Other falls are caused by an underlying balance disorder; such intrinsic falls typically occur during weight shifts or turning movements. These spontaneous falls are easily mistaken for those caused by LOC. In this regard, it has recently been demonstrated that about 25% of patients suffer retrograde amnesia after tilt-induced or carotid sinus massage-induced syncope.[3,4] The prevalence of retrograde amnesia after spontaneous syncope is not known; however, many of the falls that are defined by the patient as accidental may be caused by LOC, which the patient is not able to remember because of retrograde amnesia. For this reason, to make a differential diagnosis it is not useful to ask the patient "were you unconsciousness?"; rather, patients should

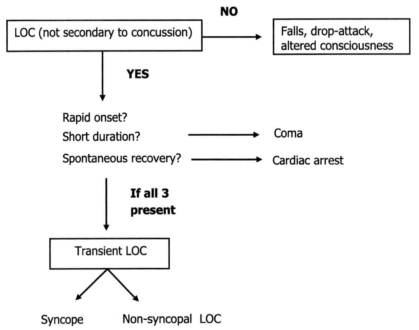

Fig. 1. Method to be used in taking clinical history. The first question to answer is whether the patient has had a real loss of consciousness; therefore, events with similar clinical features, such as falls, drop-attack, and so forth, should be ruled out. After a loss of consciousness has been diagnosed, the presence of the three features defining the presentation of transient loss of consciousness (rapid onset, short duration, spontaneous recovery) should be investigated. If one is dealing with a transient loss of consciousness, a differential diagnosis between syncope and nonsyncopal loss of consciousness should be made. After syncope has been diagnosed, one should define the cause. LOC, loss of consciousness. (*Data from* Moya A, Sutton R, Ammirati F, et al. The Task Force for the Diagnosis and Management of Syncope of the European Society of Cardiology (ESC) Guidelines for the diagnosis and management of syncope (version 2009). Eur Heart J 2009;30:2631–71.)

Questions about circumstances just prior the attack

- Position (supine, sitting, or standing)
- Activity (rest; change in posture; during or after exercise; during or immediately after urination, defecation, coughing, or swallowing)
- Predisposing factors (eg, crowded or hot places, prolonged standing, postprandial period)
- Precipitating events (eg, emotion, fear, disgust, intense pain, neck movements, flashing lights)

Symptoms preceding loss of consciousness

Dizziness, blurred vision, nausea, vomiting, abdominal discomfort, sweating, aura, palpitations, precordial pain, pain in neck or shoulders

Symptoms during loss of consciousness (eyewitness)

Way of falling (slumping or kneeling over, rigidity or flaccidity); skin color (pallor, cyanosis); movements (tonic, clonic, tonic-clonic, myoclonus, or automatisms); duration of movements; onset of movements in relation to fall; duration of loss of consciousness; tongue biting; open or closed eyes

Symptoms during recovery

Nausea, vomiting, sweating, confusion, skin color, palpitations, injury, precordial pain, muscle aches, urinary or fecal incontinence

Questions regarding background

- Family history of sudden death, congenital arrhythmogenic heart disease
- Previous major cardiac disease
- Neurologic history
- Metabolic disorders (eg, diabetes)
- Medication (antihypertensives, antianginals, antidepressants, antipsychotics, diuretics, antiarrhythmics, QT-prolonging agents) or other drugs, including alcohol
- In the case of recurrent syncope, information on recurrences, such as the time since the first syncopal episode, and on the number of spells

be asked whether they remember every part of the entire attack.[5] Likewise, witnesses should be asked whether the patient was unresponsive during part of the attack and how this unresponsiveness was established. If the patient is able to refer every part of the attack, a fall has presumably occurred, although sometimes uncertainty remains. Intrinsic falls also include the drop-attack; this is a very poorly defined entity, which mainly affects women older than 40 years. The term drop-attack is currently used to denote a particular benign syndrome of sudden, unexpected falls onto the knees, without LOC and without prodromal or postictal symptoms. Falls occur suddenly because of buckling of the legs, and the patient has no subjective sensation of vertigo or any other prior warning. Indeed, virtually all patients remember hitting the floor. Drop-attack nearly always occurs during walking, and only rarely during standing. There is no relation to changes in posture, head movements, or any other precipitating event. Patients typically fall straight down or forward onto their knees, and often suffer bruising in the patella region. The patients can usually get up immediately after the fall and resume their normal activities, unless injures have been sustained. Because the patient is able to remember every part of the entire attack, the differential diagnosis with syncope is generally easy.

DID LOC HAVE RAPID ONSET, SHORT DURATION, AND SPONTANEOUS RECOVERY?

After LOC has been diagnosed, the questions that arise are: "Did LOC have a rapid onset?", "Was LOC of short duration?" and "Was recovery spontaneous?". It must be remembered that the beginning of syncope is rapid but not necessarily sudden, because prodromal symptoms lasting up to 30 to 60 seconds may occur. During syncope, LOC generally lasts 10 to 20 seconds, but in rare cases it can go on for some minutes. If LOC is prolonged, one is dealing with a coma. If recovery is not spontaneous, but requires cardiac massage or other resuscitation maneuvers, one is dealing with cardiac arrest, although these maneuvers may sometimes be performed in patients with syncope. If the answer to these three questions is "yes," one is dealing with a "transient LOC." At this point, one should try to diagnose the cause of the LOC (see **Fig. 1**).

DIAGNOSIS OF THE CAUSE OF TRANSIENT LOC

A transient LOC can be an expression of syncope or of nonsyncopal LOC and, at this point, various

Table 1
Role of history in the differential diagnosis between syncope and epilepsy

	Epilepsy	Syncope
Trigger	Rare	Frequent
Prodromal symptoms	Sensorial or somatosensorial aura	Dizziness, blurred vision, nausea, vomiting, abdominal discomfort, sweating
Fall	Generally tonic	Generally flaccid
Skin color	Generally cyanotic	Generally pale
Movements	Tonic-clonic, rhythmic, prolonged ($\sim$1 min); onset coincides with the beginning of LOC	Myoclonus, short duration ($\sim$15 s), nonrhythmic; appear late during LOC
Automatisms	Lip smacking, chewing, fumbling, head raising	Extremely rare
Tongue biting	Frequent	Rare (localized at the tip of the tongue)
Eye deviation	Generally lateral	Generally upward
Symptoms during recovery	Prolonged confusion, aching muscles, headache	No confusion or of short duration (generally <5 min), nausea, vomiting, pallor, sweating

Abbreviation: LOC, loss of consciousness.

methods of taking the clinical history can be used. However, because there are several causes of transient LOC, it is advisable, at least for doctors with limited experience of syncope, to try to exclude a nonsyncopal LOC; therefore, the diagnosis of syncope remains basically one of exclusion.[1] Indeed, as previously reported, syncope is a transient LOC caused by global cerebral hypoperfusion but, unfortunately, there are no signs or symptoms specific to this hypoperfusion. According to this approach, the patient and witnesses, if available, should be asked questions aimed at investigating a role of nonsyncopal LOC.

CLINICAL FINDINGS OF NONSYNCOPAL LOC

In this section the clinical findings of nonsyncopal LOC are reported; these are summarized in **Tables 1 and 2**.

Epilepsy

Like syncope, epilepsy is clinically characterized by transient and (usually) short-lived attacks of a self-limited nature. It is caused by an abnormal excessive or synchronous neuronal activity in the brain. Epilepsy is rarely triggered; sometimes flashing lights or unpleasant acoustic stimuli may play a role. Typical epileptic auras, such as rising epigastric sensation, unpleasant smell or taste, or déjà vu, may precede transient LOC and provide important diagnostic clues. During the epileptic attack there are tonic-clonic movements, usually rhythmic, synchronous, and violent, which can affect the whole body; these movements last about 1 minute and, sometimes, longer. Movements may also be present in syncope and are defined as myoclonus; they are usually asynchronous, small,

Table 2
Signs and symptoms suggestive of nonsyncopal loss of consciousness

Sign/Symptom	Suggested Cause of LOC
Focal neurologic symptoms associated with transient LOC	TIA
Transient LOC preceded by tremors and intense sweating in treated patients with diabetes	Hypoglycemia
Frequent and prolonged LOCs; closed eyes during the attack; many psychosomatic disorders	Psychogenic pseudosyncope
Transient LOC, preceded by an emotional trigger in patients with narcolepsy	Cataplexy

Abbreviations: LOC, loss of consciousness; TIA, transient ischemic attack.

and nonrhythmic, and their duration is much shorter than in seizures (a few seconds). During an epileptic attack, movements often coincide with the beginning of LOC, whereas in syncope they appear later, after the fall, and are considered to be an expression of severe brain hypoxia. The timing of the movements, which may be ascertained from reliable witnesses, is very important in the differential diagnosis. It must, however, be pointed out that there are "atonic epileptic attacks," which are not accompanied by movements. These attacks do feature in the differential diagnosis of syncope, but luckily are rare and occur almost exclusively in children with learning difficulties or other neurologic abnormalities.[5] During an epileptic attack, falls are generally tonic, whereas in syncope they are flaccid; flaccidity during unconsciousness argues against epilepsy. Complex movements or automatisms (lip smacking, chewing, fumbling, head raising, and so forth) may be observed during an epileptic attack, whereas they are extremely rare in syncope.[6] Eye movements can take place in epilepsy and syncope; in epilepsy, eye deviation is lateral, whereas in syncope it is generally upward.[6] Tongue biting, which is common in epilepsy, is very rare in syncope; this occurs at the side of the tongue in seizures and at the tongue tip in syncope. During seizures, the face is generally cyanotic, whereas during syncope it is pale; however, facial cyanosis can be observed in some patients with cardiac syncope. After seizures, confusion is prolonged and is often accompanied by aching muscle and headache; by contrast, after syncope, confusion is generally of short duration (up to a few minutes), although in some patients it may be prolonged. Because injuries and urinary incontinence seem to be common in epilepsy and syncope, they are not useful to the differential diagnosis. Finally, it must be pointed out that some epileptic attacks are not associated to LOC. In such cases, however, there is no loss of postural control and the differential diagnosis with syncope is generally easy.

Transient Ischemic Attack

A transient ischemic attack (TIA) is caused by temporary regional cerebral hypoperfusion and should not be confused with syncope. LOC during TIA seems to be extremely rare and has been observed only during TIAs involving the posterior (vertebrobasilar) system. To date, no cases of LOC have been described during TIA secondary to involvement of the carotid circulation. The differential diagnosis between TIA and syncope is generally easy, because during the former some of the following neurologic symptoms are present: limb ataxia, oculomotor palsies, loss of balance, difficulty sitting without support, veering to one side, frank vertigo, unilateral hearing loss, dysphagia, laryngeal paralysis, pharyngeal paralysis, hoarseness, and facial pain. Patients with TIA of the posterior system do not have hemiparesis or hemisensory loss. At present, there are no reliable descriptions of a TIA manifesting itself as an isolated LOC.[7] For practical purposes, the following rule can be applied: a TIA concerns a focal neurologic deficit, generally without LOC, whereas syncope represents LOC without a focal neurologic deficit.[5] Even steal syndromes (the most frequent being subclavian steal syndrome) can manifest themselves as LOC associated with focal neurologic symptoms. When their history is taken, patients should always be asked whether they felt focal neurologic symptoms, to exclude a TIA or a steal syndrome. However, it must be pointed out that a neurologic symptom, such as paresthesia, is referred by about 20% of patients with reflex syncope.[8]

Hypoglycemia

Hypoglycemia can induce LOC, generally long-lasting, which takes on the clinical appearance of coma. Sometimes, however, the LOC is of short duration, and in this case a differential diagnosis must be made with syncope. In patients with diabetes treated with insulin or oral antidiabetic drugs, hypoglycemia should be suspected as a cause of transient LOC when the LOC is preceded by symptoms caused by sympathetic activation, particularly tremors and intense sweating. During recovery, prolonged confusion may be present.

Psychogenic Pseudosyncope

Psychogenic pseudosyncope is a simulation of LOC, even if involuntary; it mainly affects women. The patient does not lose consciousness, but because postural tone and responsiveness to external stimuli are lost, a differential diagnosis must be made with syncope. There are some features that help differentiate this state from true LOC. There are no triggers and the attack always occurs in the presence of other people. The attacks are frequent, sometimes several in a day, and are often prolonged, from a few minutes up to 15 minutes. If the patient can be examined, there are no gross abnormalities except for a lack of responsiveness. The eyes are generally closed, whereas during syncope and seizures they are commonly open.[5] If the eyes are opened passively, the patient may tend actively to close them or to avert the gaze away from the examiner. Lifted limbs that are suddenly released may hesitate in mid-air before falling. Sometimes there are movements that consist of asynchronous convulsion-like movements, often with pelvic thrusts and tremors.[5] During the attack, blood pressure and heart rate are normal. Contrary to what has been reported in the past, minor traumas can occur. There is no postictal confusion, but patients often become emotional and cry at the end of the attack.

Cataplexy

During cataplexy there is no LOC but patients lose postural control and are unresponsive to external stimuli. Cataplexy occurs only in the context of the disease narcoplepsy, and this is the most important finding that points to cataplepsy. The loss of muscle tone is caused by emotions, particularly mirth associated with laughing out loud. In complete attacks, patients slump flaccidly to the ground. Partial attacks are more common and are restricted to dropping of the jaw and sagging or nodding of the head. Attacks may develop slowly enough to allow the patient to stagger and break the fall before hitting the floor; such attacks therefore look rather unreal and psychogenic.

If signs and symptoms suggestive of nonsyncopal LOC (see **Tables 1** and **2**) emerge when the patient's history is taken, evaluation by a neurologist, psychiatrist, or specialist in internal medicine is indicated. If a nonsyncopal cause can reasonably be excluded, the next step is to investigate the cause of syncope.

DIAGNOSIS OF THE CAUSE OF SYNCOPE

Syncope can be reflex or cardiovascular or caused by orthostatic hypotension. There is a consensus that some types of syncope can be diagnosed after the initial evaluation, without further examinations.[1] The diagnostic criteria of these types of syncope are summarized in **Box 3**.

Typical Vasovagal Syncope

Typical vasovagal syncope can be diagnosed when transient LOC is precipitated by triggers, such as emotional distress (emotion, fear, severe pain, blood phobia, instrumentation) or orthostatic stress (prolonged standing, particularly in hot environments), and is associated with symptoms caused by activation of the autonomic system, such as nausea, vomiting, abdominal discomfort, pallor, and sweating. Other symptoms caused by activation of the autonomic system, such as palpitations, yawning, sighing, pupillary dilatation, and urinary incontinence, may be present. Besides autonomic symptoms, prodromal symptoms

---

> **Box 3**
> **Types of syncope that can be diagnosed on initial evaluation**
>
> *Typical vasovagal syncope* is diagnosed if transient loss of consciousness is precipitated by emotional distress or orthostatic stress and is associated with autonomic prodromes.
>
> *Situational syncope* is diagnosed if loss of consciousness occurs during or immediately after urination, defecation, coughing, or swallowing.
>
> *Orthostatic syncope* is diagnosed when presyncope/syncope occurs during orthostatic testing and is associated with hypotension.
>
> *Arrhythmia-related syncope* is diagnosed by electrocardiography when there is
>
> - Persistent sinus bradycardia <40 beats/min while awake or repetitive sinoatrial block or sinus pauses ≥3 seconds
> - Mobitz II second- or third-degree atrioventricular block
> - Alternating left and right bundle branch block
> - Ventricular tachycardia or rapid paroxysmal supraventricular tachycardia
> - Nonsustained episodes of polymorphic ventricular tachycardia and long or short QT interval
> - Pacemaker malfunction with cardiac pauses
>
> *Cardiac ischemia-related syncope* is diagnosed when transient loss of consciousness presents with electrocardiographic evidence of acute ischemia, with or without myocardial infarction.
>
> *Cardiovascular syncope* is diagnosed when transient loss of consciousness presents in patients with severe aortic stenosis, pulmonary embolus, severe pulmonary hypertension, or acute aortic dissection.

---

caused by cerebral hypoperfusion, such as dizziness and blurred vision, are commonly reported by the patient. Unfortunately, none of these symptoms is specific to vasovagal syncope; however, there is a consensus that when an emotional or orthostatic trigger is associated with autonomic symptoms, the diagnosis of typical vasovagal syncope can be made. Typical vasovagal syncope is mainly observed in young subjects and rarely in the elderly.

Situational Syncope

Situational syncope is diagnosed when syncope occurs during or immediately after specific triggers, such as micturition, defecation, swallowing, coughing, and, more rarely, after sneezing, laughing, or brass instrument playing. Autonomic symptoms are present in about 50% of patients.[9] There is a consensus that when a transient LOC occurs after these triggers, situational syncope can be diagnosed without further examination.

Syncope Caused by Orthostatic Hypotension

Orthostatic hypotension is caused by inadequate sympathetic vasoconstriction during upright standing, which may be responsible for syncope or presyncope. Autonomic failure can be primary, secondary, or medication-induced. Examples of primary autonomic failure include pure autonomic failure and multiple system atrophy. Secondary autonomic failure refers to autonomic dysfunction caused by diseases that primarily affect organs other than the autonomic nervous system, such as diabetic or amyloid neuropathy. In terms of the number of patients, drugs are probably the principal cause of autonomic failure. Common culprits include antihypertensives, diuretics, and antidepressants. In autonomic failure, not only standing in the upright position but also the cessation of exercise may precipitate hypotension.

Orthostatic hypotension is defined as a decrease in systolic blood pressure of at least 20 mm Hg and/or diastolic blood pressure of 10 mm Hg within 3 minutes of standing. Because asymptomatic orthostatic hypotension is frequent not only in the elderly but also in adolescents,[10] orthostatic syncope can be diagnosed only when the decrease in blood pressure during the orthostatic test is associated with syncope or presyncope. There is a consensus that, in this case, orthostatic syncope can be diagnosed without further examinations.

CLINICAL FINDINGS THAT ARE ONLY SUGGESTIVE OF A CAUSE OF SYNCOPE

In many other situations, the findings of the initial evaluation do not enable a definite diagnosis to be made, but suggest a cause of syncope (**Box 4**).

Reflex syncope should be suspected when there are no triggers, but the autonomic symptoms, particularly nausea, vomiting, and abdominal discomfort, are marked before and/or after LOC. These symptoms may also be present, although less pronounced, in cardiac syncope, whereas they are not present in orthostatic syncope, in which there is autonomic failure and not activation of the autonomic system. The absence of signs and symptoms of heart disease during the initial evaluation strongly suggests a reflex syncope. In this regard, in an Italian multicenter study

---

Box 4
Clinical features suggestive of a diagnosis on initial evaluation

Reflex syncope
- Absence of heart disease
- Long history of recurrent syncope (>4 years)
- Nausea, vomiting associated with syncope
- Prolonged standing or crowded, hot places
- During a meal or postprandially (within 2 hours)
- With head rotation or pressure on carotid sinus (tumors, shaving, tight collars)

Syncope caused by orthostatic hypotension
- After standing up
- Prolonged standing
- Pain in the shoulders or neck
- Standing after exertion
- Temporal relationship with start or changes in dosage of vasodepressive drugs
- Presence of autonomic neuropathy or parkinsonism
- After volume depletion

Cardiovascular syncope
- Presence of definite structural heart disease
- Sudden-onset palpitation followed by loss of consciousness
- During exertion or supine position
- Abnormal electrocardiogram
- Family history of unexplained sudden death or channelopathy

Electrocardiographic findings suggesting arrhythmic syncope
- Left bundle branch block or bifascicular block
- Mobitz I second-degree atrioventricular block
- Asymptomatic inappropriate sinus bradycardia (<50 beats/min)
- Nonsustained ventricular tachycardia
- Pre-excited QRS complexes
- Long or short QT intervals
- Early repolarization
- Right bundle branch block pattern with ST elevation in leads V1-V3 (Brugada syndrome)
- Negative T waves and epsilon waves suggestive of arrhythmogenic right ventricular cardiomyopathy
- Q waves suggesting myocardial infarction

the absence of heart disease allowed us to exclude a cardiac cause of syncope in 97% of patients.[11] A long history of syncope (>4 years) suggests a reflex syncope; indeed, the time between the first and the last syncopal episode is generally short in cardiac and orthostatic syncope.[11] Other findings suggestive of reflex syncope are LOC during a meal or the postprandial period (within 2 hours), or during head rotation or pressure on the carotid sinus (as caused by tumors, shaving, or tight collars); in this latter case, carotid sinus syncope should be suspected. Finally, a LOC appearing just after exercise suggests both reflex and orthostatic syncope; in young subjects, a reflex syncope is more likely, whereas in the elderly an orthostatic syncope is more likely.[5] In all the previously mentioned situations, autonomic tests should be performed first.

Orthostatic syncope should be suspected when LOC occurs after standing up or, as previously mentioned, after cessation of exercise, if the patient remains upright. Postexercise hypotension results from the drop in blood pressure that normally occurs after exercise; whereas patients with autonomic failure have difficulty in increasing their blood pressure during exercise, the physiologic drop afterward does, unfortunately, take place. Postexercise hypotension commonly leads to falls, for example when patients take a rest after reaching the top of a staircase.[5] Prodromal symptoms caused by cerebral hypoperfusion (dizziness, blurred vision) are commonly present, whereas the autonomic prodromes seen in reflex syncope are distinctly absent in orthostatic syncope; this feature is important in the differential diagnosis. Moreover, patients may report pain in the neck or shoulders at the onset of the attack ("coat-hanger pain"); this is caused by ischemia of the muscles in the upper part of the body. By contrast, "coat-hanger pain" is very rarely reported in reflex syncope.[8] Finally, orthostatic syncope should be suspected in subjects who are dehydrated as a result of hot environments; diuretics; or inadequate fluid intake in patients taking commonly prescribed drugs, such as antihypertensives, antidepressants, and antipsychotics; and in patients affected by an autonomic neuropathy. When an orthostatic syncope is suspected, autonomic tests, including tilt testing to investigate the possibility of late orthostatic hypotension, should be performed first.

Cardiac syncope should be suspected in the presence of definite structural heart disease, a history of bradyarrhythmia or tachyarrhythmia, and a family history of unexplained sudden death or channelopathy. Sudden-onset palpitations preceding LOC suggest a tachyarrhythmic cause of syncope; however, it must be pointed out that an acceleration in heart rhythm is reported by 10% to 25% of patients with vasovagal syncope.[8,11] The appearance of LOC in the supine position suggests a cardiac syncope or an epileptic attack, because reflex syncope is very rare in this position (discussed next). Syncope occurring during exercise also suggests a cardiac cause, whereas postexercise syncope, as previously mentioned, suggests a reflex or an orthostatic cause. Finally, some electrocardiogram findings, as reported in **Box 4**, suggest an arrhythmic cause of syncope. In these situations, cardiologic examinations should be performed first.

SLEEP SYNCOPE

Sleep syncope has recently been proposed as a new form of vasovagal syncope, which occurs in the supine position during the sleeping hours.[12,13] Most of these patients are middle-aged women; they report a history of waking from sleep with abdominal discomfort, an urge to defecate and nausea, followed by LOC. These symptoms always begin in the supine position, but LOC occurs in this position only in a third of patients; in two-thirds it occurs after standing up to go to the bathroom. Most of these patients also refer typical episodes of vasovagal syncope during the day. Sleep syncope must be investigated during clinical history only when the prodromal symptoms begin in the supine position. The differential diagnosis must mainly be made with epilepsy and cardiac syncope. The absence of tonic-clonic movements, automatisms, tongue biting, and mental confusion after the event, and the presence of a history of typical vasovagal syncope, are at variance with epilepsy. A history of typical vasovagal syncope is also against cardiac syncope, as is abdominal discomfort, which seems to be very rare in cardiac syncope.[11]

REFERENCES

1. Moya A, Sutton R, Ammirati F, et al. Guidelines for the diagnosis and management of syncope (version 2009). The Task Force for the Diagnosis and Management of Syncope of the European Society of Cardiology (ESC). Eur Heart J 2009;30:2631–71.
2. Van Dijk N, Boer KR, Colman R, et al. High diagnostic yield and accuracy of history, physical examination, and ECG in patients with transient loss of consciousness in FAST: the Fainting Assessment Study. J Cardiovasc Electrophysiol 2008;19:48–55.
3. Parry SW, Steen N, Baptist M, et al. Amnesia for loss of consciousness in carotid sinus syndrome.

Implications for presentation with falls. J Am Coll Cardiol 2005;45:1840–3.

4. O'Dwyer C, Bennett K, Langan Y, et al. Amnesia for loss of consciousness is common in vasovagal syncope. Europace 2011;13:1040–5.

5. Thijs RD, Bloem BR, Van Dijk JG. Falls, faint and funny turns. J Neurol 2009;256:155–67.

6. Duplyakov D, Golovina G, Garkina S, et al. Is it possible to accurately differentiate neurocardiogenic syncope from epilepsy? Cardiol J 2010;4:420–7.

7. Savitz SJ, Kaplan LR. Vertebrobasilar disease. N Engl J Med 2005;352:2618–26.

8. Romme JJ, Van Dijk N, Boer KR, et al. Influence of age and gender on the occurrence and presentation of reflex syncope. Clin Auton Res 2008;18:127–33.

9. Alboni P, Brignole M, Menozzi C, et al. Clinical spectrum of neurally mediated syncope. Europace 2004; 6:55–62.

10. Wieling W, Ganzeboom KS, Saul JP. Reflex syncope in children and adolescents. Heart 2004;90: 1094–100.

11. Alboni P, Brignole M, Menozzi C, et al. Diagnostic value of history in patients with syncope with or without heart disease. J Am Coll Cardiol 2001;37: 1921–8.

12. Jardine DL, Krediet CT, Cortelli P, et al. Fainting in your sleep? Clin Auton Res 2006;16:76–8.

13. Busweiler L, Jardine DL, Frampton CM, et al. Sleep syncope: important clinical association with phobia and vagotonia. Sleep Med 2010;11:929–33.

The Value of Tilt Testing and Autonomic Nervous System Assessment

Richard Sutton, DSc

KEYWORDS

- Syncope • Tilt testing • Implantable loop recorder • Autonomic nervous system function tests

KEY POINTS

- Tilt testing has been and remains valuable to study patients with syncope and related conditions, including the making of correct and precise diagnoses.
- Tilt testing has some shortcomings, some of which are overcome by the use of the implantable loop recorder.

HISTORY

Syncope was seldom studied in the 30 years before the advent of tilt testing in 1986.[1] The discovery of tilt testing as a means of precipitating syncope in the laboratory was serendipitous. An investigation was in progress into the hormonal changes of upright posture in carotid sinus syndrome but it proved difficult because most patients lost consciousness on the tilt table. This difficulty prompted the application of the tilt protocol to a group of syncope patients, who, at the end of exhaustive investigations, had no diagnosis. They also lost consciousness. Ultimately, an age-matched control group with no history of syncope was tilt tested when a tiny minority of them lost consciousness. The original Lancet paper[1] was written on this experience. At this time, there was a small but growing interest in using the tilt table to simulate upright posture. The Mayo Clinic had published results of using the upright posture during electrophysiological studies[2] and investigation of hypertensive and hypotensive patients with upright posture was ongoing at the Cleveland Clinic.[3] In Denmark a group was using tilt whereby the subject was sitting astride a bicycle saddle supported by the footplate of the tilt table. Thus, the subject was erect but with legs dangling without support. The research group had close to 100% syncope in their subjects to study hormonal changes before and at syncope so as to try to gain a better understanding of the fainting phenomenon.[4] If the Cleveland Clinic were not already working on this technique for clinical syncope induction, they quickly presented data on the subject in 1988.[5]

IMPACT OF TILT TESTING

The impact on the nascent electrophysiological community in the late 1980s was profound. Presentations on the subject of tilt-induced syncope were striking and generated considerable interest. The test received enthusiasm and spread in its application. During this time, efforts were made to establish it, define its methodology,[6] and gain experience in the technique.[7] Recognition of the value of the test first came with an American College of Cardiology Consensus document on tilt testing for syncope.[8]

The series of European Society of Cardiology Guidelines on the diagnosis and management of syncope followed beginning in 2001 and was updated in 2004 and 2009.[9–11] These documents

This article originally appeared in Cardiac Electrophysiology Clinics, Volume 5, Issue 4, December 2013.
The author has nothing to disclose.
Imperial College, 59-61 North Wharf Road, ICCH Building St Mary's Hospital Campus, London W2 1LA, UK
E-mail address: r.sutton@imperial.ac.uk

Cardiol Clin 33 (2015) 357–360
http://dx.doi.org/10.1016/j.ccl.2015.04.003
0733-8651/15/$ – see front matter © 2015 Elsevier Inc. All rights reserved.

were broad in concept and contained information on performance and interpretation of tilt tests. It could, however, be claimed that without the advent of tilt there would have been little to discuss. Gradually, in the 20 years since the introduction of the test in 1986, syncope has emerged as a subspecialty of electrophysiology with a considerable following sufficient to demand a minimum of several sessions at all electrophysiology meetings and contribute a substantial body of literature in major cardiology journals.

Tilt testing has been adopted by many neurologists with equal enthusiasm to that of cardiologists. However, the bulk of neurologists are not so involved and they prefer to refer when they deem necessary. The difference in selection of this test between the 2 specialties reflects the different personalities and training among the 2 groups. Most of those interested in this subject think that the fundamental problem is in the brain not in the heart. Cardiologists are doers; neurologists are more speculative. Thus, the former group thought in tilt testing that they had a means of making a diagnosis and having achieved that, therapy could follow. As is so often the case in medicine, the reality is far less clear.

NEGATIVITY TOWARD TILT TESTING

At the same time that tilt testing was becoming established in the early 2000s, evidence began to emerge that the test was certainly fallible. The series of studies now known as ISSUE 1[12–14] was published in 2001. The first of these was particularly challenging for tilt testing. The investigators' group of patients with syncope but no evidence of heart disease was termed, "Isolated Syncope." Some of these patients experienced recurrent syncope with an implanted electrocardiogram (ECG) loop recorder and a surprising number had asystole or severe bradycardia not shown at tilt testing. Approximately half the Isolated Syncope group had negative tilt tests. Thus, this ISSUE 1 study[12] demonstrated that tilt testing could not always induce syncope in those that would have recurrences and that the rhythm disturbance during syncope was also not well predicted by the tilt test, there being a large number of severe bradycardias not seen on tilt. Until this time, investigators, generally, had been clinging to the idea that a patient's collapse pattern on tilt was reproduced spontaneously, despite there being little evidence to support this concept. This series of studies was followed by ISSUE 2,[15] the findings of which, in this context, were very similar to ISSUE 1, only raising the possibility that asystole on tilt may give a high positive predictive value

for spontaneous recurrence of asystole. Since 2000, publications on the findings of implanted ECG loop recorder have been numerous[16–18] and it was obvious that the diagnostic accuracy of what actually happens during a spontaneous attack was much more precise than tilt testing whereby syncope is forced.

In 2010, the United Kingdom body, the National Institute for Healthcare and Clinical Excellence, suggested that tilt testing should not be performed for the diagnosis of syncope.[19] Their rather radical view stemmed from the evidence presented above. This professional and administrative body paid little attention to the widespread ability to undertake tilt testing, its remaining residual value, and its low cost.

It is true that a specialist in syncope is usually able to make a confident diagnosis of vasovagal syncope from the history of the patient and an observer of an attack, providing physical examination, 12-lead ECG, and orthostatic blood pressure measurements are normal.[11] Thus, tilt testing is then unnecessary. However, this ignores the fact that syncope is seen by a plethora of different kinds of physicians, many of whom are not experts in the field and unable to make the confident diagnosis referred to above. Requesting a tilt test is a facility considered valuable by many of these physicians. Moreover, it is a test, which is not costly, brings some expertise to bear on the patient's symptoms, is noninvasive, and often increases the patient's confidence in the diagnosis by precipitating an attack in front of a medical witness.

There are even more potent reasons not to abandon tilt testing now. Other diagnoses can be made by tilt testing than simple reflex or vasovagal syncope (VVS). These conditions can have similar presentations and can be very difficult for most physicians to separate from VVS on clinical grounds alone. The first of these is postural orthostatic tachycardia syndrome (POTS). This condition has an overlap with vasovagal syncope of up to 30%[20–22] and its management is different from VVS. The second of these is orthostatic hypotension whereby tilt testing shows the immediate (within the first 3 minutes of tilt) blood pressure decrease that does not occur in VVS. Again the management of this condition is different from VVS with neurologic input being mandatory except in those cases where the cause is iatrogenic by excessive hypotensive medication. The third condition for which tilt testing is required is psychogenic pseudosyncope.[23–25] These patients appear to collapse on tilt with normal and largely unchanged physiologic parameters, a finding that not only determines the diagnosis

Table 1
Conditions in which tilt testing is valuable

Condition	Physiologic Changes	Value
Vasovagal syncope	Delayed BP fall, brady	Diagnostic if usual symptoms
Orthostatic hypotension	Immediate BP fall, No brady	Diagnostic
POTS	Modest prog BP fall, tachy	Diagnostic if usual symptoms
Psychogenic pseudosyncope	No physiol change (tachy)	Apparent LOC is diagnostic

Abbreviations: BP, blood pressure; brady, bradycardia; LOC, loss of consciousness; prog, progressive; tachy, tachycardia.

but also provides grounds for beginning the psychological therapy.[26] Carefully and sympathetically applied psychology and/or cognitive behavioral therapy can restore these patients to full healthy lives.

THE PLACE OF TILT TESTING TODAY

Tilt testing continues to have an important role in making diagnoses (**Table 1**) that are difficult for nonexperts and in some cases also for experts in syncope. VVS remains the most common of these diagnoses. As expertise in syncope diagnosis improves, it can be anticipated that the requirement for tilt testing will diminish but it cannot be expected to disappear because of its value in diagnosing POTS, orthostatic hypotension, and psychogenic pseudosyncope plus some cases of clinically difficult VVS.

AUTONOMIC NERVOUS SYSTEM FUNCTION TESTS

Autonomic nervous system assessment is an area of neurology poorly understood by most cardiologists but falls into the expertise of a subspecialty of neurology. These physicians are well trained to perform and assess the autonomic nervous system and, further, to diagnose these patients and offer prognosis and treatment where appropriate. A full assessment includes heart rate and blood pressure control, respiratory control, effect of respiration on the heart, effect of vagal discharge on heart rate and gastrointestinal function, sweating, and sphincter control. The assessment is valuable in characterizing the severity of autonomic nervous system compromise. Although tests such as the Valsalva maneuver are familiar to cardiologists, many others of these autonomic assessments will not be. The full assessment is both time-consuming and difficult to perform well. Thus, it is recommended that autonomic function tests other than orthostatic blood pressure and tilt testing be performed by neurologists.[11,27] In making this recommendation, the

emphasis is on cooperative and shared care to achieve the best possible outcome for the patient.

SUMMARY

Tilt testing has been and remains valuable to study patients with syncope and related conditions including the making of correct and precise diagnoses. It must be recognized that tilt testing has some shortcomings and that some of these are overcome by use of the implantable loop recorder.

REFERENCES

1. Kenny RA, Ingram A, Bayliss J, et al. Head-up tilt: a useful test for investigating unexplained syncope. Lancet 1986;1:1352–5.
2. Hammill SC, Holmes DR Jr, Wood DL, et al. Electrophysiological testing in the upright position: improved evaluation of patients with rhythm disturbances using a tilt table. J Am Coll Cardiol 1984;4:65–71.
3. Fouad FM, Tarazi RC, Ferrario CM, et al. Assessment of parasympathetic control of heart rate by a noninvasive method. Am J Physiol 1984;246:H838–42.
4. Sander-Jensen K, Secher NH, Astrup A, et al. Hypotension induced by passive head-up tilt: endocrine and circulatory mechanisms. Am J Physiol 1986;251:R742–8.
5. Abi-Samra F, Maloney JD, Fouad-Tarazi FM, et al. The usefulness of head-up tilt testing and hemodynamic investigations in the workup of syncope of unknown origin. Pacing Clin Electrophysiol 1988;11:1202–14.
6. Fitzpatrick A, Theodorakis G, Vardas P, et al. Methodology of head-up tilt testing in patients with unexplained syncope. J Am Coll Cardiol 1991;17:125–30.
7. Fitzpatrick A, Sutton R. Tilting towards a diagnosis in recurrent unexplained syncope. Lancet 1989;1:658–60.
8. Benditt DG, Ferguson DW, Grubb BP, et al. Tilt table testing for assessing syncope. J Am Coll Cardiol 1996;28:263–75.
9. Brignole M, Alboni P, Benditt D, et al, Task Force on Syncope, European Society of Cardiology.

Guidelines on management (diagnosis and treatment) of syncope. Eur Heart J 2001;22:1256–306.

10. Brignole M, Alboni P, Benditt DG, et al. Guidelines on management [diagnosis and treatment] of syncope – update 2004. Europace 2004;6:467–537.

11. Moya A, Sutton R, Ammirati F, et al. Guidelines for the diagnosis and treatment of syncope (version 2009). Eur Heart J 2009;30:2631–71.

12. Moya A, Brignole M, Menozzi C, et al, International Study on Syncope of Uncertain Etiology (ISSUE) Investigators. Mechanism of syncope in patients with isolated syncope and in patients with tilt-positive syncope. Circulation 2001;104:1261–7.

13. Menozzi C, Brignole M, Garcia-Civera R, et al, International Study on Syncope of Uncertain Etiology (ISSUE) Investigators. Mechanism of syncope in patients with heart disease and negative electrophysiologic test. Circulation 2002;105:2741–5.

14. Brignole M, Menozzi C, Moya A, et al, International Study on Syncope of Uncertain Etiology (ISSUE) Investigators. Mechanism of syncope in patients with bundle branch block and negative electrophysiological test. Circulation 2001;104:2045–50.

15. Brignole M, Sutton R, Menozzi C, et al, International Study on Syncope of Uncertain Etiology 2 (ISSUE 2). Early application of an implantable loop recorder allows effective specific therapy in patients with recurrent suspected neurally mediated syncope. Eur Heart J 2006;27:1085–92.

16. Krahn AD, Klein GJ, Yee R, et al. Randomized assessment of syncope trial: conventional diagnostic testing versus a prolonged monitoring strategy. Circulation 2001;104:46–51.

17. Farwell DJ, Freemantle N, Sulke AN. Use of implantable loop recorders in the diagnosis and management of syncope. Eur Heart J 2004;25:1257–63.

18. Edvardsson N, Frykman V, van Mechelen R, et al, PICTURE Study Investigators. Use of an implantable loop recorder to increase the diagnostic yield in unexplained syncope: results from the PICTURE registry. Europace 2011;13:262–9.

19. NICE clinical guideline 109. Transient loss of consciousness ('blackouts') management in adults and young people. August 2010. Available at: www.nice.org.uk/guidance/CG109.

20. Fu Q, Vangundy TB, Galbreath MM, et al. Cardiac origins of the postural orthostatic tachycardia syndrome. J Am Coll Cardiol 2010;55:2858–68.

21. Ohja A, McNeeley K, Heller E, et al. Orthostatic syndromes differ in syncope frequency. Am J Med 2010;123:245–9.

22. Kanjwal K, Sheikh M, Karabin B, et al. Neurocardiogenic syncope coexisting with postural orthostatic tachycardia syndrome in patients suffering from orthostatic intolerance: a combined form of autonomic dysfunction. Pacing Clin Electrophysiol 2011;34:549–54.

23. Petersen ME, Williams TR, Sutton R. Psychogenic syncope diagnosed by prolonged head-up tilt testing. QJM 1995;88:209–13.

24. Benbadis SR, Chichkova R. Psychogenic pseudosyncope: an underestimated and provable diagnosis. Epilepsy Behav 2006;9:106–10.

25. Hall-Patch L, Brown R, House A, et al, for the Nest Collaborators. Acceptability and effectiveness of a communication strategy for the diagnosis of non-epileptic attacks. Epilepsia 2010;51:70–8.

26. Sutton R, Brignole M, Benditt DG. Key challenges in the current management of syncope. Nat Rev Cardiol 2012;9:590–8.

27. van Dijk JG, Thijs RD, Benditt DG, et al. A guide to disorders causing transient loss of consciousness: focus on syncope. Nat Rev Neurol 2009;5:438–48.

Value of Ambulatory Electrocardiographic Monitoring in Syncope

Franco Giada, MD[a],*, Angelo Bartoletti, MD[b]

KEYWORDS

- Implantable loop recorders • Transient loss of consciousness • Syncope • Electrocardiogram
- Arrhythmia

KEY POINTS

- Implantable loop recorders (ILRs) continuously monitor electrocardiographic signals and perform real-time analysis of heart rhythm for up to 36 months.
- ILRs are used to evaluate transitory loss of consciousness of possible arrhythmic origin, particularly unexplained syncope.
- ILRs can also be used to evaluate difficult cases of epilepsy and unexplained falls, although current indications for their application in these entities are less clearly defined.
- Subcutaneous implantation of ILRs is a minimally invasive procedure and may carry a risk of minor complications at the implantation site; oversensing is another potential limitation of ILRs.

INTRODUCTION

Ambulatory electrocardiographic (AECG) monitoring devices (if the diagnostic functions of pacemakers and implantable cardioverter defibrillators are excluded) include the following: Holter devices, event recorders, external loop recorders, mobile cardiac outpatient telemetry, and implantable loop recorders (ILRs). **Table 1** shows the advantages, limits, and indications for various AECG monitoring devices.

AECG monitoring in syncope has long been hampered by the lack of suitable equipment and inadequate patient compliance. The use of external recorders over extended periods has been limited by patient discomfort and complexity, and by a low diagnostic value.[1,2] In principle, ILRs do not have these disadvantages. Smaller than a pacemaker, once implanted and correctly programmed, these devices can continuously monitor electrocardiographic signals and perform long-term continuous analysis and classification of the heart rhythm.

This article analyzes the current indications of ILRs according the European Society of Cardiology guidelines on the management of syncope[3] and the European Heart Rhythm Association guidelines on the use of implantable and external electrocardiographic loop recorders,[4] and their limitations.

TECHNICAL ASPECTS, IMPLANTING TECHNIQUE, AND FOLLOW-UP OF ILR

ILRs are equipped with a memory loop and, once activated by the patient at the time of symptoms through an external activator, store a one-lead electrocardiographic tracing, both retrospectively and prospectively, for several minutes. The loop memory enables the device to be activated even after symptoms have resolved; therefore, these devices

This article originally appeared in Cardiac Electrophysiology Clinics, Volume 5, Issue 4, December 2013.
Conflict of Interest: All authors have read and approved the submission of the article. All authors declare under their own responsibility that they do not have any conflict of interest.
[a] Cardiovascular Rehabilitation and Sports Medicine Service, Cardiovascular Department, PF Calvi Hospital, Via Largo San Giorgio 3, Noale 30033, Venice, Italy; [b] Cardiology Division and Syncope Centre, San Giovanni di Dio Hospital, Nuovo Ospedale S. Giovanni di Dio, Florence, Italy
* Corresponding author.
E-mail address: francogiada@hotmail.com

cardiology.theclinics.com

Table 1
Advantages, limitations, and indications of AECG monitoring devices

	Holter Monitoring	Event Recorders	External Loop Recorders/MCOT	Implantable Cardiac Monitors
Advantages	Low cost; possibility to record asymptomatic arrhythmias	Low cost; easy to use	Retrospective and prospective ECG records; possibility to record asymptomatic arrhythmias automatically	Retrospective and prospective ECG records; good ECG records; monitoring capability up to 36 mo; possibility to record asymptomatic arrhythmias automatically
Limits	Monitoring limited to 24–48 h; size may prevent activities that may trigger the arrhythmias	Monitoring capability up to 3–4 wk; only prospective ECG records; short-lasting arrhythmias are not recorded; arrhythmic triggers are not revealed; poor ECG records	Monitoring cannot be performed for more than 3–4 wk; continual maintenance is required; devices are uncomfortable; poor ECG records	Invasiveness; risk of local complications at the implantation site
Indications	Intersymptom intervals <1 wk; noncompliant patients	Infrequent, fairly long-lasting, and noninvalidating symptoms; compliant patients	Intersymptom intervals ≤4 wk, short-lasting and/or invalidating symptoms (ie, syncope); very compliant patients	Infrequent, short-lasting and/or invalidating symptoms (ie, syncope); noncompliant patients

Abbreviations: ECG, electrocardiogram; MCOT, mobile cardiac outpatient telemetry.

can be used even in the presence of incapacitating symptoms, such as syncope, which normally prevents the activation of other electrocardiographic monitoring devices that do not have this feature.

Through implementing dedicated algorithms and sensing parameters similar to those of implantable cardioverter defibrillators and pacemakers, the new-generation ILRs are also able to automatically detect (ie, without any active intervention by the patient) any kind of arrhythmic event, from bradycardia to asystole, and atrial fibrillation to ventricular tachycardia.[5–7] Finally, the new-generation devices now have a monitoring life of at least 36 months.

The implantation of an ILR is a simple and minimally invasive procedure. The standard method follows a few fundamental steps: external electrocardiographic mapping to determine the optimal implantation site and device position, corresponding to a sufficient R-wave amplitude; insertion of the ILR, through a small skin incision, into a subcutaneous pocket; anchoring of the device to the muscular plane to avoid mechanical instability, displacement, and migration; and inspection of electrocardiographic tracing recorded by the

device with the external programmer at the end of the procedure.

The typical location of an ILR is in the left parasternal area of the chest (**Fig. 1**). This position guarantees good R-wave amplitude and clearly analyzable P, QRS, and T waves on the stored electrocardiogram,[5–7] and, in the authors' experience, makes mapping not always strictly necessary. Other locations have been suggested, especially in younger patients, to minimize the aesthetic and psychological impact of the surgical scar in the anterior chest region, without impairing the performance of the device. One of these is the so-called left axillary location,[8] involving a small incision at the fourth intercostal space at the level of the left anterior axillary line, and insertion of the ILR into a submuscular pocket parallel to the intercostal space. The inframammary location has been proposed in young girls,[9] in which the ILR is implanted through a 2-cm transverse incision at the inferior and medial border of the left or right breast. Recently, a new location was proposed in the left upper chest area, midway between the supraclavicular notch and the left breast area.[5] Finally, ILRs are easily

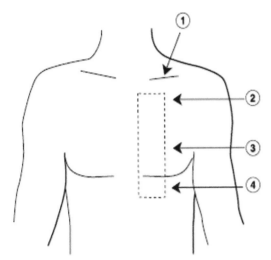

Fig. 1. Implant location of ILRs. (1) Midclavicular line, (2) 1st rib, (3) 4th rib, and (4) V3 implant site. (*From* Giada F, Bertaglia E, Reimers B, et al. Current and emerging indications for implantable cardiac monitors. Pacing Clin Electrophysiol 2012;35:1169–78; with permission.)

explanted once the diagnosis has been made or the battery has depleted.

All of the stored data are analyzed through interrogating the device. The follow-up of the ILRs can be performed periodically in-office through the external programmer similar to that of pacemakers, or remotely through an automatic transmitter and Web-based software. Furthermore, in the case of a symptomatic event, the patient is asked to come as soon as possible to the hospital, have an in-office check of the device, or transmit the data stored in the ILR via the remote monitoring system. This last feature is very promising, in that it can significantly reduce both costs and the time to diagnosis and therapy, and increase patient compliance.[10]

ILRS IN THE DIAGNOSTIC EVALUATION OF TRANSIENT LOSS OF CONSCIOUSNESS

In current clinical practice, ILRs are used as diagnostic tools to evaluate transient loss of consciousness of possible arrhythmic origin, particularly unexplained syncope. Moreover, ILRs can also be used in the field of difficult cases of epilepsy and unexplained falls, although current indications for their application in these sectors are less clearly defined.

Unexplained Syncope

In patients with syncope that remain unexplained after the initial clinical evaluation (clinical history, physical examination and standard 12-lead electrocardiogram), electrocardiographic recording is considered the diagnostic gold standard.[3,4,11] Thus, when syncopes are clinically relevant (ie, recurrent, accompanied by reduced quality of life and/or trauma), and/or when a high probability exists of an arrhythmic cause (ie, the patient has heart disease), long-term AECG monitoring via ILRs is often necessary.

Several studies have shown that in unexplained syncope patients with or without structural heart disease, both in older and in pediatric subjects, using an ILR yields more diagnosis than conventional testing does (**Table 2**).[3,12–22] Moreover, Krahn and colleagues[23] showed that a strategy of primary monitoring is more cost-effective than conventional testing in establishing a diagnosis in recurrent unexplained syncope. The European Society of Cardiology guidelines on the management of syncope[3] and the European Heart Rhythm Association guidelines on the use of implantable and external ECG loop recorders[4] provide a class I indication for the use of ILRs in patients with infrequent (ie, with less than monthly frequency) unexplained syncope of possible arrhythmic origin, or in high-risk patients when all other investigations prove inconclusive. However, an early use of ILRs in the diagnostic work-up can be safely adopted, provided that patients at high risk of life-threatening arrhythmic events are excluded. Finally, a recent study also suggests the use of ILRs to select patients with recurrent asystolic vasovagal syncope, before embarking on pacemaker implantation.[24]

Difficult Cases of Epilepsy

In clinical practice, epilepsy is sometimes difficult to distinguish from syncope occurring with myoclonic movements,[25] and ILRs may contribute to the diagnosis in this setting also.[26–30] Zaidi and colleagues[26] showed that, in patients with drug-refractory epilepsy, cardiovascular evaluation via ILRs may yield an alternative diagnosis in many patients. In a more recent prospective study, ILRs showed a high incidence of asystole in patients misdiagnosed as epileptic, or when the diagnosis of epilepsy was in doubt.[27] Studies by Petkar and colleagues[27] and Ho and colleagues[31] have also demonstrated the usefulness of ILRs in diagnosing typical epilepsy through the pattern of muscle artifacts associated with tonic-clonic seizures, as stored in the memory of the devices.

Finally, increasing interest is being shown in the evaluation of cardiac arrhythmias in patients with epilepsy, because epilepsy per se, and the drugs used for its treatment, may trigger arrhythmic disorders. Although whether epilepsy-related arrhythmias are always clinically relevant is not yet clear,

Table 2
Diagnostic value of ILRs in unexplained syncope

Studies	Patients (n)	Age (y)	Clinical Characteristics	Time to Diagnosis (mo)	Diagnostic Yield[a] (%)
Krahn et al,[12] 1999	60	66 ± 14 (mean ± SD)	SHD = 23	4 ± 3 (mean ± SD)	55
Solano et al,[13] 2004	103	69 ± 11 (mean ± SD)	SHD = 63	13, 6–23 (median, IQR)	50
Farwell et al,[14] 2006	101	74, 62–81 (median, IQR)	Unselected	17, 9–23 (median, IQR)	43
Brignole et al,[21] 2006	392	66 ± 14 (mean ± SD)	Suspected neurally mediated syncope	3, 1–7 (median, IQR)	27
Frangini et al,[15] 2008	27	15, 2–25 (median, IQR)	SHD = 8; long QT = 3; ventricular tachycardia = 5	3, 1–20 (median, IQR)	70
Kabra et al,[16] 2009	86	55 ± 19 (mean ± SD)	SHD = 24	3 ± 4 (mean ± SD)	62
Al Dhahri et al,[17] 2009	42	12, 1–19 (median, IQR)	SHD = 18; long QT = 7; family history of sudden death = 8	14, 1–24 (median, IQR)	63
Brignole et al,[4] 2009	506	Not available	Unselected	Not available	35
Edvardsson et al,[22] 2011	570	61 ± 17 (mean ± SD)	Unselected	Not available	32

Abbreviations: IQR, interquartile range; Long QT, long QT syndrome; SD, standard deviation; SHD, structural heart disease.
[a] Number of diagnoses/number of implanted patients.

some cases of sudden death in patients with epilepsy—so-called sudden unexpected death in epilepsy (SUDEP)—have already been reported.[29,32] The dysregulation of respiratory physiology, cardiac factors, dysfunction of systemic and cerebral circulation, seizure-induced hormonal and metabolic changes, and multiple antiepileptic drugs might all contribute to SUDEP. Cardiac factors include not only ictal bradyarrhythmias and asystole but also tachyarrhythmias and alterations of ventricular repolarization. Thus, ILR application in patients with epilepsy at high risk of SUDEP might be an interesting area of investigation in the near future.[32]

In conclusion, ILRs may have a diagnostic role in difficult or dubious cases of epilepsy, in drug-resistant epilepsy, and whenever the presence of potentially harmful arrhythmias must be excluded. The European Heart Rhythm Association guidelines on the use of implantable and external electrocardiogram loop recorders provide a class IIb indication for the use of implantable cardiovascular monitors in "patients in whom epilepsy is suspected but the treatment has proved ineffective and in patients with established epilepsy in order to detect peri-ictal cardiac arrhythmias that require treatment."[4]

Unexplained Falls

Falls remain a major health and socioeconomic problem. Each year, 30% of individuals older than 65 years experience falls. Up to 5% of falls result in a fracture and 1% in hip fractures.[33] Growing evidence suggests an overlap between syncope and unexplained falls in the elderly.[34,35] Moreover, patients with unexplained falls who present to the emergency room display a high prevalence of carotid sinus hypersensitivity. Thus, ILRs may also play a role in this population, especially in patients who have recurrent unexplained falls and clinical and/or ECG features at high risk for arrhythmic events.[3,4] In this regard, however, the Safepace 2 trial, a study in which patients with unexplained falls and/or syncope and cardioinhibitory carotid sinus hypersensitivity were randomized to dual-chamber pacing or ILR implantation, showed disappointing results.[36] The syncopal recurrence rate was not statistically different in the active and placebo arms of the study. The European Heart Rhythm Association guidelines on the use of implantable and external electrocardiographic loop recorders provide a class IIb indication for using implantable cardiovascular monitors in "older patients with non-accidental falls to establish the syncopal nature of the event."[4]

LIMITATIONS OF ILRS

The subcutaneous implantation of ILRs is a minimally invasive procedure and may carry a risk of minor complications at the implantation site. The literature reports this complication in fewer than 1% of patients.[21] Miniaturization of the devices might promote their use through reducing their aesthetic impact and making the implantation procedure safer, easier, and faster.

Although several steps forward have been taken in the new-generations devices, one of the major limitations of ILRs remains the sensing. It is not uncommon to have a significant part of automatically detected events reflect only artifacts. To help overcome the problem of oversensing, it is recommended that attention be paid to the implanting technique (creating a tight subcutaneous pocket and anchoring the device to the muscular plane) and to periodically check, particularly in the first weeks after implantation, the autoactivation algorithms and sensing parameters.

The various forms of supraventricular tachycardia are not always easy to distinguish in the rhythms recorded by ILRs, nor is ventricular tachycardia easy to distinguish from supraventricular tachycardia with aberrant conduction. Thus, an electrophysiologic evaluation may be necessary to clarify the nature of recorded rhythm disorders. Moreover, another potential limit of ILRs, which has been partially overcome by the electrocardiographic classification of spontaneous syncope proposed by Brignole and colleagues,[4] is the difficulty in differentiating reflex bradyarrhythmias, which have a benign prognosis, from those related to intrinsic cardiac conduction disease, which have a poor prognosis. Finally, ILRs do not provide information regarding blood pressure or electroencephalogram, which are potentially useful data for the study of patients with problematic syncope or transient loss of consciousness.

REFERENCES

1. Zimetbaum PJ, Kim KY, Josephson ME, et al. Diagnostic yield and optimal duration of continuous-loop event monitoring for the diagnosis of palpitations. Ann Intern Med 1998;28:890–5.

2. Bass EB, Curtiss EI, Arena VC, et al. The duration of Holter monitoring in patients with syncope: is 24 hours enough? Arch Intern Med 1990;150:1073–8.

3. Moya A, Sutton R, Ammirati F, et al, The Task Force for the Diagnosis and Management of Syncope, European Society of Cardiology (ESC), Developed in collaboration with, European Heart Rhythm Association (EHRA), Heart Failure Association (HFA), Heart Rhythm Society (HRS). Guidelines for the diagnosis and management of syncope (version 2009). Eur Heart J 2009;30(21):2631–71.

4. Brignole M, Vardas P, Hoffman E, et al. Indications for the use of diagnostic implantable and external ECG loop recorders. Europace 2009;11:671–87.

5. Grubb BP, Welch M, Kanjwal K, et al. An anatomic-based approach for the placement of implantable loop recorders. Pacing Clin Electrophysiol 2010;33:1149–52.

6. Jacob S, Kommuri NV, Zalawadiya SK, et al. Sensing performance of a new wireless implantable loop recorder: a 12-month follow-up study. Pacing Clin Electrophysiol 2010;33:834–40.

7. Hindricks G, Pokushalov E, Urban L, et al, for the XPECT Trial investigators. Performance of a new implantable cardiac monitor in detecting and quantifying atrial fibrillation. Results of the XPECT trial. Circ Arrhythm Electrophysiol 2010;3:141–7.

8. Miracapillo G, Costoli A, Addonisio L, et al. Left axillary implantation of loop recorder. Pacing Clin Electrophysiol 2010;33:999–1002.

9. Kannankeril PJ, Bibeau DA, Fish FA. Feasibility of the inframammary location for insertable loop recorders in young women and girls. Pacing Clin Electrophysiol 2004;27(4):492–4.

10. Furukawa T, Maggi R, Bertolone C, et al. Effectiveness of remote monitoring in the management of syncope and palpitations. Europace 2011;13(3):431–7.

11. Giada F, Gulizia M, Francese M, et al. Recurrent Unexplained Palpitations (RUP) study. Comparison of implantable loop recorder versus conventional diagnostic strategy. J Am Coll Cardiol 2007;49:1951–6.

12. Krahn AD, Klein GJ, Yee R, et al, for the Reveal Investigators. Use of an extended monitoring strategy in patients with problematic syncope. Circulation 1999;99:406–10.

13. Solano A, Menozzi C, Maggi R, et al. Incidence, diagnostic yield and safety of the implantable loop-recorder to detect the mechanism of syncope in patients with and without structural heart disease. Eur Heart J 2004;25:1116–9.

14. Farwell DJ, Freemantle N, Sulke N. The clinical impact of implantable loop recorders in patients with syncope. Eur Heart J 2006;27:351–6.

15. Frangini PA, Cecchin F, Jordao L, et al. How revealing are insertable loop recorders in pediatrics? Pacing Clin Electrophysiol 2008;31:338–43.

16. Kabra R, Gopinathannair R, Sandesara C, et al. The dual role of implantable loop recorder in patients with potentially arrhythmic symptoms: a retrospective single-center study. Pacing Clin Electrophysiol 2009;32:908–12.

17. Al Dhahri KN, Potts JE, Chiu CC, et al. Are implantable loop recorders useful in detecting arrhythmias in children with unexplained syncope? Pacing Clin Electrophysiol 2009;32:1422–7.

18. Brignole M, Menozzi C, Moya A, et al. Mechanism of syncope in patients with bundle branch block and negative electrophysiological test. Circulation 2001; 104:2045–50.

19. Menozzi C, Brignole M, Garcia-Civeira R, et al. Mechanism of syncope in patients with heart disease and negative electrophysiological test. Circulation 2002;105:2741–5.

20. Moya A, Brignole M, Menozzi C, et al. Mechanism of syncope in patients with isolated syncope and in patients with tilt-positive syncope. Circulation 2001; 104:1261–7.

21. Brignole M, Sutton R, Menozzi C, et al. Early application of an implantable loop recorder allows effective specific treatment in patients with recurrent suspected neurally mediated syncope. Eur Heart J 2006;27:1085–92.

22. Edvardsson M, Frykman V, van Mechelen R, et al. Use of an implantable loop recorder to increase the diagnostic yield in unexplained syncope: results from the PICTURE registry. Europace 2011;13:262–9.

23. Krahn AD, Klein GJ, Yee R, et al. Cost implications of testing strategy in patients with syncope. Randomized Assessment of Syncope Trial. J Am Coll Cardiol 2003;42:495–501.

24. Brignole M, Menozzi C, Moya A, et al, for the International Study on Syncope of Uncertain Etiology 3 (ISSUE-3) Investigators. Pacemaker therapy in patients with neurally mediated syncope and documented asystole: third international study on syncope of uncertain etiology (ISSUE-3): a randomized trial. Circulation 2012;125:2566–71.

25. Fitzpatrick AP, Cooper P. Diagnosis and management of patients with blackouts. Heart 2006;92: 559–68.

26. Zaidi A, Clough P, Cooper P, et al. Misdiagnosis of epilepsy: many seizure-like attacks have a cardiovascular cause. J Am Coll Cardiol 2000;36:181–4.

27. Petkar S, Iddon P, Bell W, et al. REVISE (Reveal in the Investigation of Syncope and Epilepsy) study [abstract]. Eur Heart J 2009;30(Suppl 1):15 [abstract: 245].

28. Rodrigues TD, Sternick EB, Moreira MD. Epilepsy or syncope? An analysis of 55 consecutive patients with loss of consciousness, convulsions, falls, and no EEG abnormalities. Pacing Clin Electrophysiol 2010;33:804–13.

29. Surges R, Thijs RD, Tan HL, et al. Sudden unexpected death in epilepsy: risk factors and potential pathomechanisms. Nat Rev Neurol 2009;5: 492–504.

30. Standridge SM, Holland KD, Horn PS. Cardiac arrhythmias and ictal events within an epilepsy monitoring unit. Pediatr Neurol 2010;42:201–5.

31. Ho RT, Wicks T, Wyeth D, et al. Generalized tonic-clonic seizures detected by implantable loop recorder devices: diagnosing more than cardiac arrhythmias. Heart Rhythm 2006;3:857–61.

32. Rugg-Gunn FJ, Simister RJ, Squirrell M, et al. Cardiac arrhythmias in focal epilepsy: a prospective long-term study. Lancet 2004;364:2212–9.

33. O'Loughlin JL, Robitaille Y, Boivin JF, et al. Incidence of and risk factors for falls and injurious falls among the community-dwelling elderly. Am J Epidemiol 1993;137:342–5.

34. Kenny RA, for the SAFE PACE 2 study group. SAFE PACE 2: syncope and falls in the elderly — pacing and carotid sinus evaluation a randomized controlled trial of cardiac pacing in older patients with falls and carotid sinus hypersensitivity. Europace 1999;1:69–72.

35. Richardson DA, Bexton RS, Shaw FE, et al. Prevalence of cardioinhibitory carotid sinus hypersensitivity (CICSH) in accident and emergency attendances with falls or syncope. Pacing Clin Electrophysiol 1997;20:820–3.

36. Ryan DJ, Nick S, Colette SM, et al. Carotid sinus syndrome, should be pace? A multicentre, randomised control trial (Safepace 2). Heart 2010;96(7): 550–60.

Value of EP Study and Other Cardiac Investigations

CrossMark

Mark Preminger, MD[a], Suneet Mittal, MD, FHRS[a,b],*

KEYWORDS

- Electrophysiology study • Syncope • Bradyarrhythmia • Tachyarrhythmia

KEY POINTS

- Syncope is a common condition that, at some point, affects a large portion of the population.
- Early assessment in the emergency department with a comprehensive history, physical examination, use of simple blood tests, and careful assessment of the 12-lead electrocardiogram (ECG) is often sufficient to identify patients who are at highest risk.
- An electrophysiology (EP) study to assess the integrity of the His-Purkinje system is reasonable in patients with bifascicular block who present with syncope. Patients with an HV interval of >70 msec warrant pacemaker implantation. Patients with a normal HV interval should undergo loop recorder implantation given the poor negative predictive value of EP studies for the diagnosis of a significant bradyarrhythmia.
- In patients with preserved left ventricular function and a history of palpitations preceding the syncopal episode, EP studies can identify an SVT (or VT) that may be amenable to curative therapy with catheter ablation.
- Patients with significant structural heart disease presenting with syncope rarely require EP studies because current guidelines advocate ICD implantation in this cohort for prevention of sudden death.

INTRODUCTION

With the advent of implantable loop recorders (ILRs) capable of prolonged electrocardiographic monitoring, and following studies demonstrating the benefit of implantable cardioverter-defibrillator (ICD) therapy in subgroups of patients with structural heart disease and depressed left ventricular function, the role of invasive cardiac electrophysiologic (EP) studies in patients with unexplained syncope has been substantially reduced. Nonetheless, in select high-risk patients presenting with unexplained syncope, EP studies still play an important role in identifying a diagnosis in these patients and assessing long-term risk of mortality.

IDENTIFICATION OF HIGH-RISK PATIENTS

Syncope is a common condition that, at some point, affects a large portion of the population. In the Framingham study, which evaluated and followed a cohort of 7800 patients over a 17-year period, the 10-year cumulative incidence of syncope was 6%, with 22% of patients reporting recurrent events.[1] The incidence increases sharply with age, particularly for those older than 70 years. Syncope itself is associated with a decreased survival compared with the general population, and this holds true for all forms of syncope, with the exception of neutrally mediated syncope. Multiple studies have shown that a cardiac cause for

This article originally appeared in Cardiac Electrophysiology Clinics, Volume 5, Issue 4, December 2013.
Disclosures: None.
[a] Arrhythmia Institute, Valley Health System, 223 North Van Dien Avenue, Ridgewood, NJ 07450, USA; [b] The Valley Hospital, 223 North Van Dien Avenue, Ridgewood, NJ 07450, USA
* Corresponding author. The Valley Hospital, 223 North Van Dien Avenue, Ridgewood, NJ 07450.
E-mail address: mittsu@valleyhealth.com

syncope is associated with a high risk for subsequent mortality; in fact, the 6-month mortality in these patients is in excess of 10%. This risk is twice that of the general population.[2,3] It is therefore essential to distinguish between patients likely to have a cardiac cause for syncope, and who are therefore at high risk, from low-risk patients with a neutrally mediated or noncardiac cause of syncope (**Fig. 1**).

Early assessment in the emergency room with a comprehensive history, physical examination, use of simple blood tests, and careful assessment of the 12-lead electrocardiogram (ECG) are often sufficient to identify those patients who are at highest risk. These patients warrant in-hospital and potentially invasive additional evaluation. Current practice guidelines suggest prompt hospitalization when syncope occurs in the setting of severe structural or coronary artery disease (signs and symptoms of aortic stenosis, heart failure, prior myocardial infarction, known left ventricular dysfunction), when clinical or ECG criteria suggest arrhythmic syncope (**Box 1**) or important comorbidities (severe anemia, electrolyte disturbance) are present.[4] Patients in whom a decision is made to pursue hospitalization should undergo at least 24 hours of continuous ECG (telemetry or Holter) monitoring, as well as baseline echocardiography.

In a patient (especially in a younger patient) with a normal ECG and no structural heart disease, vasovagal syncope should be strongly considered. Additionally, micturition, defecation, deglutition, and post-tussive syncope are common "situational" forms of the same disorder. A carefully obtained history remains the gold standard for diagnosis of vasovagal syncope. In patients with no underlying structural heart disease, the Calgary Syncope Symptom Score can distinguish (based on the history alone) between vasovagal and another etiology of syncope with excellent sensitivity and specificity (**Table 1**).[5] In clinical practice, tilt table testing is widely used to "diagnose" patients with vasovagal syncope; however, many fundamental limitations exist to the routine use of tilt table testing. First and foremost, there is no standardized tilt test protocol. A second major problem with tilt testing is its poor sensitivity when using a protocol that maintains high specificity. This limitation is acknowledged in the recent American Heart Association/American College of Cardiology Foundation scientific statement on the evaluation of syncope.[6] In patients without structural heart disease, the pretest probability that the diagnosis is vasovagal syncope is high, *irrespective* of the tilt test result. Therefore, it is generally more important to exclude the possibility of a serious bradyarrhythmia or tachyarrhythmia as the etiology for syncope.

When the cause for syncope remains elusive, the practitioner has to determine whether an EP study is warranted. These studies can be performed safely with a very low risk of complications.[7] **Table 2**

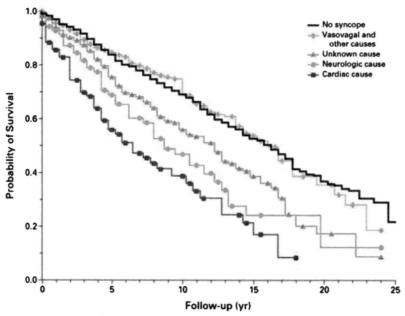

Fig. 1. Overall survival of participants with syncope, according to cause, and participants without syncope. (*From* Soteriades ES, Evans JC, Larson MG, et al. Incidence and prognosis of syncope. N Engl J Med 2002:347;978–885; with permission.)

<table>
<tr><td colspan="2">

Box 1
Features suggesting arrhythmic syncope

- Syncope during exertion or while supine
- Palpitations at the time of syncope
- Family history of sudden cardiac death
- Nonsustained ventricular tachycardia
- Bifascicular block (LBBB or RBBB combined with left anterior or left posterior fascicular block) or other intraventricular conduction abnormalities with QRS duration ≥120 msec
- Severe sinus bradycardia
- Manifest preexcitation
- Short or long QT interval
- RBBB pattern with coved ST-elevation in leads V1–V2 (Brugada pattern)
- Negative T waves in right precordial leads and epsilon waves (ARVC)

Abbreviations: ARVC, arrhythmogenic right ventricular cardiomyopathy; LBBB, left bundle branch block; RBBB, right bundle branch block.
Data from Moya A, Sutton R, Ammirati F, et al. Guidelines for the diagnosis and management of syncope (version 2009): the Task Force for the Diagnosis and Management of Syncope of the European Society of Cardiology. Eur Heart J 2009;30:2631–71.
</td></tr>
</table>

Table 1
Calgary Syncope Symptom Score

History	Point Score
Is there a history of one of the following: bifascicular block, asystole, supraventricular tachycardia, diabetes?	(−) 5
At times have bystanders noted you to be blue during your faint?	(−) 4
Did your syncope start when you were 35 y of age or older?	(−) 3
Do you remember anything about being unconscious?	(−) 2
Do you have lightheaded spells or faint with prolonged sitting or standing?	(+) 1
Do you sweat or feel warm before a faint?	(+) 2
Do you have lightheaded spells or faint with pain or in medical settings?	(+) 3

The patient has vasovagal syncope if the point score is ≥−2.
Data from Sheldon R, Rose S, Connolly S, et al, for the Syncope Symptom Study Investigators. Diagnostic criteria for vasovagal syncope based on a quantitative history. Eur Heart J 2006;27:344–50.

summarizes current recommendations for an EP study in patients with unexplained syncope. **Table 3** summarizes criteria that establish a definitive diagnosis at EP study.

ELECTROPHYSIOLOGY STUDY
Bradyarrhythmia

Often, a bradyarrhythmia is suspected but not overtly manifest on the presenting ECG. Historically, an EP study has been considered the gold standard for the evaluation of the sinus node, atrioventricular (AV) node, and His-Purkinje system function in these patients. These EP studies are most useful when the patient's baseline ECG demonstrates sinus bradycardia or conduction system disease (prolonged PR interval and/or bundle branch block). In general, EP studies have high specificity but poor sensitivity for the diagnosis of a bradyarrhythmia. Thus, they can help establish a diagnosis but cannot exclude significant pathology.

The corrected sinus node recovery time (CSNRT), a measure of the automaticity of the sinus node, is commonly determined to assess sinus node function. Typically, rapid pacing at a fixed cycle length (600 msec, then 500 msec, and then 400 msec; separated by 60 seconds) for 30 to 60 seconds is initiated in the high right atrium. The interval from the cessation of pacing to the first intrinsic return sinus beat is defined as the sinus node recovery time (SNRT). To "correct" for the influence of underlying sinus rate, the CSNRT is determined by subtracting the sinus cycle length from the SNRT. A CSNRT of more than 525 msec is considered indicative of sinus node dysfunction (see **Table 3**).

AV node and His Purkinje function is best assessed by measurements obtained on a catheter placed across the tricuspid valve on the membranous septum adjacent to the penetrating bundle of His.[8] A sharp His bundle recording provides the means of differentiating AV block occurring above, at, or below this level. Type I second-degree AV block (Wenckebach) represents a normal physiologic property of the AV node, namely decremental conduction. AV nodal Wenckebach block usually occurs during incremental atrial pacing at rates of more than 110 beats per minute. However, at EP study, the pacing rate at which Wenckebach block occurs is markedly affected by autonomic tone, making interpretations about "abnormal" AV node function in a patient with unexplained syncope difficult. Not surprisingly, no cutoff criteria are considered diagnostic of an abnormal response (see **Table 3**).

Table 2
Indications for electrophysiology study in patients with unexplained syncope

Indication	Class of Recommendation	Level of Evidence
In patients with ischemic heart disease, EPS is indicated when initial evaluation suggests an arrhythmic cause for syncope (see **Table 4**) unless there is already an established indication for ICD	I	B
In patients with BBB, EPS should be considered when noninvasive tests have failed to make the diagnosis	IIa	B
In patients with syncope preceded by sudden and brief palpitations, EPS may be performed when other noninvasive tests have failed to make the diagnosis	IIb	B
In patients with Brugada syndrome, ARVC, and hypertrophic cardiomyopathy, an EPS may be performed in selected cases	IIb	C
In patients with high-risk occupations, in whom every effort to exclude a cardiovascular cause of syncope is warranted, an EPS may be performed in selected cases	IIb	C
EPS is not recommended in patients with normal ECG, no heart disease, and no palpitations	III	B

Abbreviations: ARVC, arrhythmogenic right ventricular cardiomyopathy; BBB, bundle branch block; ECG, electrocardiogram; EPS, electrophysiology study.
Data from Moya A, Sutton R, Ammirati F, et al. Guidelines for the diagnosis and management of syncope (version 2009): the Task Force for the Diagnosis and Management of Syncope of the European Society of Cardiology. Eur Heart J 2009;30:2631–71.

Table 3
Criteria that establish a definitive diagnosis of syncope at electrophysiology study

Indication	Class of Recommendation	Level of Evidence
EPS is diagnostic, and no additional tests are required, in the following cases:		
Sinus bradycardia and prolonged CSNRT (>525 msec)	I	B
BBB and either a baseline HV interval of ≥100 msec, or second-degree or third-degree His-Purkinje block is demonstrated during incremental atrial pacing or with pharmacologic challenge	I	B
Induction of sustained monomorphic VT in patients with previous myocardial infarction	I	B
Induction of rapid SVT that reproduces hypotensive or spontaneous symptoms	I	B
An HV interval between 70 and 100 msec should be considered diagnostic	IIa	B
The induction of polymorphic VT or ventricular fibrillation in patients with Brugada syndrome, ARVC, and patients resuscitated from cardiac arrest may be considered diagnostic	IIb	B
The induction of polymorphic VT or ventricular fibrillation in patients with ischemic cardiomyopathy or DCM cannot be considered a diagnostic finding	III	B

Abbreviations: ARVC, arrhythmogenic right ventricular cardiomyopathy; BBB, bundle branch block; CSNRT, corrected sinus node recovery time; DCM, dilated cardiomyopathy; EPS, electrophysiology study; SVT, supraventricular tachycardia; VT, ventricular tachycardia.
Data from Moya A, Sutton R, Ammirati F, et al. Guidelines for the diagnosis and management of syncope (version 2009): the Task Force for the Diagnosis and Management of Syncope of the European Society of Cardiology. Eur Heart J 2009;30:2631–71.

On the other hand, the His bundle and its distal extensions, the bundle branches, and the Purkinje network are not influenced by autonomic tone. Thus, conduction delay or block at or below the level of the His bundle is a more ominous finding. Abnormal conduction within the His bundle is reflected either by prolongation of the His bundle duration to a width of greater than 25 msec or the emergence of a "split" His electrogram. In this case of a split His electrogram, both type I and type II patterns of block between H1 and H2 can be observed. Intra-His block accounts for up to 20% of heart block cases and usually requires implantation of a permanent pacemaker.

A properly measured HV interval measures 35 to 55 msec. An HV interval of shorter than 60 msec is associated with a low incidence (2%–4%) of progression to complete AV block, whereas an

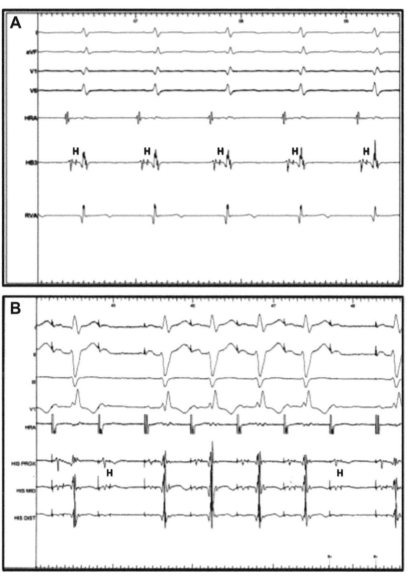

Fig. 2. Normal His-Purkinje conduction and infra-Hisian atrioventricular (AV) block during rapid atrial pacing. (*A*) Shown are surface ECG leads I, avF, V1, and V6 along with intracardiac recordings from the high right atrium (HRA), His-bundle region (HBE3), and right ventricular apex (RVA). The rhythm is sinus; there is 1:1 AV conduction with a normal HV interval. (*B*) Shown are surface ECG leads I, II, III, and V1, along with intracardiac recordings from the HRA and His-bundle region (His prox, mid, and dist). During rapid atrial pacing from the HRA, there is evidence of right bundle branch block. In addition, there is intermittent type II infra-Hisian AV block. Specifically, the His-bundle electrogram (H) is not followed by ventricular depolarization. This is a sign of significant His-Purkinje system dysfunction.

HV interval of longer than 100 msec has been associated with progression to complete AV block in nearly one-quarter of patients, and death in nearly one-fifth of patients over an average follow-up period of 2 years.[9,10] Current guidelines state that an HV interval of 100 msec or longer is a class I indication for pacemaker implantation, *even in the absence of symptoms*.[3] In patients presenting with syncope, an HV interval between 70 and 100 msec is considered a class IIb indication for cardiac pacing.[3] Alternatively, provocative testing can be performed.[11–13] An increment in HV interval of longer than 10 msec or development of infra-His block during either rapid atrial pacing or following administration of a class IA antiarrhythmic drug (eg, procainamide 10 mg/kg intravenously) is associated with a 30% to 40% incidence of progression to complete AV block over a 2-year to 4-year period (**Fig. 2**). Unfortunately, an HV interval shorter than 70 msec, especially in patients

Table 4
Characteristics of implantable loop recorders

ILR Device	Reveal XT	Confirm ICM	Sleuth AT
Manufacturer	Medtronic	St. Jude	Transoma Medical
Indication approved by the Food and Drug Administration	• Patients with clinical syndromes or situations at increased risk of cardiac arrhythmias • Patients who experience transient symptoms that may suggest a cardiac arrhythmia		
Size and comparable item	8 cc Similar to memory stick drive	6.5 cc Similar to memory stick drive	8 cc Similar to 50-cent piece or small pacemaker, with flexible antenna
Additional components	• Hand-held, personal diagnostic manager (PDM) • Home transmitter/ base station	• Hand-held, activator box • Home transmitter/ base station • Programming device/ portable computer (for doctor only)	• Hand-held, personal diagnostic manager (PDM) • Home transmitter/ base station
Monitoring service	Medtronic CareLink Network for data storage and physician notification of events	St. Jude Merlin Network for data storage and physician notification of events	Medicomp: 24/7 monitoring by certified cardiac technicians with alert to physicians of substantive events
Placement	Subcutaneous, chest area	Subcutaneous, chest area	Subcutaneous, chest toward shoulder
Data collection modes	• Patient triggered storage • Automatic programmed storage at predetermined heart rates • 49.5 min of stored electrograms • Transtelephonic monitoring	• Patient triggered storage • Automatic programmed storage at predetermined heart rates • 48 min of stored electrograms • Transtelephonic monitoring	• Patient triggered storage • Automatic programmed storage at predetermined heart rates • Automatic capture every 20 s, 7.5 min, 15 min, or 4 h • 43 min of stored electrograms • Wireless transmission of data to PDM and transtelephonic delivery to Medicomp Service
Longevity (battery life)	3 y	3 y	2.3 y

The Reveal XT and Confirm devices remain commercially available. The Sleuth AT device is no longer available, as the manufacturer went out of business.

with underlying bundle branch block, cannot be considered a reassuring finding in patients with syncope. For example, with use of an implanted loop recorder, it has been possible to demonstrate that in one-third of patients with bundle branch block (specifically, right bundle branch and fascicular block or left bundle branch block), recurrent syncope results from paroxysmal AV block, even though the EP study is "normal" (HV <70 msec).[14]

The disappointing yield of EP studies in patients with syncope in the absence of structural heart disease has necessitated the use of alternative diagnostic strategies. The most promising is the implantable loop recorder. This has been shown to be superior to a more conventional strategy of EP and tilt testing in making a definitive diagnosis (which is usually a form of bradycardia) in patients without structural heart disease presenting with syncope.[15] The appeal of the implantable loop recorder has been greatly enhanced by the release of second-generation devices that can be interrogated remotely from a patient's home and have a near 3-year battery longevity (**Table 4**). These devices are implanted subcutaneously in the left parasternal region; storage of ECG data can be triggered by either the patient (in response to symptoms) or automatically if the heart rate falls below or exceeds a physician-programmed detection rate. The captured data can be retrieved either remotely or in-office using a standard device programmer.[16,17]

Tachyarrhythmia

Although syncope occurs in up to 15% to 20% of patients with a supraventricular tachycardia (SVT), *unexplained* syncope is rarely caused by an SVT. Symptoms of palpitations typically precede episodes of syncope in patients with an underlying SVT; however, in elderly patients, the onset of an SVT can be associated with marked hemodynamic compromise that can result in an abrupt syncopal episode without prodrome (**Fig. 3**). In patients with Wolff-Parkinson-White (WPW) syndrome, syncope is associated with a faster cycle length of orthodromic tachycardia and shorter refractory periods of the accessory pathway. As a result, EP study (and catheter ablation) is a class I indication in patients with WPW with unexplained syncope.

In the past, an EP study was used routinely to assess a patient's risk for developing a ventricular tachyarrhythmia. The greatest yield of EP testing was demonstrated in patients with underlying structural heart disease, those in whom syncope occurred *during* exercise, those who experienced chest pain or palpitations before syncope, and those with a family history of sudden death. Sustained monomorphic ventricular tachycardia is inducible in approximately 40% of patients with an ischemic cardiomyopathy who present with unexplained syncope.[18] Because these patients are at high risk for sudden cardiac death, an ICD is

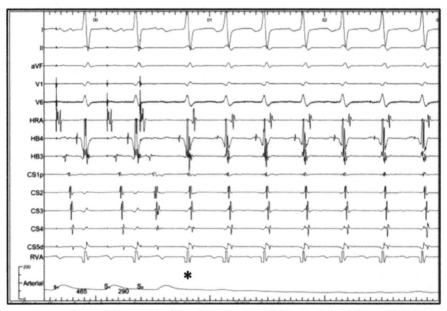

Fig. 3. Hemodynamic collapse during induced supraventricular tachycardia (SVT). Shown are surface ECG leads I, II, avF, V1 and V6, intracardiac electrograms from the high right atrium (HRA), His-bundle (HB3 and HB4), coronary sinus (CS), and right ventricular apex (RVA), and continuous blood pressure recordings. There is immediate hemodynamic collapse at the onset of induced SVT (*asterisk*). This patient presented with an episode of syncope preceded by palpitations.

Box 2
Indications for ICD implantation in patients with unexplained syncope

Class I indication

- ICD therapy is indicated in patients with syncope of undetermined origin with clinically relevant, hemodynamically significant sustained ventricular tachycardia or fibrillation induced at EP study (*Level of Evidence: B*).

Class IIa indications

- ICD implantation is reasonable for patients with unexplained syncope, significant left ventricular dysfunction, and nonischemic dilated cardiomyopathy (*Level of Evidence: C*).
- ICD implantation is reasonable for patients with hypertrophic cardiomyopathy who have 1 or more major[a] risk factors for sudden cardiac death (*Level of Evidence: C*).
- ICD implantation is reasonable for the prevention of sudden cardiac death in patients with arrhythmogenic right ventricular dysplasia/cardiomyopathy who have 1 or more risk factors for sudden cardiac death (*Level of Evidence: C*).
- ICD implantation is reasonable to reduce sudden cardiac death in patients with long-QT syndrome who are experiencing syncope and/or ventricular tachycardia while receiving β blockers (*Level of Evidence: B*).
- ICD implantation is reasonable for patients with Brugada syndrome who have had syncope (*Level of Evidence: C*).

Class IIb indication

- ICD therapy may be considered in patients with syncope and advanced structural heart disease in whom thorough invasive and noninvasive investigations have failed to define a cause (*Level of Evidence: C*).

Class III indication

- ICD therapy is not indicated for syncope of undetermined cause in a patient without inducible ventricular tachyarrhythmias and without structural heart disease (*Level of Evidence: C*).

[a] See Section 3.2.4 in Ref.[21] for definition of major risk factors.

Adapted from Epstein AE, DiMarco JP, Ellenbogen KA, et al. ACC/AHA/HRS 2008 guidelines for device-based therapy of cardiac rhythm abnormalities: A report of the American College of Cardiology/American Heart Association Task Force on Practice Guidelines (writing committee to revise the ACC/AHA/NASPE 2002 guideline update for implantation of cardiac pacemakers and antiarrhythmia devices) Developed in collaboration with the American Association for Thoracic Surgery and Society of Thoracic Surgeons. J Am Coll Cardiol 2008;51:e1–62.

usually inserted. Within 15 months of ICD implantation, approximately 40% of these patients receive an appropriate therapy from the ICD for management of recurrent ventricular tachycardia or fibrillation. (The risk of recurrent events is greatest in patients with a prolonged QRS duration [$\geq$120 msec].[19]) Surprisingly, inducible patients, despite treatment with an ICD, have a higher overall mortality than noninducible patients.[18]

In patients with a nonischemic cardiomyopathy, it is unlikely to be able to induce monomorphic ventricular tachycardia. However, the negative predictive value of an EP study in this population is poor. Knight and colleagues[20] studied 14 patients with nonischemic cardiomyopathy, unexplained syncope, and a negative EP study, and compared their 2-year survival to 19 cardiac arrest survivors with nonischemic cardiomyopathy. All patients were implanted with an ICD. Fifty percent of patients with syncope received appropriate ICD, similar to the 40% incidence of appropriate ICD therapy in the cardiac the arrest group (P = NS). Patients with a nonischemic cardiomyopathy whose left ventricular ejection fraction is less than 30% appear to have particularly high mortality. Therefore, ICD implantation has been advocated in all of these patients who present with syncope, irrespective of the findings at EP testing.[21]

In practice, EP testing has largely been abandoned in patients with underlying structural heart disease presenting with unexplained syncope. Several randomized clinical trials have shown that these patients benefit from an ICD on the basis of their underlying left dysfunction alone, irrespective of the history of syncope. Current practice guidelines advocate a similar approach in patients with high-risk conditions, such as hypertrophic cardiomyopathy, Brugada syndrome, and congenital short-QT and long-QT syndrome who present with syncope.[21] **Box 2** summarizes current guidelines for ICD implantation in patients with unexplained syncope.

SUMMARY

EP studies have long been used as a diagnostic tool in patients presenting with unexplained syncope. However, recent data suggest that EP studies have only a limited role in a select group of these patients (see **Table 2**). In our laboratory, we routinely assess the HV interval in patients with bifascicular block to determine a patient's need for permanent pacing. However, given the poor negative value of EP studies, a loop recorder is generally indicated in patients with suspected bradycardia due to sinus node, AV node, or His-

Purkinje system dysfunction. Another role for an EP study is in those patients with suspected SVT (or VT) that may be amenable to catheter ablation. In patients with advanced structural hart disease, EP study is rarely required because these patients require ICD implantation for prevention of sudden death. However, because EP studies cannot provide a concurrent correlation between the abnormal finding and its relationship to the syncopal episode, it is imperative that *diagnostic* abnormal findings (see **Table 3**) are well understood by the practitioner.

REFERENCES

1. Soteriades ES, Evans JC, Larson MG, et al. Incidence and prognosis of syncope. N Engl J Med 2002;347:878–85.
2. Kappor WN. Syncope. N Engl J Med 2000;343:1856–62.
3. Maisel WH, Stevenson WG. Syncope—getting to the heart of the matter. N Engl J Med 2002;347:931–3.
4. Moya A, Sutton R, Ammirati F, et al. Guidelines for the diagnosis and management of syncope (version 2009): the Task Force for the Diagnosis and Management of Syncope of the European Society of Cardiology. Eur Heart J 2009;30:2631–71.
5. Sheldon R, Rose S, Connolly S, et al, for the Syncope Symptom Study Investigators. Diagnostic criteria for vasovagal syncope based on a quantitative history. Eur Heart J 2006;27:344–50.
6. Strickberger SA, Benson DW, Biaggioni I, et al. AHA/ACCF scientific statement on the evaluation of syncope. J Am Coll Cardiol 2006;47:473–84.
7. Horowitz LN, Kay HR, Kutalek SP, et al. Risks and complications of clinical cardiac electrophysiologic studies: a prospective analysis of 1,000 consecutive patients. J Am Coll Cardiol 1987;9:1261–8.
8. Scherlag BJ, Lau SH, Helfant RH, et al. Catheter technique for recording His bundle activity in man. Circulation 1969;39:13–8.
9. Scheinman MM, Peters RW, Sauve MJ, et al. Value of the H-Q interval in patients with bundle branch block and the role of prophylactic permanent pacing. Am J Cardiol 1982;50:1316–22.
10. McAnulty JH, Rahimtoola SH, Murphy ES, et al. A prospective study of sudden death in "high-risk" bundle-branch block. N Engl J Med 1978;299:209–15.
11. Haft JI, Weinstock M, DeGuia R, et al. Assessment of atrioventricular conduction in left and right bundle branch block using His-bundle electrograms and atrial pacing. Am J Cardiol 1971;27:474–80.
12. Dhingra RC, Wyndham C, Bauernfeind R, et al. Significance of block distal to the His bundle induced by atrial pacing in patients with chronic bifascicular block. Circulation 1979;60:1455–64.
13. Tonkin AM, Heddle WF, Tornos P. Intermittent atrioventricular block: procainamide administration as a provocative test. Aust N Z J Med 1978;8:594–602.
14. Brignole M, Menozzi C, Moya A, et al, on behalf of the International Study on Syncope of Uncertain Etiology (ISSUE) Investigators. Mechanism of syncope in patients with bundle branch block and negative electrophysiological test. Circulation 2001;1004:2045–50.
15. Krahn AD, Klein GJ, Yee R, et al. Randomized assessment of syncope trial: conventional diagnostic testing versus a prolonged monitoring strategy. Circulation 2001;104:46–51.
16. Paruchuri V, Adhaduk M, Garikipati NV, et al. Clinical utility of a novel wireless implantable loop recorder in the evaluation of patients with unexplained syncope. Heart Rhythm 2011;8:858–63.
17. Mittal S, Steinberg JS, editors. Remote patient monitoring in cardiology: a case-based guide. 1st edition. New York: Demos Medical; 2012. p. 31–50.
18. Mittal S, Iwai S, Stein KM, et al. Long-term outcome of patients with unexplained syncope treated with an electrophysiologic-guided approach in the implantable cardioverter-defibrillator era. J Am Coll Cardiol 1999;34:1082–9.
19. Guttigoli AB, Wilner BF, Stein KM, et al. Usefulness of prolonged QRS duration to identify high-risk ischemic cardiomyopathy patients with syncope and inducible ventricular tachycardia. Am J Cardiol 2005;95:391–4.
20. Knight BP, Goyal R, Pelosi F, et al. Outcome of patients with nonischemic dilated cardiomyopathy and unexplained syncope treated with an implantable defibrillator. J Am Coll Cardiol 1999;33:1964–70.
21. Epstein AE, DiMarco JP, Ellenbogen KA, et al. ACC/AHA/HRS 2008 guidelines for device-based therapy of cardiac rhythm abnormalities: a report of the American College of Cardiology/American Heart Association task force on practice guidelines (Writing committee to revise the ACC/AHA/NASPE 2002 guideline update for implantation of cardiac pacemakers and antiarrhythmia devices) Developed in Collaboration With the American Association for Thoracic Surgery and Society of Thoracic Surgeons. J Am Coll Cardiol 2008;51:e1–62.

How to Differentiate Syncope from Seizure

Robert Sheldon, MD, PhD

KEYWORDS

- Syncope • Convulsive syncope • Epileptic seizures • Tilt tests

KEY POINTS

- Although differences exist in the presentations of syncope and epileptic convulsions, some patients present as diagnostic dilemmas.
- Estimates of the prevalence of convulsive activity during syncope have a wide range (about 4%–40% of spells), and the differences between epileptic convulsions and convulsive syncope may be difficult for observers to distinguish.
- A careful, perceptive, evidence-based history is essential, and bystander observations are important.
- Tilt tests, despite their limitations, seem to be useful in many patients.
- Excellent communication between neurologists and internists or cardiologists probably offers the best chance for accurate diagnoses.

INTRODUCTION

The diagnosis of transient loss of consciousness poses practical challenges. The first causes to be considered are syncope and epileptic seizures, and the distinction between the two is not always made accurately.[1] Other less common possibilities, such as narcolepsy, cataplexy, arrhythmias, and pseudoseizures and pseudosyncope, should be remembered. The United Kingdom All Party Parliamentary Group on Epilepsy in 2007 reported that 74,000 UK patients were being treated for epilepsy that they did not require. Part of the problem is the frequent association of convulsive activity with syncope.[2] The investigation of loss of consciousness can be costly and intrusive and is often inconclusive.[3–7] We first review the presentations of epilepsy, syncope, and convulsive syncope, and then review how to distinguish syncope from epilepsy in patients who are diagnostic dilemmas.

EPILEPTIC SEIZURES

Epileptic seizures usually do not resemble syncopal spells. The most common epileptic seizures that are also associated with loss of consciousness are generalized tonic-clonic convulsions (**Box 1**). Atonic epileptic seizures are uncommon and occur only in children.[8] The prevalence and incidence of syncope and epilepsy are important when considering misdiagnosis rates. Banerjee and colleagues[9] reported a narrative review of world-wide publications of the epidemiology of epilepsy. The estimates vary considerably depending on the location, the method of detection and diagnosis, and the definition of prevalence. On the whole, the age-adjusted prevalence is 2 to 20 per 1000 people, and the age-adjusted incidence is 0.15 to 0.5 per 1000. In contrast to syncope, which has a lifetime cumulative incidence of more than 50%, epilepsy is much less common.

This article originally appeared in Cardiac Electrophysiology Clinics, Volume 5, Issue 4, December 2013.
The author has nothing to disclose.
Department of Cardiac Science, Libin Cardiovascular Institute of Alberta, University of Calgary, 3280 Hospital Drive Northwest, Calgary, Alberta T2N 4N1, Canada
E-mail address: sheldon@ucalgary.ca

cardiology.theclinics.com

Box 1
Common presentations in adults of epileptic convulsions and syncope

Epilepsy	Syncope
Generalized tonic-clonic epilepsy	Vasovagal syncope: blood/injury exposure
Partial complex epilepsy with collapse	Vasovagal syncope: orthostatic stress
	Initial orthostatic hypotension
	Cardiac arrhythmias
	Classic orthostatic hypotension

The presentation of epilepsy depends to some extent on the specific type, but when considering a diagnosis of syncope versus epileptic seizures the most important point is that the patient while fainting is usually limp, whereas the patient with epilepsy usually convulses. Specific triggers are less common in epilepsy than in syncope, although some memorable ones include strobe lights and sudden arousal. Similarly, specific auras are less common than are generally appreciated. Epileptic convulsions tend to last considerably longer than syncopal spells, and are followed by significant postictal confusion and disorientation. This diagnostic point requires careful questioning, because many patients with syncope also report postspell confusion. The latter is minor and brief. The convulsions tend to be rhythmic, severe, and bilateral. Useful diagnostic clues include a history of lateral tongue biting and bedwetting.[10]

SYNCOPE

Syncope is a transient loss of consciousness caused by transient global cerebral hypoperfusion characterized by rapid onset, short duration, and spontaneous complete recovery.[1] It is quite common, although in contrast to epilepsy there are fewer epidemiologic data. Savage and colleagues[11] studied middle-aged Framingham adults to estimate a lifetime prevalence of syncope of 3%, an estimate now known to be extremely low. Two estimates[12,13] of vasovagal syncope indicate that the likelihood of syncope by age 60 is about 37%, and many more faint for the first time in their later years. For many, syncope seems to occur in clusters, and the 5-year prevalence in adolescents is probably around 15% to 20%.[14] Therefore, syncope probably has a lifetime prevalence exceeding 500 per 1000 people, with correspondingly high values for incidence and prevalence over 1 to 5 years.

Syncope has numerous potential causes and classifications abound (see **Box 1**). A particularly useful one appears in the European Society Guidelines 2009,[1] whose highest level classification includes reflex syncope, syncope caused by orthostatic hypotension, and cardiac syncope, almost always caused by abrupt bradycardia or abrupt tachycardia. In the community at large vasovagal syncope is by far the most common diagnosis.[15] It is generally benign and usually does not require specific treatment. Conversely, syncope secondary to such causes as cardiac tachyarrhythmias, heart block, or valvular disease may forebode a fatal or nonfatal outcome that might be avoided with appropriate management.[1,16]

Therefore, the distinction between syncope and epilepsy depends to some extent on the cause of the syncope. One easily recognizable cause is initial orthostatic hypotension.[17] Typically the history is one of syncope either within 30 seconds of standing up, or while walking to a nearby destination, such as the kitchen, bathroom, or nearby room. The patient manages to walk only a few feet before collapse. A second easily recognizable cause is vasovagal syncope caused by exposure to needles, blood, carnage, and so forth (the so-called blood/injury fear syndrome).[18] The third very common cause is vasovagal syncope that occurs when the subject has been sitting, standing, or walking quietly for at least several minutes.[18] Memorable examples include patients who faint in church; while standing at attention; or in hot environments, such as showers. Syncope caused by classic orthostatic hypotension usually is accompanied by a history of frequent presyncope that is worsened by longer periods of upright posture, and syncope itself is much less common than presyncope. Patients with syncope caused by cardiac arrhythmias usually have no prodrome other than very brief palpitations[19,20] and usually have a history of some form of electrical or structural heart disease and electrocardiogram (ECG) abnormalities.[15,18]

Depending on the cause of syncope there may or may not be a prodrome, which most commonly consists of diaphoresis and a sense of flushing warmth.[18] True loss of consciousness usually lasts less than a minute, although some patients may take several minutes to fully regain consciousness. There is often a period, occasionally quite prolonged, of fatigue.[21] The most important feature that distinguishes syncope from seizures is that patients with syncope are usually limp, whereas patients who seize have convulsive activity, other than in rare childhood cases.

CONVULSIVE SYNCOPE

Convulsive syncope is probably quite common, is a cause of referral for epilepsy assessment and care, and is a persistent cause of misdiagnosis by specialists (**Table 1**). It has been documented clinically,[22] during tilt table testing,[23,24] and on recordings from implantable loop recorders (ILRs).[25–27] The most common kind of convulsive syncope is myoclonus, usually lasting less than a minute. Often convulsive syncope is preceded by presyncope and its associated symptoms, such as warmth and sweating, and followed by nausea and mild confusion and fatigue. Prolonged convulsions and marked postictal confusion are uncommon.

Lin and colleagues[22] reported a fascinating study of syncope and convulsions during blood donations, with documentation of the type of convulsion and hemodynamics during the event. The study had a retrospective and prospective component. Convulsions occurred in 12% and 42% of syncopal spells in the retrospective and prospective studies, respectively. Tonic spasms were seen in 66% of convulsive syncopal spells in the prospective group, accompanied by pallor, diaphoresis, fixed staring gaze, upward eye deviation, and nuchal rigidity (**Table 2**). The elbows were often flexed. Recovery occurred in less than 30 seconds and was followed by mild confusion. A minority of patients had brief clonic convulsions, violent myoclonic jerks, and rarely severe convulsive activity causing injury and requiring restraint.

Table 1
Estimated prevalence of convulsions during syncope

Clinical Scenario	Observation Type	Seizure Estimate (%)
Healthy subjects		
Blood donor clinic[22]	Chart review	12
Blood donor clinic[22]	Prospective observation	42
Physiology study[28]	Syncope induction and observation	90
Patients with syncope		
Tilt testing[23]	Syncope induction and observation	4.4
Tilt testing[24]	Syncope induction and observation	8

Chart reviews of reported convulsive activity and tilt test serendipitous observations are probably more relevant to clinical experience.

Table 2
Clinical observations during convulsive syncope

Clinical Sign Cluster	Observation
Typical syncope findings	Pallor Diaphoresis Postictal fatigue
Head and neck	Fixed gaze Upward eye deviation Nuchal rigidity
Convulsive activity	Tonic spasms Myoclonic jerks, focal or multifocal Brief clonic convulsions Focal seizures or deficits Tonic-clonic convulsions Generalized convulsions

There is a wealth of presentations of convulsive activity during syncope.[22–24,28]

The magnitudes of hypotension and bradycardia were similar in convulsive and nonconvulsive syncope.

Lempert and colleagues[28] deliberately induced transient cerebral hypoxia and syncope in a "fainting lark" maneuver in 42 healthy subjects. They used a combination of orthostasis, hyperventilation, and the Valsalva maneuver. Myoclonus occurred in 90%, featuring multifocal arrhythmic jerks in proximal and distal muscles (see **Table 2**). Generalized myoclonus was common accompanied by head turns, oral automatisms, and righting movements. Frequently the eyes remained open with initial upward deviation. Although these were arguably unusual physiologic circumstances the pattern of events does resemble that seen in convulsive syncope in blood donor clinics. Song and colleagues[23] reported that 10 (4.4%) of 226 patients who fainted on tilt testing had seizure-like activity at the time (see **Table 2**). Five had multifocal myoclonic jerky movements, and five had focal myoclonic jerky movements. Passman and colleagues[24] reported that 18 (8%) of 222 positive tilt tests had associated convulsive activity. Eleven patients (5%) had tonic-clonic activity; three had focal seizures; and one each had dysarthria, aphasia, unilateral extremity dysesthesia, and temporal lobe epilepsy symptoms (see **Table 2**).

These studies in relatively controlled circumstances attest to the common and pleiomorphic convulsive activity during syncope. The reported prevalence varies widely, depending on the situation. About 6% of syncope induced by tilt testing is associated with convulsions,[23,24] and 12% of blood donor patients in a retrospective analysis had convulsive syncope.[22] The higher prevalence during the fainting lark maneuvers and the prospective observation may reflect increased observer awareness, clinical irrelevance, or both. Not surprisingly, convulsive syncope leads to diagnostic challenges.

Several groups have examined the misdiagnosis rate in populations of patients thought to be epileptics (**Table 3**). Josephson and colleagues[29] reviewed 1506 consecutive out-patient referrals to an epilepsy clinic in Nova Scotia and found that 13% ultimately had a clinical diagnosis of vasovagal syncope. Smith and colleagues[30] reported the true diagnoses of 184 patients referred for management of treatment-refractory epilepsy. The misdiagnosis rate was 26%, of whom 7% (of the total) in fact had syncope. Chowdhury and colleagues[31] reviewed six publications that reported misdiagnosis rates between 1998 and 2007. The clinical venues that were studied included family practices and epilepsy clinics. The overall misdiagnosis rate was 20%, with patients diagnosed by neurologists as having definite epilepsy having the least reclassification rate. The causes of misclassification varied widely, although where reported syncope accounted for 25% to 35% of the true diagnoses.

From the previous discussion, it is clear that the prevalence of convulsive activity during syncope is high, as is the rate of misdiagnosis of epilepsy. Some of the misdiagnosis is caused by diagnosing convulsive syncope as epilepsy.

THE ROLE OF THE HISTORY

The history is the foundation of an accurate diagnosis.[1] However, physicians frequently disagree about diagnoses, and patients vary greatly in their presentations. Some diagnostic factors are present more often than others, and patients have variable combinations of them. The diagnosis of syndromes of loss of consciousness has been particularly troublesome because the principal symptom is unconsciousness, and bystander histories are often not available. In the Fainting Assessment Study,[32] whose investigators had deep physiologic and diagnostic experience with syncope, only 24% of patients had a definite diagnosis based on expert bedside assessment.

Another difficulty may be the lack of structured, evidence-based histories and diagnostic criteria. van Donselaar and colleagues[32] reported that agreement about seizure diagnosis among three neurologists was improved by structured diagnostic criteria. Two groups[21,33] then established the importance of historical features in distinguishing among causes of syncope. However, the results were not easily useable, and the populations did not specifically address syncope versus seizures. Accordingly, diagnostic point scores were developed to address these questions.

A comprehensive questionnaire was administered to 671 patients in three academic centers in Canada and Wales, and point scores developed with logistic regression analysis.[10,18,34] The cause of loss of consciousness was known in 539 patients (according to gold standard criteria), and included various types of epilepsy, vasovagal syncope, and cardiac arrhythmias. The point score (**Table 4**) distinguished between syncope and seizures[10] with a sensitivity of 94% and a specificity of 94%. Significant historical aspects suggestive of seizure activity included preceding emotional stress, déjà vu or jamais vu, head turning or unusual posturing or motor activity during an event, confusion on awakening, or tongue laceration. Syncope was favored by separate episodes of presyncope, preceding diaphoresis, or events precipitated by prolonged standing or sitting. The point score was independent of the number of losses of consciousness and length of history, suggesting that it could be used early in the patient's clinical course. The point score functioned in the same fashion as a skilled clinician, weighing the evidence for and against competing diagnostic possibilities.

There were some potential limitations. This score, like all others, was developed based on the kinds of patients in the study, and only patients with diagnostic electroencephalograms (EEGs)

Table 3 Misdiagnosis rates in epilepsy because of syncope	
Clinical Setting	**Misdiagnosis Rate Because of Syncope**
Epilepsy clinic[29]	13% on case review
Family practice and epilepsy clinics[30]	7% on case review
Treatment-refractory epilepsy[31]	6% on case review
Questionable epilepsy[35]	65% positive tilt tests
Questionable epilepsy[36]	67% positive tilt tests
Questionable or refractory epilepsy[25]	42% cardiovascular, of whom 27% vasovagal syncope
Questionable or refractory epilepsy[26]	21% asystolic or bradycardic on ILR during seizure

Table 4
Diagnostic questions to determine whether loss of consciousness is caused by epileptic seizures or syncope

Question	Points (*if Yes*)
At times do you wake with a cut tongue after your spells?	2
At times do you have a sense of déjà vu or jamais vu before your spells?	1
At times is emotional stress associated with losing consciousness?	1
Has anyone ever noted your head turning during a spell?	1
Has anyone ever noted that you are unresponsive, have unusual posturing or have jerking limbs during your spells, or have no memory of your spells afterward? (*Score as yes for any positive response*)	1
Has anyone ever noted that you are confused after a spell?	1
Have you ever had lightheaded spells?	−2
At times do you sweat before your spells?	−2
Is prolonged sitting or standing associated with your spells?	−2

The patient has seizures if the point score is ≥1, and syncope if the point score is <1. The overall accuracy is 94%, with a sensitivity of 94% for seizures and specificity of 94%.
From Sheldon R, Rose S, Ritchie D, et al. Historical criteria that distinguish syncope from seizures. J Am Coll Cardiol 2002;40:142–8; with permission.

and either generalized convulsions or complex seizures were included. The study did not include patients with convulsive activity during definite syncopal spells, and there is a risk of overfitting the data. Nonetheless, it has proved useful in complex cases where the diagnosis of syncope or epileptic convulsions has been difficult.

Despite the difficulties, there are some simple clinical observations that can distinguish between convulsive syncope and epileptic convulsions. These are presented in **Box 2**.

TILT TESTS FOR QUESTIONABLE EPILEPSY

Tilt tests can help provide diagnostic clarity in patients with a questionable history of epileptic seizures, according to the consistent findings of three studies (see **Table 3**). Sabri and colleagues[35] studied 40 patients younger than 21 years old who had an initial diagnosis of epilepsy (mainly partial complex seizures), but whose diagnosis was challenged after a neurologic chart review. Tilt testing was positive in 65% of patients. Remarkably, almost all patients whether they had positive or negative tilt tests had clinical factors suggestive of either vasovagal syncope or initial orthostatic hypotension. Similarly, Grubb and colleagues[36] subjected 15 patients with recurrent unexplained seizure-like episodes to tilt testing. The seizures were unresponsive to antiepileptic medication. Fully 67% had tonic-clonic seizure activity during tilt testing associated with hypotension and

Box 2
Clinical tips for distinguishing convulsive syncope from epilepsy

	Convulsive Syncope	Epilepsy
Occurs supine	Uncommon	Common
Also has syncope and presyncope	Common	Uncommon
Typical prodrome: diaphoresis, presyncope, warmth	Common	Uncommon
Pallor	Common	Uncommon
Tongue biting	Uncommon	Common
Tongue bite location	Tongue tip	Tongue side
Prodromal cry	Uncommon	Common
Eye deviation	Fixed or upward	Lateral deviation
Incontinence	Uncommon	Common
Muscle movement	Pleiomorphic (see **Table 2**)	Rhythmic and generalized
Convulsion duration	Less than a minute	Often a few minutes
Postictal symptoms	Brief haziness, fatigue, diaphoresis, nausea	Confusion

bradycardia. The EEG showed diffuse brain wave slowing (not typical of epileptic seizures) in five patients during the convulsive episode. These are the typical findings observed during syncope induced by tilt testing.[37] In the largest study to date Zaidi and colleagues[25] subjected 74 adult patients with an established diagnosis of epilepsy who were either refractory to antiepileptic drug treatment, or whose diagnosis was subsequently challenged on clinical grounds. A cardiovascular diagnosis was established in 42% of patients, including vasovagal syncope in 27%. Taken together these studies estimate that 50% of patients with either questionable or drug-refractory epilepsy have positive tilt tests. Given the imperfect sensitivity of tilt tests,[38] most patients with questionable or drug-refractory epilepsy may have syncope as their true diagnosis.

VIDEO RECORDING

Direct video recordings of transient losses of consciousness at first blush offer considerable promise. It has proved accurate in diagnosing epilepsy and pseudoseizures. Might video recordings offer similar hope? Of the five case series that reported the use of video recordings, four were concerned solely with establishing the diagnosis of pseudo-syncope or pseudoseizures,[39–42] both of which are functional disorders. The fifth actually established the diagnosis of syncope with a combination of EEG recordings and tilt test results.[43] Therefore, there is no evidence one way or the other that video recording helps distinguish between syncope and true epileptic seizures.

ILR FOR QUESTIONABLE EPILEPSY

ILRs document the ECG findings of events that occur sporadically and infrequently, such as syncope. Other technologies, such as ambulatory electrocardiography and external event recorders, have a low rate of diagnosis because of the infrequent nature of events such as syncope. The European Heart Rhythm Association issued guidelines for the indications for ILRs in the assessment of syncope.[44] These were informed by the efficacy, safety, and cost utility demonstrated in studies of ILRs for syncope, particularly the EASYAS[45] and RAST[6] studies. The guidelines, recognizing the paucity of evidence of the ability of ILRs to distinguish syncope from epileptic seizures, recommended their use here as class IIB, level C.

Given that much of syncope is associated with sinus rhythm or sinus bradycardia, and epilepsy associated with sinus rhythm, using an ILR might not seem a promising approach. However,

Kanjwal and colleagues[27] reported three patients with recurrent and drug-refractory convulsive episodes who actually had prolonged episodes of asystole or complete heart block. As part of a larger study Zaidi and colleagues[25] studied 10 adult patients with an established diagnosis of epilepsy who were either refractory to antiepileptic drug treatment, or whose diagnosis was subsequently challenged on clinical grounds. All received an ILR, and two had seizures associated with either complete heart block or sinus pauses. The largest study to date is Reveal in the Investigation of Syncope and Epilepsy (REVISE),[26] which reported the results of ILR assessment of 103 adult patients with definite or probable epilepsy. The patients were included if they were drug-refractory or if clinical reassessment cast doubt on their diagnoses. Fully 65% had a transient loss of consciousness that was associated with ECG documentation, and 22 patients (21%) had asystole or profound bradycardia. Given that at least half of syncopal spells documented by ILR in patients with syncope are associated with normal sinus rhythm, the total misdiagnosis rate in the REVISE study might be 60% to 70%. Therefore, the accumulated ILR data indicate that at least 20% of patients with a questionable diagnosis of epileptic seizures may actually have convulsive syncope caused by bradycardias, and the true prevalence of convulsive syncope in this population might be much higher.

HEALTH SERVICES DELIVERY

Many patients present with symptoms at the interface between cardiology and neurology, yet there is relatively little information available on how clinicians can best organize to provide care. The European Society of Cardiology 2009 syncope guidelines[1] recognized this by framing their recommendations in the context of transient loss of consciousness, classifying these as syncope, epileptic seizures, psychogenic disorders, and other rare causes. The guidelines[1] also recommended the establishment of formal multidisciplinary syncope units, either virtual or geographically contained, staffed by a core of syncope experts, and having easy access to other consultants and diagnostic tools.

There are several models of multidisciplinary service units for assessing the causes of transient losses of consciousness, although all those reported have an emphasis on syncope. Successful models of an entirely outpatient assessment of older patients has been reported by a UK center.[46–49] A causal diagnosis was reached in almost all patients, but almost none had a diagnosis of epilepsy established. Three small subsequent studies showed that similar dedicated units achieved a diagnosis in almost all elderly patients,[47,48] and achieved a dramatic reduction in bed occupancy and length of stay. Ammirati and colleagues[3] reported in a retrospective observational study that a syncope unit seemed to increase the diagnostic yield from 75% to 82%, and reduce hospital costs by 85%.

In contrast, six Italian hospitals with organized syncope units[50] showed only a weak trend to fewer admissions and tests, and only 11% of eligible patients with syncope were referred to the unit. The only randomized study evaluating the efficiency and accuracy of the investigation of syncope with a dedicated syncope clinic/unit is the SEEDS trial.[51] This study reported a much higher diagnostic yield in those patients seen in an emergency department syncope unit arm, mostly because of increased detection of vasovagal syncope, with lower hospital admission rates.

The common factors in these models were access to diagnostic tools, but in particular easy access to specialists who could make rapid, efficient, accurate diagnoses. What could be learned from these for differentiating between syncope and epilepsy in patients who present as diagnostic dilemmas? Here the needs are more focused and the patient volume much lower. More formalized interdisciplinary interactions could be established in which difficult cases could be assessed jointly and optimal investigation pathways and standards enacted. Both cardiologists and neurologists could provide seamless access to investigations, such as tilt tests and ILRs, and EEGs and occasionally video monitoring facilities to provide help with distinguishing among difficult symptoms. Such interactions might also facilitate the routine assessment of patients with seizure who are either atypical or who are not responding to antiepileptic therapy. Finally, both specialties should work together to create diagnostic and therapeutic tools for use with patients with possible autonomic neuropathies, pseudosyncope, and pseudoseizures.

SUMMARY

Despite the evident differences in the presentations of syncope and epileptic convulsions there will always be patients who present as diagnostic dilemmas. There is a wide range of estimates of the prevalence of convulsive activity during syncope (about 4%–40% of spells), and the differences between epileptic convulsions and convulsive syncope may be difficult for observers.

A careful, perceptive, evidence-based history is essential, and bystander observations are important. Tilt tests despite their limitations seem to be useful in many patients. Finally, excellent communication between neurologists and internists or cardiologists probably offers the best chance for accurate diagnoses.

REFERENCES

1. Moya A, Sutton R, Ammirati F, et al. Guidelines for the diagnosis and management of syncope (version 2009): the Task Force for the Diagnosis and Management of Syncope of the European Society of Cardiology (ESC). Eur Heart J 2009;30: 2631–71.
2. McKeon A, Vaughan C, Delanty N. Seizure versus syncope. Lancet Neurol 2006;5:171–80.
3. Ammirati F, Colaceci R, Cesario A, et al. Management of syncope: clinical and economic impact of a syncope unit. Europace 2008;10:471–6.
4. Baron-Esquivias G, Moreno SG, Martinez A, et al. Cost of diagnosis and treatment of syncope in patients admitted to a cardiology unit. Europace 2006;8:122–7.
5. Bartoletti A, Fabiani P, Adriani P, et al. Hospital admission of patients referred to the emergency department for syncope: a single-hospital prospective study based on the application of the European Society of Cardiology Guidelines on syncope. Eur Heart J 2006;27:83–8.
6. Krahn AD, Klein GJ, Yee R, et al. Cost implications of testing strategy in patients with syncope: randomized assessment of syncope trial. J Am Coll Cardiol 2003;42:495–501.
7. Sun BC, Emond JA, Camargo CA. Direct medical costs of syncope-related hospitalizations in the United States. Am J Cardiol 2005;95:668–71.
8. Hirano Y, Oguni H, Osawa M. Epileptic negative drop attacks in atypical benign partial epilepsy: a neurophysiological study. Epileptic Disord 2009; 11:37–41.
9. Banerjee PN, Filippi D, Hauser WA. The descriptive epidemiology of epilepsy: a review. Epilepsy Res 2009;85:31–45.
10. Sheldon R, Rose S, Ritchie D, et al. Historical criteria that distinguish syncope from seizures. J Am Coll Cardiol 2002;40:142–8.
11. Savage DD, Corwin L, McGee DL, et al. I - epidemiologic features of isolated syncope: the Framingham Study. Stroke 1985;16:626–9.
12. Ganzeboom KS, Mairuhu G, Reitsma JB, et al. Lifetime cumulative incidence of syncope in the general population: a study of 549 Dutch subjects aged 35-60 years. J Cardiovasc Electrophysiol 2006;17:1172–6.

13. Serletis A, Rose S, Sheldon AG, et al. Vasovagal syncope in medical students and their first-degree relatives. Eur Heart J 2006;27:1965–70.

14. Ganzeboom KS, Colman N, Reitsma JB, et al. Prevalence and triggers of syncope in medical students. Am J Cardiol 2003;91:1006–8 A8.

15. Sheldon RS, Morillo CA, Krahn AD, et al. Standardized approaches to the investigation of syncope: Canadian Cardiovascular Society position paper. Can J Cardiol 2011;27:246–53.

16. Soteriades ES, Evans JC, Larson MG, et al. Incidence and prognosis of syncope. N Engl J Med 2002;347:878–85.

17. Wieling W, Krediet CT, van Dijk N, et al. Initial orthostatic hypotension: review of a forgotten condition. Clin Sci (Lond) 2007;112:157–65.

18. Sheldon R, Rose S, Connolly S, et al. Diagnostic criteria for vasovagal syncope based on a quantitative history. Eur Heart J 2006;27:344–50.

19. Sud S, Massel D, Klein GJ, et al. The expectation effect and cardiac pacing for refractory vasovagal syncope. Am J Med 2007;120:54–62.

20. Kanjwal K, Kanjwal Y, Karabin B. Clinical symptoms associated with asystolic or bradycardic responses on implantable loop recorder monitoring in patients with recurrent syncope. Int J Med Sci 2009;6:106–10.

21. Calkins H, Shyr Y, Frumin H, et al. The value of the clinical history in the differentiation of syncope due to ventricular tachycardia, atrioventricular block, and neurocardiogenic syncope. Am J Med 1995; 98:365–73.

22. Lin JT, Ziegler DK, Lai CW, et al. Convulsive syncope in blood donors. Ann Neurol 1982;11:525–8.

23. Song PS, Kim JS, Park J, et al. Seizure-like activities during head-up tilt test-induced syncope. Yonsei Med J 2010;51:77–81.

24. Passman R, Horvath G, Thomas J, et al. Clinical spectrum and prevalence of neurologic events provoked by tilt table testing. Arch Intern Med 2003; 163:1945–8.

25. Zaidi A, Clough P, Cooper P, et al. Misdiagnosis of epilepsy: many seizure-like attacks have a cardiovascular cause. J Am Coll Cardiol 2000;36:181–4.

26. Petkar S, Hamid T, Iddon P, et al. Prolonged implantable electrocardiographic monitoring indicates a high rate of misdiagnosis of epilepsy: REVISE study. Europace 2012;14:1653–60.

27. Kanjwal K, Karabin B, Kanjwal Y, et al. Differentiation of convulsive syncope from epilepsy with an implantable loop recorder. Int J Med Sci 2009;6: 296–300.

28. Lempert T, Bauer M, Schmidt D. Syncope: a videometric analysis of 56 episodes of transient cerebral hypoxia. Ann Neurol 1994;36:233–7.

29. Josephson CB, Rahey S, Sadler RM. Neurocardiogenic syncope: frequency and consequences of its misdiagnosis as epilepsy. Can J Neurol Sci 2007; 34:221–4.

30. Smith D, Defalla BA, Chadwick DW. The misdiagnosis of epilepsy and the management of refractory epilepsy in a specialist clinic. QJM 1999;92: 15–23.

31. Chowdhury FA, Nashef L, Elwes RD. Misdiagnosis in epilepsy: a review and recognition of diagnostic uncertainty. Eur J Neurol 2008;15:1034–42.

32. van Donselaar CA, Geerts AT, Meulstee J, et al. Reliability of the diagnosis of a first seizure. Neurology 1989;39:267–71.

33. Alboni P, Brignole M, Menozzi C, et al. Diagnostic value of history in patients with syncope with or without heart disease. J Am Coll Cardiol 2001;37: 1921–8.

34. Sheldon R, Hersi A, Ritchie D, et al. Syncope and structural heart disease: historical criteria for vasovagal syncope and ventricular tachycardia. J Cardiovasc Electrophysiol 2010;21:1358–64.

35. Sabri MR, Mahmodian T, Sadri H. Usefulness of the head-up tilt test in distinguishing neurally mediated syncope and epilepsy in children aged 5-20 years old. Pediatr Cardiol 2006;27:600–3.

36. Grubb BP, Gerard G, Roush K, et al. Differentiation of convulsive syncope and epilepsy with head-up tilt testing. Ann Intern Med 1991;115:871–6.

37. Sheldon RS, Koshman ML, Murphy WF. Electroencephalographic findings during presyncope and syncope induced by tilt table testing. Can J Cardiol 1998;14:811–6.

38. Sheldon R. Tilt testing for syncope: a reappraisal. Curr Opin Cardiol 2005;20:38–41.

39. Benbadis SR, Chichkova R. Psychogenic pseudosyncope: an underestimated and provable diagnosis. Epilepsy Behav 2006;9:106–10.

40. Chung SS, Gerber P, Kirlin KA. Ictal eye closure is a reliable indicator for psychogenic nonepileptic seizures. Neurology 2006;66:1730–1.

41. Hubsch C, Baumann C, Hingray C, et al. Clinical classification of psychogenic non-epileptic seizures based on video-EEG analysis and automatic clustering. J Neurol Neurosurg Psychiatr 2011;82: 955–60.

42. Luzza F, Di Rosa S, Pugliatti P, et al. Syncope of psychiatric origin. Clin Auton Res 2004;14:26–9.

43. Yilmaz S, Gokben S, Levent E, et al. Syncope or seizure? The diagnostic value of synchronous tilt testing and video-EEG monitoring in children with transient loss of consciousness. Epilepsy Behav 2012;24:93–6.

44. Brignole M, Vardas P, Hoffman E, et al. Indications for the use of diagnostic implantable and external ECG loop recorders. Europace 2009;11: 671–87.

45. Farwell DJ, Freemantle N, Sulke AN. Use of implantable loop recorders in the diagnosis and

management of syncope. Eur Heart J 2004;25: 1257–63.

46. Allcock LM, O'Shea D. Diagnostic yield and development of a neurocardiovascular investigation unit for older adults in a district hospital. J Gerontol A Biol Sci Med Sci 2000;55:M458–62.

47. Dey AB, Bexton RS, Tyman MM, et al. The impact of a dedicated "syncope and falls" clinic on pacing practice in northeastern England. Pacing Clin Electrophysiol 1997;20:815–7.

48. Kenny RA, O'Shea D, Walker HF. Impact of a dedicated syncope and falls facility for older adults on emergency beds. Age Ageing 2002;31:272–5.

49. McIntosh S, Da Costa D, Kenny RA. Outcome of an integrated approach to the investigation of dizziness, falls and syncope in elderly patients referred to a 'syncope' clinic. Age Ageing 1993; 22:53–8.

50. Brignole M, Disertori M, Menozzi C, et al. Management of syncope referred urgently to general hospitals with and without syncope units. Europace 2003;5:293–8.

51. Shen WK, Decker WW, Smars PA, et al. Syncope Evaluation in the Emergency Department Study (SEEDS): a multidisciplinary approach to syncope management. Circulation 2004;110:3636–45.

Risk Stratification of Patients Presenting with Transient Loss of Consciousness

Venkata Krishna Puppala, MD, MPH[a,b], Mehmet Akkaya, MD[c],
Oana Dickinson, MD[c], David G. Benditt, MD, FACC, FRCPC, FHRS[d],*

KEYWORDS

- Syncope • Risk stratification • Transient loss of consciousness • Syncope clinic

KEY POINTS

- Transient loss of consciousness (TLOC) has many possible causes, and syncope is among the most frequent.
- Important goals in initial evaluation of patients with TLOC include determining whether the episode was true syncope (vs other causes of TLOC, such as seizures or head trauma) and ascertaining the appropriate venue for subsequent care.
- At present, 30% to 50% of patients with syncope are admitted to hospital for evaluation, although many of these individuals could be safely and more cost-effectively managed outside of hospital.
- To reduce unnecessary admissions, several recent studies have focused on development of risk stratification tools to assist frontline clinicians in making a disposition decision.
- Although there is not yet consensus regarding an optimum decision process, the various available risk stratification recommendations provide direction in assessing short-term and long-term risks associated with syncope.
- Patients who have high short-term risk of adverse outcomes need prompt hospitalization for diagnosis and/or treatment, whereas others may be safely referred for outpatient evaluation (preferably at a clinic specializing in syncope evaluations).

INTRODUCTION

Syncope is a syndrome in which transient loss of consciousness (TLOC) occurs as a consequence of a self-limited, brief, and spontaneously self-terminating period of inadequate cerebral oxygen delivery.[1,2] The most common cause is a transient, but spontaneously reversible, decrease of systemic arterial pressure to a level less than the minimum needed to sustain cerebral blood flow (ie, less than the cerebrovascular autoregulatory range).[1–3] Other causes, such as acute hypoxemia (eg, abrupt aircraft decompression) or major, but transient,

This article originally appeared in Cardiac Electrophysiology Clinics, Volume 5, Issue 4, December 2013.
The authors have nothing to disclose.
Dr O. Dickinson and Dr V.K. Puppala were supported by the Bakken family fund, Minnesota Medical Foundation, Minneapolis, Minnesota.
[a] St Joseph Hospital, Healtheast Care System, Department of Medicine, St Paul, MN 55101, USA; [b] Cardiac Arrhythmia Center, University of Minnesota Medical School, MMC 508, 420 Delaware Street Southeast, Minneapolis, MN 55455, USA; [c] Cardiovascular Division, Department of Medicine, Cardiac Arrhythmia Center, University of Minnesota Medical School, Minneapolis, MN 55455, USA; [d] Cardiovascular Division, Department of Medicine, Cardiac Arrhythmia Center, University of Minnesota Medical Center, University of Minnesota Medical School, MMC 508, 420 Delaware Street Southeast, Minneapolis, MN 55455, USA
* Corresponding author.
E-mail address: bendi001@umn.edu

Cardiol Clin 33 (2015) 387–396
http://dx.doi.org/10.1016/j.ccl.2015.04.007
0733-8651/15/$ – see front matter © 2015 Elsevier Inc. All rights reserved.

metabolic derangements affecting neuronal activation, are rare.

Whether the cause of transient systemic hypotension is innocent in nature (eg, the vasovagal [common] faint), or potentially life threatening (eg, torsades de pointes ventricular tachycardia), syncope may lead to physical injury, accidents, diminished quality of life, and economic loss. As a result, it is essential to recognize and evaluate patients with possible syncope, and differentiate true syncope from other nonsyncope causes of TLOC (eg, seizures, concussions, metabolic derangements), identify the specific causes(s) of the faints, and develop a treatment plan designed to prevent recurrences.[1,3]

CLASSIFICATION OF SYNCOPE

The classification of syncope is mainly based on the underlying mechanisms, which ultimately lead to global hypoperfusion. A table summarizing the diagnostic classification of the causes of syncope based on the European Society of Cardiology (ESC) syncope practice guidelines is given elsewhere in this issue.[1]

Reflex Syncope (Also Termed Neurally Mediated Reflex Syncope)

Reflex syncope includes several conditions in which neural reflex activity initiates a period of inappropriate vasodilation and relative or marked bradycardia. The most important, and the most common, among the reflex syncopes is vasovagal syncope (VVS), also known as the common faint. The second most frequently encountered form (although principally in older individuals and primarily in men) is carotid sinus syncope (CSS).[3–6] CSS must be distinguished from carotid sinus hypersensitivity, a finding that may be elicited by carotid sinus massage in many older individuals. CSS is only diagnosed if carotid sinus massage reproduces symptoms or, in the absence of other diagnoses, a sinus pause longer than 6 seconds is triggered by carotid sinus massage (previously 3 seconds was considered diagnostic, but that value is probably too nonspecific a criterion).

The other forms of reflex syncope tend to be classed as situational faints because they accompany certain specific activities (eg, syncope triggered by cough, micturition, or defecation).[1,3] In each of these cases, the reflex is triggered by the specific stimulus in a given patient. As in the case of VVS and CSS, the initial trigger event in situational faints (eg, micturition syncope, cough syncope) initiates either a slow heart rate (or at least slow for the degree of accompanying hypotension), or depressed vascular tone, or both. The result is

systemic hypotension causing transient cerebral hypoperfusion and loss of consciousness. Lesser degrees of hypotension may cause disturbance of cerebral function without complete syncope. The resulting near-syncope symptoms may include nonspecific lightheadedness, visual spots or blinking lights or gray-out, and/or loss of hearing or abnormal hearing (eg, tinnitus), and often a vague sense of lightheadedness.

Orthostatic Syncope

Orthostatic hypotension leading to syncope occurs as result of the body's inability to maintain blood pressure and consequently adequate cerebral perfusion; this in turn results in TLOC.[1,7,8] The causes may be related to inadequate circulatory volume, as occurs with dehydration; excessive diuresis leading to volume depletion; or drug-induced vasodilation. Orthostatic hypotension may alternatively be a reflection of inadequate or delayed autonomic vasoconstrictor response.

Orthostatic syncope, as the name suggests, is usually initiated by a movement from supine or seated to an upright posture (although symptoms may be delayed for several minutes). Such a change in posture results in shift of 500 to 1000 mL of blood away from the chest to the venous capacitance system below the diaphragm. Absent an effective neurovascular constriction response, the sequestration of blood below the diaphragm reduces venous return to the heart with consequent reduction of cardiac filling pressure and stroke volume; if sufficiently severe, the resulting hypotension may lead to symptomatic cerebral hypoperfusion.

The human body has physiologic defenses against postural hypotension; these include baroreflex-initiated increase in heart rate, arterial and venous vasoconstriction (particularly in the splanchnic bed and lower extremities), and (albeit delayed) neuroendocrine adjustments operating through the renin-angiotensin-aldosterone system.[7] However, these defenses could be undermined if there is superimposed excessive volume depletion, or loss of cardiac chronotropic response, or impaired reflex vasoconstriction caused by autonomic dysfunction or medications such as β-blockers. Loss of skeletal muscle tone (a problem more often encountered in elderly individuals) may also contribute by reducing the effectiveness of muscle pump activity.

Physical counterpressure maneuvers such as leg crossing with tensing of thigh and buttock muscles may be helpful acutely for delaying symptoms by enhancing muscle pump activity and increasing venous return.[1] Longer-term physical rehabilitation should focus on restoring effective neurovascular reactivity to postural change.

Syncope Caused by Cardiac Arrhythmias

Syncope can occur as a result of either bradyarrhythmias or tachyarrhythmias. Bradycardia is the more common cause of syncope in this category; symptomatic hypotension can occur as a result of sinus pauses, high-grade atrioventricular (AV) block, or asystole (prolonged pause) that occurs at the termination of an atrial tachyarrhythmia (particularly at the end of an episode of atrial fibrillation). In such cases, cardiac pacemaker therapy may be indicated.

Syncope that occurs as a direct consequence of tachyarrhythmia may be caused by supraventricular or ventricular arrhythmias. Neurally mediated hypotension is thought to play an important contributory role in these patients. Patients with autonomic dysfunction (whether reflex in nature or caused by neurologic disease) are at greatest risk for arrhythmia-related syncope. In essence, protective reflexes that support the circulation when faced by tachycardic stress fail to act, or do so excessively sluggishly. The result is a period of symptomatic systemic hypotension.

In patients with ventricular tachyarrhythmia, the occurrence of syncope portends an increased risk of sudden cardiac death. In particular, patients with poor left ventricular function and syncope are at higher mortality risk.[9] Patients with channelopathy (ie, long QT syndrome, Brugada syndrome, catecholaminergic paroxysmal ventricular tachycardia) with documented tachyarrhythmias and syncope should be deemed to be at high mortality risk. Whether the presence of syncope per se increases risk is not certain in many of these conditions, but the occurrence of syncope may bring the previously undiagnosed patient to medical attention. These patients need prompt referral to cardiac electrophysiology for further evaluation and management, often entailing placement of an implantable cardioverter-defibrillator.

Syncope Caused by Structural Cardiac and Cerebrovascular Disease

Structural cardiac and vascular disease is only infrequently the direct cause of syncope. The most common conditions in this group are acute myocardial infarction/ischemia or pulmonary embolism. However, valvular heart disease (eg, severe aortic stenosis, severe mitral stenosis, and large left atrial myxoma) and pulmonary hypertension are well-known and potentially treatable causes of syncope. In all of these conditions, the cerebral hypoperfusion is in part a result of the direct hemodynamic impact of the anatomic anomaly, but is also importantly contributed to by neural reflex mechanisms. Perhaps the hypotension and bradycardia often associated with inferior wall myocardial ischemia is the best known of the reflex effects. However, inappropriate vascular dilation with exertion in patients with severe aortic stenosis is well documented and an accepted basis for symptomatic hypotension.[10]

True syncope almost never occurs as a result of cerebrovascular disease alone because the brain has a well-protected circulation with multiple vessels feeding the circle of Willis. However, on rare occasions, a transient ischemic attack (TIA) in the distribution of the vertebrobasilar distribution may trigger syncope. However, these cases are not only rare but also tend to be identifiable because of their association with symptoms of posterior circulation problems such as loss of balance and vertigo. Subclavian stenosis with so-called steal syndrome is another rare condition that may cause various neurologic symptoms triggered by vigorous use of the ipsilateral arm muscles; syncope as a solitary presentation is extremely unusual.[11]

SYNCOPE MIMICS

Several conditions may seem to cause a syncopal event. However, unlike true syncope, or even nonsyncope TLOC such as seizures, concussions, or intoxications, these syncope mimics do not cause true loss of consciousness and their basis is not cerebral hypoperfusion. They are considered here primarily because they cause diagnostic confusion.

The most common condition in the syncope mimic category is psychogenic pseudosyncope (neurologists tend to use the term psychogenic pseudoseizure). These pseudosyncopes may be difficult to differentiate from true faints, but an important clue is their frequency; psychogenic events are usually numerous and often occur many times a day. They also tend to last for a longer time than real faints. True syncope almost never occurs with such a frequency or lasts for more than a minute or two. Tilt testing may help identify these patients and permit discussion with them regarding the diagnosis.[12]

Other syncope mimics include cataplexy (which usually occurs in conjunction with narcolepsy), and certain types of akinetic or minimally kinetic seizures. Minimally kinetic seizures are rare, but may not be as uncommon as was previously thought.[13] In addition, accidental falls with or without TLOC caused by concussion may be misdiagnosed as syncope events, especially in the elderly.

DIAGNOSTIC PATHWAY

Syncope by itself is only infrequently an immediately life-threatening condition; nonetheless, it may result in untoward consequences of physical injury and/or diminished quality of life. In some cases, syncope may be a symptomatic manifestation of potentially life-threatening underlying conditions (particularly severe structural heart disease) that predispose to arrhythmias and heart failure.

Fig. 1 provides an overview, based on the ESC Syncope Task Force guidelines,[1] of an approach to assessment of a patient who presents with TLOC/collapse. The starting point is the initial evaluation (**Box 1**). The physician initially responsible for evaluating patients with TLOC is most often an emergency department (ED) or urgent care physician.

A confident diagnosis may or may not be determined in the ED or clinic. If the cause of the collapse is established with clinical certainty, then the subsequent step is usually clear. However, more often the diagnosis is uncertain or unknown. In uncertain or unknown cases, the practitioner must choose between immediate hospitalization versus timely outpatient evaluation; this decision has historically favored a conservative safe course of action, with many more patients being admitted than is warranted (various reports indicate that current admission rates tend to be 30%–50%). This high admission rate seems to persist even when physicians are tutored in the ESC guidelines. For instance, a single-hospital prospective study by Bartoletti and colleagues,[14] based on the ESC guidelines for management of syncope, looked at the admission rates among patients referred to

ED with syncope. A total of 1124 patients were diagnosed with syncope; 440 (39.1%) met at least 1 criterion for admission to hospital based on ESC guidelines,[1] and 680 (60.9%) were without any indication for admission. The hospital admission percentages were 89.3% among patients with an indication and 25.3% among patients without any indication. The high admission rates among low-risk patients despite being backed up by guidelines shows that ED physicians remain concerned about patient safety after discharge. However, unnecessary inpatient admissions add to the cost of care for patients with syncope and, given a typical 2 to 3 days of observation, may not be expected to improve either safety or diagnostic outcomes in the absence of a clearly life-threatening condition (eg, acute myocardial infarction, pulmonary embolism, recurrent symptomatic ventricular tachyarrhythmias). In the Evaluation of Guidelines in Syncope Study 2 (EGSYS2) study,[15] despite expert on-line assistance to frontline physicians, the admission rate was still 39% (although less than the historical control of 47%).

RISK STRATIFICATION OF PATIENTS WITH SUSPECTED SYNCOPE

Recent efforts designed to risk stratify patients with TLOC/syncope are directed toward development of criteria that permit effective hospital admission versus syncope clinic outpatient assessment decision making.[16] The most important objectives

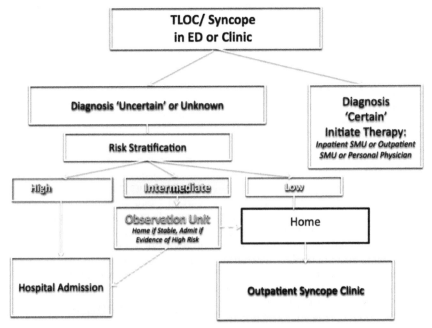

Fig. 1. Strategy for managing patients with TLOC/syncope in the emergency department (ED) or urgent care setting. SMU, syncope management unit; ED, emergency department.

Box 1
Essential questions to be addressed during the initial evaluation

1. Is loss of consciousness attributable to syncope versus other causes, including accidental falls?

2. Are there important clinical features in the history that suggest the diagnosis (eg, premonitory symptoms in vasovagal fainters, postural change in orthostatic syncope)?

3. Was injury sustained by the collapse that may require further directed assessment?

4. Is there evidence of underlying cardiac, vascular, or respiratory disease?

5. Are there residual neurologic deficits that suggest cerebrovascular disease or primary autonomic disorder?

6. Are there signs of frailty or instability that may contribute to accidental falls?

7. Does the patient have findings that suggest emotional lability accompanied by frequent collapses that may favor a psychogenic component to the problem?

8. Is there a history of drug abuse (including alcohol)?

9. Is there a history of diabetes?

Data from Moya A, Sutton R, Ammirati F, et al. The Task Force for the Diagnosis and Management of Syncope of the European Society of Cardiology (ESC). Guidelines for the diagnosis and management of syncope (version 2009). Eur Heart J 2009;30:2631–71.

of risk stratification are to assess the immediate-term (usually defined as 1 week to 1 month) and longer-term (approximately 1 year) risk of:

1. Death or life-threatening events
2. Recurrence, which in turn may lead to physical injury or diminished quality of life

If immediate risk of adverse events is deemed to be high, this should prompt the evaluating physician to admit the patient to hospital for further evaluation. In contrast, absent an excessive short-term risk, timely outpatient assessment (preferably in a clinic dedicated to the evaluation of syncope and collapse) can be scheduled. The initial outpatient clinic visit should generally be within 3 to 5 days of the ED/urgent care visit. In the case of an intermediate risk, the physician may elect to place the patient in an observation unit if one is available, as was done in the Syncope Evaluation in Emergency Department Study, in which the observation unit was in the ED (see **Fig. 1**).[17]

In some patients with syncope, the immediate risk may not be high, but clinical findings suggest longer-term increased risk of life-threatening events. This patient may need hospitalization in order to further assess risk. The nature of the testing is determined by the specific presenting features.

Several clinical studies have begun to provide the needed risk stratification guidance for frontline health care providers. However, there is as yet no consensus on the short-term and longer-term risk factors. Developing such a consensus remains an important goal for the future.[16]

Short-term or Immediate Risk

Several clinical studies have focused on determining the patients who are at increased risk of adverse events in the 30 days after initial presentation. The findings from these reports are summarized briefly here and in **Box 2**.

1. San Francisco rule[18]:
   In this study the risk factors that predicted the increased risk of an adverse event within 7 days in patients who presented after a syncopal event include the following:
   a. An abnormal electrocardiogram (ECG; eg, new rhythm changes or nonsinus rhythm, new conduction disease)
   b. Systolic blood pressure less than 90 mm Hg.
   c. Hematocrit less than 30%
   d. Congestive heart failure (either present at the time of presentation or a history of congestive heart failure [CHF]).

The adverse events included the occurrence of death, myocardial infarction, malignant arrhythmia, pulmonary embolism, stroke, subarachnoid hemorrhage, significant hemorrhage, or any other serious

Box 2
Short-term risk (1 week–1 month)

Study	Clinical Markers
San Francisco Quinn et al,[18] 2004	Abnormal electrocardiogram, low blood pressure, chronic heart failure, SOB, hematocrit <30%
Rose rule Reed et al,[19] 2010	Abnormal electrocardiogram, increased BNP, chest pain, fecal blood
STePS Costantino et al,[21] 2008	Abnormal electrocardiogram, trauma, no warning, male gender

Abbreviation: SOB, shortness of breath.

event that required a return to ED and subsequent hospitalization.

2. The Rose rule[19]:

This single-center ED study was designed to identify risk factors that predicted the likelihood of adverse events within 1 month of presentation to the ED after an episode of syncope. The adverse events in this case were defined as the occurrence of death, acute myocardial infarction, life-threatening arrhythmia, being diagnosed with any arrhythmia that required implantation of a cardiac pacemaker or defibrillator, pulmonary embolism, cerebrovascular accident, hemorrhage or profound anemia requiring blood transfusion, and any return to ED within 1 month that required urgent surgical or endoscopic intervention. The findings that predicted the likelihood of these adverse outcomes included:

a. Brain natriuretic peptide (BNP) greater than or equal to 300 pg/mL
b. Stool positive for occult blood
c. Oxygen saturation less than or equal to 94% on room air on initial presentation
d. Hemoglobin less than or equal to 90 g/L
e. Chest pain at the time of syncope
f. Bradycardia (heart rate ≤50 beat per minute)

At 1 month only 7.1% of the study population met with an end point. The sensitivity and specificity of the Rose rule were 87.2% and 65.5% respectively.

3. The Boston study[20]:

A total of 293 patients were followed for 30 days after their initial presentation to the ED with syncope. Adverse outcomes included death, serious illness that required hospitalization, or acute interventions. Sixty-eight patients met with an adverse outcome (23% of the population). The risk factors identified in this study that predicted the likelihood of an adverse event (with a sensitivity and specificity of 97% and 62% respectively) were:

a. Acute coronary syndrome
b. Conduction system disease
c. History of cardiac disease
d. Valvular heart disease
e. Family history of sudden death
f. Abnormal vital signs in ED
g. Volume depletion
h. Primary central nervous system event

4. Short-Term Prognosis of Syncope study (STePS)[21]:

This study from northern Italy included 676 patients after screening 2700 patients with presumed syncope, and assessed adverse outcomes within 10 days of initial presentation with syncope. The statistically significant risk factors were:

a. Age greater than 65 years
b. Male gender
c. Structural heart disease
d. Heart failure
e. Trauma
f. Absence of symptoms of impending syncope
g. An abnormal ECG

The study had a low rate of adverse events, and therefore had a low positive predictive value of only 11% to 14%.

Overall, the studies discussed earlier tried to identify the risk factors that predicted the likelihood of an adverse outcome. The identified risk factors tended to have a high sensitivity but not high specificity.

SHORT-TERM HIGH-RISK TLOC/SYNCOPE MARKERS

The risk factors that were consistently associated with increased risk of adverse outcomes in almost all of the studies are:

1. Acute coronary syndrome or symptoms that suggest ACS associated with syncope (ie, chest pain or shortness of breath)
2. Evidence (or a history) of congestive heart failure at the time of presentation
3. History of structural heart disease
4. Abnormal ECG
5. Anemia
6. Hemodynamic instability

When identified on initial evaluation, these risk factors almost always result in the decision to hospitalize the patient.

Hospitalization of patients presenting with syncope is a decision that should be carefully considered after initial assessment. The ESC guidelines on management of syncope published in 2001 listed criteria for hospitalization of patients with syncope[22] and these have been modified in subsequent guideline versions (**Box 3**).[1]

LONGER-TERM RISK

The risk of an adverse event in a year or more after an episode of syncope is categorized as long-term risk, which has been the subject of several studies (**Table 1**).

1. Martin and colleagues[23]

This University of Pittsburgh medical center study consisted of 2 prospective studies.

Box 3
High-risk criteria for short-term morbidity and mortality that require prompt hospitalization or intensive evaluation

Severe structural heart disease or coronary heart disease:

- Heart failure
- Low left ventricular ejection fraction
- Previous myocardial infarction

Clinical features that suggest arrhythmic syncope:

- Syncope in supine position
- Syncope during exertion
- Palpitations associated with syncope
- Family history of sudden cardiac death

ECG findings suggesting arrhythmic syncope:

- Nonsustained ventricular tachycardia
- Bifascicular block (left bundle branch block or right bundle branch block combined with left anterior or posterior fascicular block)
- Other intraventricular conduction abnormalities with QRS complex duration greater than or equal to 120 milliseconds
- Sinus bradycardia (<50 bpm) or sinoatrial block in absence of negative chronotropic medications (like β-blockers or nondihydropyridine calcium channel blockers) or physiologic bradycardia associated with physical training
- Preexcited QRS complex
- Prolonged or short QT interval
- Right bundle branch block patter with ST elevation in leads V1 to V3 (Brugada pattern)
- Negative T waves in right precordial leads, epsilon waves, and ventricular late potentials that suggest arrhythmogenic right ventricular dysplasia

Important comorbidities:

- Severe anemia
- Electrolyte abnormalities

Adapted from Moya A, Sutton R, Ammirati F, et al. The Task Force for the Diagnosis and Management of Syncope of the European Society of Cardiology (ESC). Guidelines for the diagnosis and management of syncope (version 2009). Eur Heart J 2009;30:2631–71; with permission.

Table 1
Long-term risk

Study	Clinical Markers
Martin et al,[23] 1997	Abnormal ECG, CHF, SOB, ventricular arrhythmia, age >45 y
Osservatorio Epidemiologico sula Sincope nel Lazio score Colivicchi et al,[24] 2003	Abnormal ECG, age >65 y, history of CV disease, no warning
EGSYS Del Rosso et al,[22] 2008	Palpitation before event; abnormal ECG or heart disease; syncope during effort or supine

Abbreviations: CV, cardiovascular; ECG, electrocardiogram.

and ECG obtained in the ED were used to identify predictors of arrhythmias or mortality within the first year. The second study consisted of 374 patients with syncope in order to validate the system (validation cohort). The objective was to identify the predictors of adverse outcomes (death or serious arrhythmias) at 1-year follow-up. The study identified 4 principal multivariate risk factors:

a. Abnormal ECG (odds ratio [OR] 3.2, 1.6–6.4) defined as rhythm abnormalities, conduction disorders, hypertrophy, old myocardial infarction, or AV block
b. History of ventricular arrhythmia (OR 4.8, 1.7–13.9)
c. History of congestive heart failure (OR 3.1, 1.3–7.4)
d. Age greater than 45 years (OR 3.2, 1.3–8.1)

Arrhythmias or death at less than 1 year occurred in 7.3% of the derivation cohort and 4.4% of the validation cohort without any risk factors, versus 80.4% (derivation cohort) to 57.6% (validation cohort) with 3 or 4 risk factors.

2. STePS Study[21]:

The risk factors associated with adverse outcomes in this study identified through a multivariate analysis included age greater than 65 years, history of neoplasm, cerebrovascular disease, structural heart disease, or ventricular arrhythmia. A total of 676 patients were included in this study. Of these patients 9.3% had a long-term adverse outcome, which included 40 (6%) deaths and 22

The first included 252 patients with syncope who were enrolled in a risk assessment scheme (derivation cohort) wherein data from the patient's history, physical examination,

(3.3%) requiring major therapeutic procedures. The risk factors that correlated with these adverse outcomes were:

a. Age greater than 65 years
b. History of neoplasms
c. Cerebrovascular diseases
d. Structural heart diseases
e. Ventricular arrhythmias

The risk of mortality at 1 year was higher (P<.05) in patients who were admitted to the hospital (14.7%) compared with the patients who were discharged home (1.8%).

3. Osservatorio Epidemiologico sula Sincope nel Lazio (OESIL) Study[24]:
    The risk factors identified as predictors of 1-year mortality in this study include:

a. Age greater than 65 years
b. History of cardiovascular disease
c. Lack of prodrome
d. Abnormal ECG, defined as rhythm abnormalities, conduction disorders, hypertrophy, old myocardial infarction, possible acute ischemia, or AV block

It was also noted in OESIL that mortality within 1 year increased progressively from 0% in patients with none of the risk factors discussed earlier, to approximately 57% for 4 factors.

4. EGSYS score[22]:
    This EGSYS study identified 6 risk factors that predicted adverse outcomes:

a. History or evidence of ischemic heart disease
b. Valvular heart disease
c. Cardiomyopathy
d. Congenital heart disease

e. Congestive heart failure
f. Abnormal ECG (sinus bradycardia, AV block of greater severity than first degree, bundle branch block, acute or old myocardial infarction, supraventricular or ventricular tachycardia, evidence of left or right ventricular hypertrophy, ventricular preexcitation, long QT or Brugada pattern)

The 2-year mortality was 2% in patients with a score of less than 3% and 21% for a score greater than or equal to 3.

RISK STRATIFICATION BASED ON CARDIAC VERSUS NONCARDIAC CAUSES OF SYNCOPE

Cardiac causes of syncope have been associated with both short-term and long-term risk of adverse outcomes in all the risk stratification studies discussed earlier. The morbidity and mortality associated with cardiac versus noncardiac causes of syncope have been the subject of several studies. One of the largest of these[25] evaluated the incidence and prognosis among participants in Framingham Heart Study from 1971 to 1998. This report has an inherent weakness in its diagnostic classifications because of the limited nature of the collected clinical information. Nevertheless it provides a helpful overview. Of the 7814 participants, 822 reported syncope. The cause of syncope was identified as VVS in 21.2% and cardiac in 9.4%. In 36.6% of the patients the cause was unknown. The multivariable hazard ratios among participants were significantly higher in patients with cardiac causes of syncope or mortality from any cause, death and stroke when compared with patients with syncope of other causes (Table 2).

Table 2
Syncope risk stratification

Cause of Syncope	Multivariable Adjusted Hazard Ratio for Death from Any Cause[a] (95% Confidence Intervals)	Multivariable Adjusted Hazard Ratio for Coronary Artery Disease or Acute Myocardial Infarction[a] (95% Confidence Intervals)	Multivariable Adjusted Hazard Ratio for Fatal or Nonfatal Stroke[a] (95% Confidence Intervals)
Syncope from any cause	1.31 (1.14–1.51)	1.27 (0.99–1.64)	1.06 (0.77–1.45)
Cardiac syncope	2.01 (1.48–2.73)	2.66 (1.69–4.19)	2.01 (1.06–3.80)
Neurologic origin (including seizure)	1.54 (1.12–2.12)	0.79 (0.37–1.69)	2.96 (1.69–5.18)
Vasovagal or other (eg, orthostatic, medication induced)	1.08 (0.88–1.34)	1.03 (0.71–1.49)	0.87 (0.54–1.42)

[a] Compared with patients without syncope.
Data from Soteriades ES, Evas JC, Larson MG, et al. Incidence and prognosis of syncope. N Engl J Med 2002;347:878–85.

In an earlier but smaller report from an experienced diagnostician, Kapoor[26] evaluated a total of 433 patients with syncope. Initial history, physical examination, ECG and prolonged cardiac monitoring were helpful in assigning the cause of syncope, but only in 22% of the study population. At the end of 5 years the mortality was significantly higher (50.5%) in patients with cardiac syncope compared with patients with noncardiac or unknown causes of syncope (24.1%). There was a total of 54 deaths in this population. Incidence of sudden cardiac death was significantly higher (33.1%) in patients with cardiac causes of syncope compared with noncardiac (4.9%) or unknown causes (8.5%).

More recently, albeit in a primarily older set of patients, Ungar and colleagues[27] examined the risk of cardiovascular mortality in a total of 380 patients (aged 66 ± 20 years, range 20–100 years) who were enrolled in EGSYS2. The short-term (1 month) and long-term (2 years) mortalities were examined. Syncope recurred in 63 (16.5%) of the patients. However, only 1 had recurrence in the first month. Syncope recurrence was similar in all diagnostic categories. A total of 35 deaths (9.2% of the population) occurred by the end of 2 years (614 ± 73 days). The patients who died were older, had cardiac risk factors, abnormal ECG or history of structural heart disease (82%), and sustained injuries related to syncope. Only 3% of deaths occurred in patients without an abnormal ECG and/or structural heart disease. The mortality was significantly higher in patients with cardiac or cardiopulmonary causes of syncope.

Numeroso and colleagues[28] noted similar findings in a recent study that included a total of 200 patients with syncope who were followed to evaluate the incidence of adverse events of death, recurrence of syncope, cardiovascular events, and major procedures at the end of 1 month (short term) and 1 year (long term). Cardiac syncope was associated with both short-term and long-term occurrence of at least one adverse event.

The role of syncope as a marker of increased mortality risk remains unresolved. In this regard, a large recent population study from Denmark[29] provides a provocative data set suggesting that syncope may predispose to identifying a high-risk population. This report examined retrospectively the risk of cardiovascular morbidity and mortality in patients without any apparent previous comorbidity who were admitted to hospital with a first syncope event between 2001 and 2009. A total of 37,017 patients with syncope were identified from nationwide registries in Denmark. The median age was 47 years. Approximately 5 times the number of patients without syncope were chosen as control subjects (n = 185,085) from the Danish population matched for age and sex. Multivariable Cox regression analysis showed a significantly increased all-cause mortality and cardiovascular hospitalization and event rate, recurrent syncope, stroke event rate, and/or placement of implantable cardioverter-defibrillator or pacemaker in patients with syncope compared with the control subjects without syncope. These findings cannot be considered definitive with respect to syncope as a risk marker (because, at a minimum, the factors driving admission were not controlled), but they nonetheless emphasize the importance of careful initial evaluation of all patients with syncope, and the need to develop well-considered risk assessment tools for use in the ED and clinic.

SUMMARY

Risk stratification of patients presenting with TLOC/syncope is an important part of the management strategy because it provides an opportunity to hospitalize and protect patients at immediate or short-term risk of life-threatening events while avoiding unnecessary hospitalization of low-risk patients, thereby reducing the health care burden.

A consensus on risk stratification methodology remains to be developed. Nevertheless, available risk stratification recommendations agree on the need to hospitalize new patients with TLOC/syncope with any underlying cardiac disease (structural or arrhythmic). Other important markers requiring hospitalization include anemia and hemodynamic instability. A complete summary of current criteria for hospitalization is provided in the ESC guidelines for management of syncope.[1] Patients without high-risk findings are appropriate for prompt subsequent outpatient evaluation (ideally by referral to a syncope clinic).

REFERENCES

1. Task Force for the Diagnosis and Management of Syncope, European Society of Cardiology (ESC), European Heart Rhythm Association (EHRA), Heart Failure Association (HFA), Heart Rhythm Society (HRS), Moya A, Sutton R, Ammirati F, et al. Guidelines for the diagnosis and management of syncope (version 2009). Eur Heart J 2009;30:2631–71.
2. Blanc JJ, Benditt DG. Syncope: definition, classification, and multiple potential causes. In: Benditt DG, Blanc JJ, Brignole M, et al, editors. The evaluation and treatment of syncope. A

handbook for clinical practice. Elmsford (NY): Futura Blackwell; 2003. p. 3–10.

3. Van Dijk JG, Thijs RD, Benditt DG, et al. A guide to disorders causing transient loss of consciousness: focus on syncope. Nat Rev Neurol 2009;5:438–48.

4. Ryan DJ, Nick S, Colette SM, et al. Carotid sinus syndrome, should we pace? A multicentre randomised controlled trial (SAFE PACE 2). Heart 2010; 96:347–51.

5. Parry SW, Steen N, Bexton RS, et al. Pacing in elderly recurrent fallers with carotid sinus hypersensitivity: a randomized double-blind placebo-controlled cross-over trial. Heart 2009;95:405–9.

6. Krediet CT, Parry SW, Jardine DL, et al. The history of diagnosing carotid sinus hypersensitivity: why are the current criteria too sensitive? Europace 2011;13:14–22.

7. Mathias CJ. Autonomic diseases: clinical features and laboratory evaluation. J Neurol Neurosurg Psychiatr 2003;74(Suppl 3):iii31–41.

8. Freeman R, Wieling W, Axelrod FB, et al. Consensus statement on definition of orthostatic hypotension, neurally mediated syncope and the postural tachycardia syndrome. Clin Auton Res 2011;21(2):69–72.

9. Olshansky B, Poole JE, Johnson G, et al. Syncope predicts the outcome of cardiomyopathy patients: analysis of the SCD-HeFT study. J Am Coll Cardiol 2008;51:1277–82.

10. Schwartz LS, Goldfischer J, Sprague GJ, et al. Syncope and sudden death in aortic stenosis. Am J Cardiol 1969;23:647–58.

11. Chan-Tack KM. Subclavian steal syndrome: a rare but important cause of syncope. South Med J 2001;94:445–7.

12. Petersen ME, Williams TR, Sutton R. Psychogenic syncope diagnosed by prolonged head-up tilt testing. Q J Med 1995;88:209–13.

13. Kovac S, Diehl B. Atonic phenomena in focal seizures: nomenclature, clinical findings and pathophysiological concepts. Seizure 2012;21:561–7.

14. Bartoletti A, Fabiani P, Adriani P, et al. Hospital admission of patients referred to the emergency department for syncope: a single-hospital prospective study based on the application of the European Society of Cardiology Guidelines on syncope. Eur Heart J 2006;27:83–8.

15. Brignole M, Ungar A, Casagranda I, et al. Prospective multicentre systematic guideline-based management of patients referred to the syncope units of general hospitals. Europace 2010;12:109–18.

16. Benditt DG, Can I. Initial evaluation of "syncope and collapse": the need for a risk stratification consensus. J Am Coll Cardiol 2010;55:722–4.

17. Shen WK, Decker WW, Smars PA, et al. Syncope Evaluation in the Emergency Department Study (SEEDS). A multidisciplinary approach to syncope management. Circulation 2004;110:3636–45.

18. Quinn JV, Stiell IG, McDermott DA, et al. Derivation of the San Francisco syncope rule to predict patients with short-term serious outcomes. Ann Emerg Med 2004;43:224–32.

19. Reed MJ, Newby DE, Coull AJ, et al. The ROSE (risk stratification of syncope in the emergency department) study. J Am Coll Cardiol 2010;55:713–21.

20. Grossman SA, Fischer C, Lipsitz LA, et al. Predicting adverse outcomes in syncope. J Emerg Med 2007; 33:233–9.

21. Costantino G, Perego F, Dipaola F, et al. Short- and long-term prognosis of syncope, risk factors, and role of hospital admission: results from the STePS (Short-Term Prognosis of Syncope) study. J Am Coll Cardiol 2008;51:276–83.

22. Del Rosso A, Ungar A, Maggi R, et al. Clinical predictors of cardiac syncope at initial evaluation in patients referred urgently to a general hospital: the EGSYS score. Heart 2008;94:1624–6.

23. Martin TP, Hanusa BH, Kappor WN. Risk stratification of patients with syncope. Ann Emerg Med 1997;29:459–66.

24. Colivicchi F, Ammirati F, Melina D, et al. Development and prospective validation of a risk stratification system for patients with syncope in the emergency department: the OESIL risk score. Eur Heart J 2003;24:811–9.

25. Soteriades ES, Evas JC, Larson MG, et al. Incidence and prognosis of syncope. N Engl J Med 2002;347: 878–85.

26. Kapoor WN. Evaluation and outcome of patients with syncope. Medicine (Baltimore) 1990;69:160–75.

27. Ungar A, Del Rosso A, Giada F, et al. Evaluation of Guidelines of Syncope Study 2 Group. Early and late outcome of treated patients referred for syncope to emergency department; the EGSYS 2 follow up study. Eur Heart J 2010;31:2021–6.

28. Numeroso F, Mossini G, Lippi G, et al. Evaluation of the current prognostic role of cardiogenic syncope. Intern Emerg Med 2013;8(1):69–73.

29. Ruwald MH, Hansen ML, Lamberts M, et al. Prognosis among healthy individuals discharged with a primary diagnosis of syncope. J Am Coll Cardiol 2013;61:325–32.

Syncope in Children and Adolescents

 CrossMark

Khalil Kanjwal, MD[a], Hugh Calkins, MD[b],*

KEYWORDS

- Syncope • Neurocardiogenic syncope • Children • Adolescents

KEY POINTS

- Most strategies for managing syncope in children reflect data from studies involving the adult population.
- In the future, there will be a great need for studies in children and adolescents suffering from recurrent syncope.
- To date, there has been no Food and Drug Administration (FDA)–approved therapy for neurocardiogenic syncope (NCS), which is the most common cause of syncope both in adults and children.
- None of the clinical trials of pharmacotherapy in NCS has shown benefit over placebo.
- NCS should be considered a chronic condition, and, as with other chronic diseases, the aim of the therapy should be to decrease the recurrence of syncope rather than to completely eliminate it.

INTRODUCTION

A search of the literature reveals a paucity of published data on the management of syncope in children. No separate guidelines exist for the evaluation and management of syncope in children and adolescents, and many of the management strategies are derived from data obtained from studies involving the adult population. Because the causes of syncope are discussed in detail elsewhere in this issue, this article discusses the approach to the diagnosis and management of syncope in children and how syncope in children differs from that in adults. This discussion is framed by addressing a series of questions that are pertinent to the management of syncope in children.

HOW IS SYNCOPE DEFINED?

Syncope is not a disease but a symptom of various disease processes. The word, syncope, is derived from the Greek word, synkoptein (to cut short). Syncope is defined as a transient, self-limited loss of consciousness and postural tone. The recovery is spontaneous, rapid, prompt, and complete without any neurologic sequele. Most of the time syncope leads to a fall. The mechanism invariably is insufficient blood and oxygen supply to the brain.[1–4]

HOW COMMON IS SYNCOPE IN CHILDREN?

Syncope accounts for approximately 126/100,000 children coming to medical attention in one population-based study[1–4]; 1 of every 2000 emergency department visits is due to syncope. Syncope has been reported more common in girls, and the peak incidence has been reported between the ages of 15 and 19 years. It has been reported that approximately 15% of children experience at least 1 episode of syncope before their 18th birthday.[4–8]

This article originally appeared in Cardiac Electrophysiology Clinics, Volume 5, Issue 4, December 2013.
The authors have nothing to disclose.
[a] Section of Cardiac Electrophysiology, Johns Hopkins University, Baltimore, MD 21287, USA; [b] Division of Cardiology, The Johns Hopkins Hospital, Johns Hopkins University, Sheikh Zayed Tower- Room 7125R, 1800 Orleans Street, Baltimore, MD 21287, USA
* Corresponding author.
E-mail address: hcalkins@jhmi.edu

cardiology.theclinics.com

Vasovagal syncope (VVS), also called NCS, has been reported as the most common cause of syncope (75%), followed by cardiac disease in 10% and psychogenic or unexplained syncope in 8% to 17%.

Seizure disorder can mimic syncope in children and accounts for approximately 5% of the episodes that were presumed due to syncope. This article discusses some of the most common causes of syncope in children.[8]

HOW IS SYNCOPE CLASSIFIED IN CHILDREN?

There are various terms related to syncope and familiarity with them is important to understand what these terms imply.

- Presyncope refers to the aura of syncope without actually having syncope. The symptoms may include dizziness, nausea, warmth or cold sensation, and, rarely, some visual changes.[1,7–9] Patients often report having a feeling that they "will pass out."
- Syncope can sometimes occur without aura or warning signs. These dramatic episodes with minimal or no warning signs often lead to severe injuries and morbidity.[9–12]
- Reflex syncope is frequently triggered by a stimulus like the sight of blood or pain.
- Syncope occurring only on standing is usually due to one of the many forms of orthostatic intolerance, especially vasodepressor syncope.
- Rarely, syncope can lead to convulsive movements and is often termed, convulsive syncope.[12] In children, it often is challenging to differentiate episodes of convulsive syncope from seizure disorder.

This article follows a simple classification of syncope into 3 categories: autonomic, cardiac, and noncardiac (**Box 1**).

Autonomic Syncope

The past 2 decades have witnessed a substantial growth in understanding of this category of syncope, which is by far the most common cause of syncope in children. Once considered a single entity, it is now known that this group comprises a series of abnormalities in autonomic control.[12,13]

Neurocardiogenic syncope
NCS is also referred to as a "common faint." The common triggers associated with the development of neurally mediated syncope include orthostatic stress, such as from prolonged standing or a hot shower, or emotional stress, such as from the sight of blood. It has been proposed that NCS

Box 1
Classification of syncope

Autonomic syncope
- NCS
- Dysautonomic syncope
- POTS
- Breath-holding spells
- Blood injury phobia
- Fainting lark

Cardiac syncope
- Obstructive causes
  - HCM
  - Aortic stenosis
  - Primary pulmonary hypertension
- Primary myocardial dysfunction
- Arrhythmias

Noncardiac causes of syncope
- Convulsive syncope
- Brainstem attacks

---

results from a paradoxic reflex, called Bezold-Jarisch reflex, that is initiated when ventricular preload is reduced by venous pooling.[12–18] This reduction leads to a reduction in cardiac output and blood pressure, which is sensed by arterial baroreceptors. The resultant increased catecholamine levels, combined with reduced venous filling, leads to a vigorously contracting volume-depleted ventricle. The heart itself is involved in this reflex by virtue of the presence of mechanoreceptors, or C-fibers, consisting of nonmyelinated fibers found in the atria, ventricles, and pulmonary artery. It has been proposed that vigorous contraction of a volume-depleted ventricle leads to activation of these receptors in susceptible individuals. These afferent C-fibers project centrally to the dorsal vagal nucleus of the medulla, leading to a paradoxic withdrawal of peripheral sympathetic tone and an increase in vagal tone, which, in turn, causes vasodilation and bradycardia.[18] The ultimate clinical consequence is syncope or presyncope. Not all neurally mediated syncope results from activation of mechanoreceptors. In humans, the sight of blood or extreme emotion can trigger syncope, suggesting that higher neural centers can also participate in the pathophysiology of vasovagal syncope. In addition, central mechanisms can contribute to the production of neurally mediated syncope. Anemia lowers the threshold for NCS; thus, on a physiologic basis, it is the oxygen delivery rather than mere cerebral perfusion that leads to eventual syncope. Patients suffering from NCS usually have an aura or warning signs (gray-out spells), which allows them to take evasive measure to avoid injuries from a fall that can result from syncope with minimal or no warning signs (black-out spells).

Dysautonomic syncope

Standing displaces up to 500 mL of blood to the abdomen and lower extremities due to the effect of gravity, resulting in an abrupt drop in venous return to the heart.[19–21] This drop leads to a decrease in cardiac output and stimulation of aortic, carotid, and cardiopulmonary baroreceptors that trigger a reflex increase in sympathetic outflow. As a result, heart rate, cardiac contractility, and vascular resistance increase to maintain a stable systemic blood pressure on standing. Although these disorders are often seen in adults they are also recognized in adolescents at increasing frequency.[12–17] Usually the symptoms may appear near the periods of rapid growth. Some investigators think that predominance of parasympathetic versus sympathetic tone that may coincide with the periods of rapid growth may result in predisposition for bradycardia and hypotension in the affected individuals.

Orthostatic intolerance is a term used to refer to the signs and symptoms of an abnormality in any portion of this blood pressure control system. Symptoms of orthostatic intolerance include syncope, lightheadedness, presyncope, tremulousness, weakness, fatigue, palpitations, diaphoresis, and blurred or tunnel vision. Many adolescents may also have acral cyanosis resulting from excess venous pooling. Orthostatic hypotension is defined as a 20–mm Hg drop in systolic blood pressure or a 10–mm Hg drop in diastolic blood pressure within 3 minutes of standing. Orthostatic hypotension is asymptomatic or associated with the symptoms of orthostatic intolerance (listed previously). These symptoms are often worse immediately on arising in the morning or after meals or exercise. Initial orthostatic hypotension is defined as a greater than 40–mm Hg decrease in blood pressure immediately on standing with rapid return to normal (<30 seconds). In contrast, delayed progressive orthostatic hypotension is characterized by a slow progressive decrease in systolic blood pressure on standing.[12–17]

Dysautonomic syncope has also been reported to occur in patients with joint hypermobility syndrome (JHS) and includes symptoms of syncope, presyncope, palpitations, chest discomfort, fatigue and heat intolerance, orthostatic hypotension, postural orthostatic tachycardia syndrome (POTS), and uncategorized orthostatic intolerance. JHS is one of the most common heritable collagen disorders. It is currently thought that the connective tissue laxity seen in hypermobility patients allows for a greater than normal degree of vascular dispensability, leading to an exaggerated amount of blood pooling in the lower extremity during upright posture.[22–24]

Orthostatic hypotension can also result from neurogenic causes, which are subclassified into primary and secondary autonomic failure. Primary causes are generally idiopathic, whereas secondary causes are associated with a known biochemical or structural anomaly or are seen as part of a particular disease or syndrome.[25] Another form of inherited dysautnomia usually affecting children with Ashkenazi Jewish ancestry is familial dysautnomia (FD), also called Riley-Day syndrome.[26] The FD gene has been identified as *IKBKAP*. Mutations result in tissue-specific expression of mutant IκB kinase–associated protein. It is currently thought that FD belongs to a group of hereditary sensory motor neuropathy type III. Clinical features reflect widespread involvement of sensory and autonomic neurons. Patients with FD present in infancy with failure to thrive, poor sucking and swallow difficulties, thermoregulatory disturbances, breath-holding spells, sleep disturbances, and seizures. Dysautonomic syncope as a result of postural hypotension is usually seen in adolescents. Approximately 60% of FD patients suffer from breath-holding spells during first 5 years of their life. Some patients suffer an autonomic crisis, such as hypertension, tachycardia, excessive sweating, or erythematous blotching of the skin.[27]

Postural orthostatic tachycardia syndrome

POTS is currently defined as symptoms of orthostatic intolerance associated with heart rate increases of 30 or more beats per minute (or a rate that exceeds 120 beats per minute) that occurs within the first 10 minutes of standing or upright tilt, in absence of other chronic debilitating conditions, such as protracted periods of bed rest or the use of medications known to affect vascular or autonomic function.[28–32] The estimated prevalence of those who are affected by POTS in the United States is at least 500,000.[31] Several POTS patients may have no change, a small decline, or even a modest increase in blood pressure on standing. Abnormalities of the heart rate are only one manifestation of autonomic dysfunction in such patients, who may also suffer disturbances in sweating, temperature regulation, and bowel and bladder function. The early descriptions of the disorder focused on a group of patients who had been previously healthy until a sudden febrile illness (presumably viral) brought on an abrupt onset of symptoms.[28–32] Recent research has shown that this syndrome may have multiple etiologies, and it is now known that POTS can have multiple variants resulting from these multiple causes, including partial dysautonomic, centrally mediated hyperadrenergic stimulation and norepinephrine transporter dysfunction,[33] autoimmune antibody against cholinesterase receptors,[34] POTS associated with deconditioning,[35] and hypervolemia.[36] A recently published study reported that POTS might be a manifestation of autonomic cardiac neuropathy.[37] POTS has been reported associated with trauma,[38] Lyme disease,[39] electrocution,[40] multiple sclerosis,[41] and mitochondrial cytopathy[42] and also after ablation of slow pathway for atrioventricular (AV) node reentrant tachycardia.[43]

Breath-holding spells

The breath-holding spells group of disorders is usually seen in children and are broadly subdivided into 2 groups. The cyanotic form usually occurs at approximately 6 months of age, peaks at approximately 2 years, and completely disappears by the 5th year.[44] The episode begins with a loud cry, which is followed by apnea. The child turns pale or cyanotic. There may be associated jerky or myoclonic movements or ophistonous, which is followed by limp. The whole episode may last less than 1 minute and end with the gasping breaths by the child and sudden deep inspirations with return of normal color and consciousness.[45] In some severe episodes, however, recovery is often delayed, as the child may remain drowsy for few moments. The other form is called pallid breath-holding spells or reflex anoxic seizures. It is usually seen in children between 12 and 24 months. This is similar to the cyanotic form, which is usually brought on by injury or pain, such as head bump or sudden startle. The child suddenly stops breathing and in contrast to cyanotic form there is no crying and the child loses consciousness quickly. The child becomes deadly pale and hypotonic and also develops rhythmic muscular contractions. These episodes are associated with severe bradycardia and/or asystole on a monitor. The frequency of these episodes is highly variable, from 2 to 4 episodes in a day to once every year. Almost 30% of the children have a history of similar episodes in one of their family members. There is no specific treatment for these breath-holding spells. A correct diagnosis and reassurance of the parents are all that is needed. Approximately 50% of the children have complete resolution of symptoms by age 4,

and 100% of patients never experience further episodes after their 8th year. It has been reported, however, that up to 25% of people suffering breath-holding spells as children may develop NCS and concentration problems at a later stage of their life. This association has led some investigators to believe that these breath-holding spells are infantile forms of NCS.[46]

Blood injury phobia

Most phobias usually lead to a hyperadrenergic state and patients with BIP usually have tachycardia. A specific group of children who suffer from blood injury phobia (BIP), however, have a paradoxic bradycardia or a severe asystole in response to an initial transient tachycardia,[47,48] which often leads to presyncope or syncope. These children, over a period of time, like other children who suffer from phobic disorders, learn to avoid such situations, because they perceive these injury or blood scenes as unpleasant. Unlike other phobic disorders, however, children with BIP do not have increased association with other psychiatric disorders, such as depression. Some of these children later on develop NCS and there is some evidence of clinical overlap between BIP and breath-holding spells. Deconditioning by exposure is often helpful and the tendency to have syncope can be prevented by muscle tensing and inducing anger.[49]

Fainting lark

The fainting lark is a game or trick played by older children in schools or colleges. The fainting lark starts with squatting with the knees fully bent while breathing rapidly and taking 20 deep breaths, followed by standing up suddenly and performing forced expiration against closed glottis (valsalva). In a similar version, another person pushes on the chest of a subject and pushes the subject against the wall. Some children with autism and learning disabilities suffer from compulsive valsalva and as such may develop syncope, especially convulsive syncope, which often mimics seizure disorder.[50,51]

Cardiac Syncope

Cardiac syncope is responsible for approximately 10% of syncope seen in children and young adults. Cardiovascular causes result from either obstruction to the blood flow, myocardial dysfunction, or arrhythmias.[52]

Obstructive causes

Hypertrophic cardiomyopathy Hypertrophic cardiomyopathy (HCM) affects approximately 0.2% of the general population. Although a significant number of patients suffer a spontaneous mutation, it has also been reported that both autosomal dominant and recessive variants also exist. HCM is characterized usually by asymmetric septal hypertrophy, which produces a dynamic left ventricular outflow tract obstruction.[53] Symptoms usually include dyspnea, fatigue, palpitations, near syncope, or syncope (either from abnormal blood pressure responses during exercise or from serious ventricular tachyarrhythmias). Although syncope occurs in up to 20% of patients in general, it is less common in pediatric population. When present, however, syncope carries a more ominous prognosis in children. Early onset of disease in infancy carries a worse prognosis and a majority (85%) of the infants die by age 1 year.[53–55] The aim of therapy is to provide symptomatic relief and decrease the risk of sudden cardiac death from ventricular tachycardia. Negative inotropes, such as β-blockers, calcium channel blockers, and disopyramide, may provide symptomatic relief. Surgical myotomy and myomectomy may help relieve symptoms but carry an operative mortality of almost 2%. Implantable cardioverter defibrillators (ICDs) are now commonly used in patients with recurrent syncope, ventricular arrhythmia, or family history of sudden cardiac death.[55]

Aortic stenosis Aortic valve stenosis causes a fixed obstruction to blood flow. Congenital aortic stenosis accounts for approximately 5% of congenital cardiac anomalies in children. Bicuspid aortic valve is more common and seen in up to 2% of the general population.[56] In pediatric patients, more severe cases of aortic stenosis are seen in patients suffering from unicommisural aortic valve. Approximately 25% of these patients have other cardiac anomalies, such as aortic coarctation. As the disease progresses and the stenosis become severe, these patients may develop syncope from reduction in cardiac output and cerebral perfusion. These patients are also at an increased risk of sudden cardiac death from ischemia, which results from both increased demand and decreased supply from hypotension. Therapy is aimed at either balloon valvuloplasty or surgical correction.[57,58]

Primary pulmonary hypertension Primary pulmonary hypertension is a diagnosis of exclusion. It is defined as mean pulmonary artery pressure of greater than 25 mm Hg at rest and greater than 30 mm Hg during exercise.[59] It affects approximately 1/1,000,000 to 2/1,000,000 in Western countries and has more female predominance, which may seen even at early childhood as well. Up to 50% of the children with pulmonary hypertension suffer syncope.[60] Syncope may result from both arrhythmias and obstruction to blood flow. Vasodilators, including calcium channel blockers and prostaglandins, are used to alleviate symptoms. Most of these patients are also treated with anticoagulation.[61]

Primary myocardial dysfunction

Cardiomyopathies are rarely seen in children and syncope seen in these patients may be due to ischemia, arrhythmias, or some inflammatory process.[8] Neuromuscular dystrophies, such as Duchenne, Becker, and Emery-Dreifuss muscular dystrophies, may present as myocardial dysfunction as well as bradyarrhythmias from AV block.[52] Myocarditis resulting in ventricular tachycardia may also present as syncope in children and unrecognized myocarditis may be an important cause of sudden unexplained death in children. Myocardial ischemia is rarely seen in children and usually results from anomalous left main coronary artery arising from a pulmonary trunk or to interarterial course of left coronary artery between aorta and pulmonary artery making it vulnerable to compression. These patients usually have exercise-related syncope because the blood flow to both aorta and pulmonary artery increases during exercise making the left coronary artery more vulnerable to compression. Another rare condition, seen in children of Asian descent under age 5 years, is Kawasaki disease.[62] Syncope may occur especially during acute myocarditis from ventricular arrhythmias. Arrythmogenic right ventricular dysplasia can result in ventricular tachycardia and syncope. It should be suspected in children with exercise-induced syncope and left bundle branch pattern of ventricular tachycardia. Usually this disorder becomes manifest in the 3rd to 4th decades of life and, rarely, rarely early. Cardiac MRI shows classis involvement of the right ventricle. Many of these patients may need ICDs. Other causes of syncope include patients with Eisenmenger syndrome, tetralogy of Fallot, and pulmonary stenosis and right ventricular outflow tract obstruction.[63,64]

Arrhythmias as a cause of syncope

Cardiac rhythm disturbances in the absence of structural heart disease are rarely seen as a cause of syncope in children.[63–65] Patients with long QT syndrome, Brugada syndrome, or short QT syndrome, however, essentially have a structurally normal heart but may be at a risk of syncope and sudden cardiac death.

Long QT syndrome Patients with long QT syndrome usually present with syncope associated with emotions or exercise and have a structurally normal heart. They are prone to develop a polymorphic ventricular tachycardia torsades de pointes, which can lead to hemodynamic compromise and subsequent syncope. They may also suffer abrupt-onset syncope in response to a fright or awakening by a loud noise, such as an alarm clock. Usually, patients may exhibit symptoms during second decade of life.[66–69] β-Blocker therapy may reduce mortality (from 70% in untreated patients) to 7%.[70] Some patients may be candidates for ICD implantation. Sympathetic ganglionectomy has been reserved for sever refractory cases.

Brugada syndrome Brugada syndrome is a hereditary disorder resulting from mutation in an α subunit of sodium channel protein involving the *SC5NA* gene. It manifests as incomplete right bundle branch block and ST elevation in leads V1 to V3. Patients with Brugada syndrome are at risk of syncope and sudden cardiac death from polymorphic ventricular tachycardia. Many patients with Brugada syndrome have a normal ECG and manifest typical Brugada pattern only after a drug challenge either with ajmaline or procainamide.[71] In an earlier published study on a population of children affected by Brugada syndrome, fever was found the most important precipitating factor for any arrhythmic event and the risk of fatal arrhythmias was significantly higher in previously symptomatic patients and in those demonstrating a spontaneous type I ECG (60% vs 7%). These patients should receive ICD if they have a cardiac arrest or have documented ventricular tachycardia even without cardiac arrest or a spontaneous type I ECG with syncope.[71,72]

Cathocholaminergic polymorphic ventricular tachycardia Cathocholaminergic polymorphic ventricular tachycardia is another rare inherited arrhythmic disorder affecting up to 1/10,000 people. It is an autosomal dominant disorder resulting from mutation in ryanodine receptor 2 (*RYR2*) gene. Less commonly, autosomal recessive variant has been seen resulting from *CASQ2* gene. Patients with CPVT suffer from disruption of the calcium handling within cardiac myocytes, which leads to ventricular tachycardia especially following exercise and emotional stress.[73] They may present with a bidirectional ventricular tachycardia as well. β-Blockers are the only proved therapy in these patients and ICDs have been used especially in patients with recurrent cardiac arrests on β-blockers.[73]

Arrhythmias may also result from repaired or palliated structural heart disease. Sinus node dysfunction has been reported to occur after atrial repair surgeries.[74–76] If severe enough, these patients may suffer symptomatic bradycardia and syncope. Similarly, AV block in pediatric patients is either congenital (seen in maternal lupus), which may not require pacing, or acquired from infections, such as diphtheria, endocarditis, Lyme disease, and Rocky Mountain spotted fever. Ventricular tachycardia, although rare, has been reported to occur in patients with corrected tetralogy of Fallot. Usually, these arrhythmias originate close to the ventricular path, especially in septum and outflow tract. Supraventricular tachycardia, like in adults, rarely presents as syncope in children. The most common causes of supraventricular tachycardia, including AV reciprocating tachycardia and AV reentrant tachycardia, have clinical presentation similar to that seen in adults.

Noncardiac Causes of Syncope

In some individuals, global cerebral hypoxia may result not only in loss of consciousness but also in convulsive activity. These episodes of convulsive syncope may at times be difficult to distinguish from seizures resulting from epilepsy.[77,78] Autonomically mediated forms of reflex syncope (such as neurocardiogenic or vasovagal syncope) may produce sudden episodes of profound hypotension and bradycardia resulting in loss of consciousness and, on occasion, convulsive activity. It has been reported that as many as one-third of patients initially diagnosed with epilepsy actually had a cardiovascular cause of their convulsive episodes. In contrast to convulsive syncope, however, convulsions in epileptic disorders are prolonged (>1 min), rhythmic, and usually not provoked by the stimuli that commonly provoke syncope. Similarly, many times seizures, especially neonatal seizures and complex partial seizures with minimal convulsive activity, may be confused with true syncope. It may be difficult to differentiate these 2 entities, especially when there is minimal or no convulsive activity (akinetic seizures). Ictal electroencephalogram (EEG) may be the only way to differentiate these seizures from syncope. In case of syncope, EEG may be normal or demonstrate diffuse slowing of the background activity. In case of seizure, however, there is an abnormal increase in the background activity.

Another group of disorders that may closely mimic both syncope and seizures includes loss of consciousness that results in the setting of complex migraine headaches or basilar migraines, which are sometimes referred to as brainstem attacks.[79] Loss of consciousness can also occur in patients suffering from hydrocephalus who experience sudden increase in intracranial pressure. If hydrocephalus is suspected neuroimaging for may reveal structural abnormalities, such as a tumors or brainstem herniation with dilated ventricles.[79]

Advances in understanding of the causes of syncope combined with advances in technology of the diagnostic modalities have greatly reduced the number of patients with recurrent syncope of unknown origin. In at least 10% of syncope patients, however, the cause remains unidentified after a traditional cardiac and neurologic work-up. Physicians should exercise great caution, however, before labeling any patient's syncope "psychogenic" in origin because a potential treatable cardiac cause is uncovered only by prolonged and diligent cardiac monitoring in these patients.[80]

HOW IS SYNCOPE EVALUATED IN CHILDREN AND ADOLESCENTS?

The cause of syncope is successfully identified in almost half of the patients with detailed history and a comprehensive physical examination. Unlike adults, it may be difficult to obtain history from children and often history is obtained from the parents or an eyewitnesses. When obtaining information from a patient or an eyewitness, a detailed account of circumstances and activity immediately before the event, identified triggers or precipiting factors, situations around the period of syncope, whether the syncope occurred during standing or lying down, and any symptoms or warning signs before the event should be diligently obtained. Information about the convulsive movements, loss of bladder and bowel control, tongue bite, and whether the recovery was quick or delayed may provide important clue to the diagnosis. When obtaining history, it is also important to recognize patients who may be at risk of sudden cardiac death. The group of patients who may be considered high risk and thus need further cardiac work-up include the following[81]:

- Patients having syncope during peak exercise
- Family history of sudden cardiac death
- Convulsive or traumatic syncope
- Chest pain preceding syncope
- Family history of deafness
- Syncope in children with structural heart disease
- Syncope in patients with abnormal cardiovascular examination
- Syncope in patients with focal neurologic defects

A comprehensive cardiovascular examination, including supine, sitting, and standing blood pressure and heart rate, should be recorded. It should be repeated at 2-, 5-, and 10-minute intervals in the standing position. Close and special attention should be paid to complete cardiac examinations, including murmurs, clicks, gallops, or any rhythm disturbances. A comprehensive neurologic examination should be performed and attention should be paid to focal neurologic abnormalities.

Laboratory Studies

Blood tests
The routine use of blood tests, such as serum electrolytes, cardiac enzymes, glucose, and hematocrit levels, is of low diagnostic value in syncopal patients and, therefore, is not recommended routinely.

Electrocardiogram
A 12-lead ECG should be obtained in every patient with loss of consciousness, especially after exercise. Particular attention should be paid to QT interval, pre-excitation, bundle branch block, and ventricular hypertrophy for any evidence of AV block.

ECG evaluation is particularly important if long QT syndrome is a possibility. If events seem related to exercise or stress and a standard ECG is normal, an exercise ECG should be performed.

Video-assisted recording
Video recording has allowed physicians to see real episodes and, when combined with physical monitoring, including continuous ECG and EEG, may help provide with improved diagnostic yield.[82]

Ambulatory ECG monitoring
Ambulatory ECG monitoring has allowed a greater symptom rhythm correlation in patients suffering from frequent syncope. If patients suffer frequent syncope, an external digital monitoring may help reveal the potential rhythm disturbance at the time of syncope. If the episodes are infrequent, implantable loop monitors can allow for prolonged monitoring up to 3 years.[83]

Head-up tilt table testing
Head-up tilt table testing (HUTT) is generally performed for 30 to 45 minutes after a 20-minute horizontal pretilt stabilization phase, at an angle between 60° and 80° (with 70° the most common). The sensitivity of the test can be increased, with an associated fall in specificity, by the use of longer tilt durations, steeper tilt angles, and provocative agents, such as isoproterenol or nitroglycerin.[84–86] HUTT has been safely performed in children greater than 6 years of age. If cooperative, it can also be performed in younger children. In contrast to studies in adult patients, there are few reported studies on the use of HUTT in pediatric patients.

Given the lack of extensive data on the use of HUTT in pediatric patients, most of the consensus recommendations in pediatric patients come from adult HUTT data. The issue of HUTT duration has not been assessed in the pediatric population, however. Also, the gravity-induced orthostatic stress during HUTT is less pronounced in children than in adults, given their lower size and body surface area. A more prolonged HUTT or using a provocative agent (isoproterenol) during HUTT may be necessary in pediatric patients. HUTT may not be necessary for the further evaluation of syncope in pediatric patients who present with a normal physical examination, absence of abnormal laboratory findings, and a medical history characteristic of vasovagal syncope.

Echocardiogram

Echocardiograms are commonly used to evaluate patients with syncope who have abnormal ECG or abnormal cardiovascular examination. They should be performed in all patients having suspicion of structural heart disease.

Imaging

Neuroimaging is not performed routinely when evaluating the children and young adults with syncope unless a patient has abnormality on neurologic examination, which may have signs of raised intracranial pressure or focal neurologic defects. Cardiac imaging, including cardiac MR, rarely may be needed to evaluate a person with a suspicion of anomalous coronary artery.

HOW IS SYNCOPE MANAGED IN CHILDREN?

The approach to treatment of a patient with syncope depends largely on the cause and mechanism of syncope. Management of the most common cause of syncope (NCS) in children is discussed later and outlined in **Box 2**.

Box 2
Management of neurocardiogenic syncope in children

Education and reassurance

Physical countermaneuvers

Paced breathing

Fluid therapy

Pharmacologic treatment

Pacemaker therapy

Cardioneuroablation

Education and Reassurance

Treatment of syncope due to VVS begins with a careful history, with particular attention focused on identifying precipitating factors, quantifying the degree of salt intake and current medication use, and determining whether a patient has any prior conditions that may alter the approach used for treatment. For most patients with neurally mediated syncope, particularly those with infrequent episodes associated with an identifiable precipitant, education and reassurance are sufficient.[1]

Physical Countermaneuvers

Physical maneuvers, if used early at the onset of symptoms of NCS, may help abort the episode. The easiest of these maneuvers is assumption of a supine posture. Subsequently, leg elevation may lead to increased venous return to the heart. Sitting and squatting may also augment peripheral vascular resistance and improve venous return to the heart. Increase in the venous return to the heart subsequently increases cardiac output, blood pressure, and cerebral perfusion and aborts the syncope. The combination of leg crossing and the tension of the thigh and abdominal musculature has been shown highly effective in preventing reflex syncope in young patients.[87,88] If the patients are cooperative, progressively prolonged periods of enforced upright posture or tilt training might reduce the recurrence of NCS by lowering vascular compliance in the compartments most responsible for venous pooling. Raising the head of the bed during sleep (>10°) also contributes to the improvement of the symptoms. Compression stockings can sometimes be helpful but to be effective must be waist high and provide at least 30 mm Hg of ankle counterpressure. The European Society of Cardiology Guidelines on Management Diagnosis and Treatment of Syncope identify the following physical measures as class 2 treatments for neurally mediated syncope: (1) tilt training (2) head-up tilt sleeping (>10°), (3) isometric leg and arm counterpressure maneuvers, and (4) moderate aerobic and isometric exercise.[84] It has been reported that 2 minutes of an isometric hand grip maneuvers initiated at the onset of symptoms during tilt testing rendered two-thirds of patients asymptomatic. Other studies have demonstrated that tilt (standing) training is effective in the treatment of neurally mediated syncope. Standing training involves leaning against a wall with the heel 10 inches from the wall for progressively longer periods over 2 to 3 months. Standing time initially should be 5 minutes 2 times per day with a progressive increase to 40 minutes twice daily. Although the results of nonrandomized studies of standing training have been positive, the results of randomized trials suggest that standing training may have only limited effectiveness.

Paced Breathing

In some cooperative patients, respiratory training with paced breathings has been shown to prevent tilt-induced NCS. Paced breathing is a deeper, slower way of breathing. It involves filling the lungs to full capacity when inhaling and then pushing out as much air as possible when exhaling. Paced breathing was shown to inhibit HUTT-induced syncope in one study.[89]

Fluid Therapy

Increasing oral fluid and salt intake is an effective measure to prevent an episode of VVS. Patients are also told to drink approximately 2 L of fluid a day and ingest 2 g to 4 g of salt or increase fluid intake until the urine is clear and colorless. In one study, acute oral therapy with 200 mL to 250 mL of water was found to prevent HUTT-induced syncope in 78% of patients who demonstrated a positive HUTT prior to fluid therapy.[1]

Pharmacologic Treatment

Currently, there is no therapy that is FDA approved for patients with NCS, and there is a paucity of evidence supporting any pharmacologic therapy. In contrast to the physical maneuvers, the value of pharmacologic agents is less certain. The medications that are generally relied on to treat VVS include β-blockers, fludrocortisone, serotonin reuptake inhibitors, and midodrine. Despite the widespread use of these agents, none of these pharmacologic agents has been demonstrated effective in multiple large prospective randomized clinical trials. Although many investigators previously considered β-blockers effective therapy, recent studies have reported that the β-blockers, metoptolol, propranolol, and nadolol, are no more effective than placebo.[90–92]

Pacemaker Therapy

In some patients with HUTT-induced episodes of profound bradycardia and sometimes asystole, it seems logical that permanent pacemaker placement might be of benefit in preventing syncope in this subgroup. An important concern remains, however, as to whether these tilt-induced asystolic events accurately reflected what occurred during the spontaneous episodes. Although there were questions regarding the use of pacemakers in the treatment of patients with severe NCS with documented asystole, the recent Third International Study on Syncope of Uncertain Etiology (ISSUE-3)[93] trial seems to confirm their effectiveness. When considering pacemaker implantation for patients with NCS, pacemakers that provide specialized pacing algorithms are often selected. These include rate drop hysteresis or closed loop stimulation. Closed loop stimulation is a form of rate adaptive pacing, which responds to myocardial contraction dynamics by measuring variations in right ventricular intracardiac impedance. When an incipient NCS episode is detected, pacing rate is increased. Although no prospective randomized clinical trials exist to determine which pacing feature is superior, several recent nonrandomized or retrospective trials suggest that close look stimulation may be preferable.[94,95] Further research is needed in this evolving approach to management of NCS.

Cardioneuroablation

Recently, there have been reports on the use of radiofrequency energy (similar to ablation of atrial fibrillation) in patients with refractory NCS, targeting the ganglionic plexii in right and left atrium and thus abolishing Bezold-Jarisch reflex. This procedure has been referred to as cardioneuroablation and the initial reports from few centers are encouraging and have markedly reduced the recurrences in patients with refractory syncope.[96–99] These results need to be confirmed, however, in large randomized controlled trials.

FUTURE PERSPECTIVE

There is paucity of literature in the field of syncope in children and adolescents. Most of the management strategies in children reflect data from studies involving the adult population. In the future there will be a great need for studies in children and adolescents suffering from recurrent syncope. Also, to date, there has been no FDA-approved therapy for NCS, which represents the most common cause of syncope in both adults and children. None of the clinical trials of pharmacotherapy in NCS has shown benefit over placebo. One potential reason is that most of these trials were flawed or the endpoints of the study were not reasonable. Most of these clinical trials looked at the "time to first syncope," which may not be a reasonable endpoint to assess success of any therapy. NCS should be considered a chronic condition, and, as with other chronic diseases, the aim of the therapy should be to decrease the recurrence of syncope rather than to completely eliminate it. More reasonable endpoints, such as syncope burden, are needed when new clinical trials are devised. In the future, hopefully there will be data on the pharmaco-therapy of NCS and its variants, including POTS and other forms of dysautonomic syncope.

REFERENCES

1. Brignole M, Alboni P, Benditt DG, et al, Task Force on Syncope, European Society of Cardiology. Guidelines on management (diagnosis and treat-ment) of syncope—update 2004. Europace 2004; 6:467–537.

2. Kapoor WN. Syncope. N Engl J Med 2000;343: 1856.

3. Lewis DA, Dhala A. Syncope in the pediatric pa-tient. The cardiologist's perspective. Pediatr Clin North Am 1999;46:205.

4. Pratt JL, Fleisher GR. Syncope in children and adolescents. Pediatr Emerg Care 1989;5:80.

5. Massin MM, Bourguignont A, Coremans C, et al. Syncope in pediatric patients presenting to an emergency department. J Pediatr 2004;145:223.

6. Gillette PC, Garson A Jr. Sudden cardiac death in the pediatric population. Circulation 1992;85:l64.

7. Strickberger SA, Benson DW, Biaggioni I, et al. AHA/ACCF scientific statement on the evaluation of syncope: from the American Heart Association Councils on Clinical Cardiology, Cardiovascular Nursing, Cardiovascular Disease in the Young, and Stroke, and the Quality of Care and Outcomes Research Interdisciplinary Working Group; and the American College of Cardiology Foundation: in collaboration with the Heart Rhythm Society: endorsed by the American Autonomic Society. Circulation 2006;113:316.

8. Driscoll DJ, Jacobsen SJ, Porter CJ, et al. Syncope in children and adolescents. J Am Coll Cardiol 1997;29:1039–45.

9. Stephenson JB. Fits and faints. London: Mac Keith Press; 1990.

10. Horrocks IA, Nechay A, Stephenson JB, et al. Anoxic–epileptic seizures: observational study of epileptic seizures induced by syncopes. Arch Dis Child 2005;90:1283–7.

11. Gastaut H. Syncopes: generalised anoxic cerebral seizures. In: Vinken PJ, Bruyn GW, editors. Hand-book of clinical neurology, vol. 15: the epilepsies. Amsterdam: North-Holland Publishing; 1970.

12. Grubb BP, Friedman R. Syncope in child and adoles-cent. In: Grubb BP, Olshansky B, editors. Syncope: mechanisms and management. 2nd edition. Mulden (MA): Blackwell Press; 2005. p. 273–86.

13. Grubb BP. Dysautonomic (orthostatic) syncope. In: Grubb BP, Olshansky B, editors. Syncope: mecha-nisms and management. 2nd edition. Mulden (MA): Blackwell Press; 2005. p. 72–91.

14. Stewart JM. Orthostatic intolerance in pediatrics. J Pediatr 2002;140:404–11.

15. Stewart JM, Gewitz MH, Weldon A, et al. Patterns of orthostatic intolerance: the orthostatic tachy-cardia syndrome and adolescent chronic fatigue. J Pediatr 1999;135:218–25.

16. Stewart JM. Chronic orthostatic intolerance and the postural tachycardia syndrome (POTS). J Pediatr 2004;145:725–30.

17. Wieling W. Standing, orthostatic stress and autonomic function. In: Bannister R, Mathias C, editors. Autonomic failure: a textbook of clinical disorders of the autonomic nervous system. Oxford (United Kingdom): Oxford University Press; 1992. p. 308–20.

18. Grubb BP. Clinical practice. Neurocardiogenic syncope. N Engl J Med 2005;352(10):1004–10.

19. Wieling W, VanLieshout JJ. Maintenance of postural normotension in humans. In: Low P, editor. Clinical autonomic disorders. Philadelphia: Lippincott-Williams and Wilkins; 2008. p. 57–67.

20. Thompson WO, Thompson PK, Dailey ME. The effect of upright posture on the composition and volume of the blood in man. J Clin Invest 1988;5: 573–609.

21. Consensus Committee of the American Autonomic Society and the American Academy of Neurology. Consensus statement on the definition of ortho-static hypotension, pure autonomic failure and mul-tiple system atrophy. Neurology 1996;46:1470–1.

22. Rowe PC, Barron DF, Calkins H, et al. Orthostatic intolerance and chronic fatigue syndrome asso-ciated with Ehlers-Danlos syndrome. J Pediatr 1999;135(4):494–9.

23. Rowe PC, Barron DF, Calkins H, et al. Ehlers-Danlos syndrome. J Pediatr 1999;135(4):513.

24. Gazit Y, Nahir M, Grahame R, et al. Dysautonomia in the joint hypermobility syndrome. Am J Med 2003;115:33–40.

25. Shohat M, Halpern GJ. Familial dysautonomia. 2003 Jan 21 [updated 2010 Jun 01]. In: Pagon RA, Bird TD, Dolan CR, et al, editors. GeneReviews, Ñc[Internet]. Seattle (WA): University of Washington; 1993.

26. Dong J, Edelmann L, Bajwa AM, et al. Familial dysau-tonomia: detection of the IKBKAP IVS20(+6T -> C) and R696P mutations and frequencies among Ashkenazi Jews. Am J Med Genet 2002;110(3): 253–7.

27. Axelrod F. Familial dysautonomia. Mathias C, Bannister R. Clinical features and evaluation of the primary autonomic failure syndromes. In: Mathias C, Bannister R, editors. Autonomic failure: a textbook of clinical disorders of the autonomic nervous system. 4th edition. Oxford (United Kingdom): Oxford University Press; 1999. p. 307–20.

28. Low PA, Opfer-Gehrking TL, Textor SC, et al. Postural tachycardia syndrome (POTS). Neurology 1995;45:S19–25.

29. Schondorf R, Low PA. Idiopathic postural orthostatic tachycardia syndrome: an attenuated form of acute pandysautonomia? Neurology 1993;43(1):132–7.

30. Jacob G, Biaggioni I. Idiopathic orthostatic intolerance and postural orthostatic tachycardia syndrome. Am J Med Sci 1999;317:88–101.

31. Robertson D. The Epidemic of orthostatic tachycardia and orthostatic intolerance. Am J Med Sci 1999;317:75–7.

32. Thieben M, Sandroni P, Sletten D, et al. Postural orthostatic tachycardia syndrome — Mayo Clinic experience. Mayo Clin Proc 2007;82:308–13.

33. Jordan J, Shannon JR, Diedrich A, et al. Increased sympathetic activation in idiopathic orthostatic intole- rance: role of systemic adrenoreceptor sensitivity. Hypertension 2002;39:173–8.

34. Vernino S, Low PA, Fealey RD, et al. Autoantibodies to ganglionic acetylcholine receptors in auto- immune autonomic neuropathies. N Engl J Med 2000;343:847–55.

35. Levine BD, Zuckerman JH, Pawelczyk JA. Cardiac atrophy after bed-rest deconditioning: a nonneural mechanism for orthostatic intolerance. Circulation 1997;96:517–25.

36. Raj SR, Robertson D. Blood volume perturbations in the postural tachycardia syndrome. Am J Med Sci 2007;334:57–60, 24.

37. Haensch CA, Lerch H, Schlemmer H, et al. Cardiac neurotransmission imaging with 123I-meta-iodo-benzylguanidine in postural tachycardia syndrome. J Neurol Neurosurg Psychiatry 2010;81:339–43.

38. Kanjwal K, Karabin B, Kanjwal Y, et al. Autonomic dysfunction presenting as postural tachycardia syndrome following traumatic brain injury. Cardiol J 2010;17:482–7.

39. Kanjwal K, Karabin B, Kanjwal Y, et al. Postural orthostatic tachycardia syndrome following Lyme disease. Cardiol J 2011;18:63–6.

40. Kanjwal K, Karabin B, Kanjwal Y, et al. Postural orthostatic tachycardia syndrome: a rare complication following electrical injury. Pacing Clin Electrophysiol 2010;33(7):e59–61.

41. Kanjwal K, Karabin B, Kanjwal Y, et al. Autonomic dysfunction presenting as postural orthostatic tachycardia syndrome in patients with multiple sclerosis. Int J Med Sci 2010;7:62–7. PMC2840604.

42. Kanjwal K, Karabin B, Kanjwal Y, et al. Autonomic dysfunction presenting as orthostatic intolerance in patients suffering from mitochondrial cytopathy. Clin Cardiol 2010;33(10):626–9.

43. Kanjwal K, Karabin B, Sheikh M, et al. New onset postural orthostatic tachycardia syndrome following ablation of AV node reentrant tachycardia. J Interv Card Electrophysiol 2010;29(1):53–6.

44. Lombroso CT, Lerman P. Breathholding spells (cyanotic and pallid infantile syncope). Pediatrics 1967;39:563–81.

45. Stephenson JB. Reflex anoxic seizures ('white breath-holding'): nonepileptic vagal attacks. Arch Dis Child 1978;53:193–200.

46. DiMario FJ Jr. Prospective study of children with cyanotic and pallid breath-holding spells. Pediatrics 2001;107:265–9.

47. Marks I. Blood-injury phobia: a review. Am J Psychiatry 1988;145:1207–13.

48. Connolly J, Hallam RS, Marks IM. Selective association of fainting with blood-injury-illness fear. Behav Ther 1976;7:8–13.

49. Ost LG, Lindahl IL, Sterner U, et al. Exposure in vivo vs applied relaxation in the treatment of blood phobia. Behav Res Ther 1984;22:205–16.

50. Howard P, Leathart GL, Dornhorst AC, et al. The mess trick and the fainting lark. Br Med J 1951; 2(4728):382–4.

51. Wieling W, van Lieshout JJ. The fainting lark. Clin Auton Res 2002;12(3):207.

52. Massin MM, Malekzadeh-Milani S, Benatar A. Cardiac syncope in pediatric patients. Clin Cardiol 2007;30(2):81–5.

53. Nishimura RA, Holmes DR. Hypertrophic obstructive cardiomyopathy. N Engl J Med 2004;350: 1320–7.

54. Colan SD. Hypertrophic cardiomyopathy in childhood. Heart Fail Clin 2010;6(4):433–44.

55. Ostman-Smith I. Hypertrophic cardiomyopathy in childhood and adolescence strategies to prevent sudden death. Fundam Clin Pharmacol 2010; 24(5):637–52.

56. Hoffman JI, Kaplan S. The incidence of congenital heart disease. J Am Coll Cardiol 2002;39:1890.

57. Maskatia SA, Ing FF, Justino H, et al. Twenty-five year experience with balloon aortic valvuloplasty for congenital aortic stenosis. Am J Cardiol 2011; 108(7):1024–8.

58. Karamlou T, Jang K, Williams WG, et al. Outcomes and associated risk factors for aortic valve replacement in 160 children: a competing-risks analysis. Circulation 2005;112(22):3462–9.

59. Pfammatter JP. Needle in the haystack - potentially dangerous syncope in childhood. Praxis (Bern 1994) 2011;100(24):1487–91.

60. Douwes JM, van Loon RL, Roothooft MT, et al. Pulmonary arterial hypertension in childhood [review]. Ned Tijdschr Geneeskd 2011;155(49): A3901.

61. Barst RJ, McGoon MD, Elliott CG, et al. Survival in childhood pulmonary arterial hypertension: insights from the registry to evaluate early and long-term pulmonary arterial hypertension disease management. Circulation 2012;125(1): 113–22.

62. Burns JC, Shike H, Gordon JB, et al. Sequelae of Kawasaki disease in adolescents and young adults. J Am Coll Cardiol 1996;28(1):253–7.

63. Garson A Jr. Arrhythmias in pediatric patients. Med Clin North Am 1984;68:1171.

64. Rocchini AP, Chun PO, Dick M. Ventricular tachycardia in children. Am J Cardiol 1981;47:1091.

65. Garson A Jr, Smith RT, Moak JP, et al. Ventricular arrhythmias and sudden death in children. J Am Coll Cardiol 1985;5:130B.

66. Schwartz PJ, Moss AJ. Prolonged QT interval: what does it mean? J Cardiovasc Med 1982;7:1317.

67. Priori SG, Schwartz PJ, Napolitano C, et al. Risk stratification in the long QT syndrome. N Engl J Med 2003;348(19):1866–74.

68. Schwartz PJ, Stramba-Badiale M, Segantini A, et al. Prolongation of the QT interval and the sudden infant death syndrome. N Engl J Med 1998;338(24):1709–14.

69. Vincent GM. The long-QT syndrome: bedside to bench to bedside. N Engl J Med 2003;348(19):1837–8.

70. Moss AJ, Zareba W, Hall WJ, et al. Effectiveness and limitations of beta-blocker therapy in congenital long-QT syndrome. Circulation 2000;101(6):616–23.

71. Probst V, Denjoy I, Meregalli PG, et al. Clinical aspects and prognosis of Brugada syndrome in children. Circulation 2007;115(15):2042–8.

72. Sarkozy A, Boussy T, Kourgiannides G, et al. Long-term follow-up of primary prophylactic implantable cardioverter-defibrillator therapy in Brugada syndrome. Eur Heart J 2007;28(3):334–44.

73. Sy RW, Gollob MH, Klein GJ, et al. Arrhythmia characterization and long-term outcomes in catecholaminergic polymorphic ventricular tachycardia. Heart Rhythm 2011;8(6):864–71.

74. Hamilton RM, Fidler L. Right ventricular cardiomyopathy in the young: an emerging challenge. Heart Rhythm 2009;6(4):571–5.

75. Celik M, Sarıtaş B, Tatar T, et al. Risk factors for postoperative arrhythmia in patients with physiologic univentricular hearts undergoing Fontan procedure. Anadolu Kardiyol Derg 2012;12(4):347–51.

76. Stephenson EA, Lu M, Berul CI, et al, Pediatric Heart Network Investigators. Arrhythmias in a contemporary fontan cohort: prevalence and clinical associations in a multicenter cross-sectional study. J Am Coll Cardiol 2010;56(11):890–6.

77. Joensen P. Prevalence, incidence, and classification of epilepsy in the Faroes. Acta Neurol Scand 1986;74:150–5.

78. Zaidi A, Clough P, Cooper P, et al. Misdiagnosis of epilepsy: many seizure-like attacks have a cardiovascular cause. J Am Coll Cardiol 2000;36:181–4.

79. Rossi LN. Headache in childhood [review]. Childs Nerv Syst 1989;5(3):12934 [Erratum in: Childs Nerv Syst 1990 Jan;6(1):58].

80. Kanjwal K, Kanjwal Y, Karabin B, et al. Psychogenic syncope? A cautionary note. Pacing Clin Electrophysiol 2009;32(7):862–5.

81. Strieper MJ. Distinguishing benign syncope from life-threatening cardiac causes of syncope. Semin Pediatr Neurol 2005;12:32.

82. Sheth RD, Bodensteiner JB. Effective utilization of home-video recordings for the evaluation of paroxysmal events in pediatrics. Clin Pediatr (Phila) 1994;33:578–82.

83. Al Dhahri KN, Potts JE, Chiu CC, et al. Are implantable loop recorders useful in detecting arrhythmias in children with unexplained syncope? Pacing Clin Electrophysiol 2009;32(11):1422–7.

84. Lin P, Wang C, Cao MJ, et al. Application of the head-up tilt table test in children under 6 years old. Zhongguo Dang Dai Er Ke Za Zhi 2012; 14(4):276–8.

85. Yilmaz S, Gokben S, Levent E, et al. Syncope or seizure? The diagnostic value of synchronous tilt testing and video-EEG monitoring in children with transient loss of consciousness. Epilepsy Behav 2012;24(1):93–6. http://dx.doi.org/10.1016/j.yebeh.2012.02.006. PubMed PMID: 22459868.

86. Dietz S, Murfitt J, Florence L, et al. Head-up tilt testing in children and young people: a retrospective observational study. J Paediatr Child Health 2011;47(5):292–8.

87. Krediet CT, van Dijk N, Linzer M, et al. Management of vasovagal syncope: controlling or aborting faints by leg crossing and muscle tensing. Circulation 2002;106:1684–9.

88. Moya A, Sutton R, Ammirati F, et al. Guidelines for the Diagnosis and Management of Syncope 2009. Eur Heart J 2009;30(21):2631–71.

89. Jauregui-Renaud K, Marquez MF, Hermosillo AG, et al. Paced breathing can prevent vasovagal syncope during head-up tilt testing. Can J Cardiol 2003;19(6):698–700.

90. Scott WA, Pongiglione G, Bromberg BI, et al. Randomized comparison of atenolol and fludrocortisone acetate in the treatment of pediatric neurally mediated syncope. Am J Cardiol 1995;76:400–2.

91. Qingyou Z, Junbao D, Chaoshu T. The efficacy of midodrine hydrochloride in the treatment of children with vasovagal syncope. J Pediatr 2006; 149:777–80.

92. Madrid AH, Ortega J, Rebollo JG, et al. Lack of efficacy of atenolol for the prevention of neurally mediated syncope in a highly symptomatic population: a prospective, double-blind, randomized and placebo-controlled study. J Am Coll Cardiol 2001; 37:554–9.

93. Brignole M, Menozzi C, Moya A, et al. Pacemaker therapy in patients with neurally-medicated syncope and documented asystole. Third International Study on Syncope of Uncertain Etiology (ISSUE-3): a randomized trial. Circulation 2012;125(21):2566–71.

94. Kanjwal K, Karabin B, Kanjwal Y, et al. Preliminary observations on the use of closed-loop cardiac

pacin in patients with refractory neurocardiogenic syncope. J Interv Card Electrophysiol 2010;
1:69–73.

95. Palmisano P, Zaccaria M, Luzzi G, et al. Closed-loop
cardiac pacing vs. conventional dual-chamber
pacing with specialized sensing and pacing algorithms for syncope prevention. Europace 2012;14:
1038–43.

96. Rebecchi M, de Ruvo E, Strano S, et al. Ganglion-
ated plexi ablation in right atrium to treat cardioinhibitory neurocardiogenic syncope. J Interv Card
Electrophysiol 2012;34(3):231–5.

97. Liang Z, Jiayou Z, Zonggui W, et al. Selective atrial
vagal denervation guided by evoked vagal reflex

to treat refractory vasovagal syncope. Pacing
Clin Electrophysiol 2012;35(7):e214–8. http://dx.doi.
org/10.1111/j.1540-8159.2011.03320.x.   PubMed
PMID: 22303858.

98. Yao Y, Shi R, Wong T, et al. Endocardial autonomic
denervation of the left atrium to treat vasovagal
syncope: an early experience in humans. Circ
Arrhythm Electrophysiol 2012;5(2):279–86. http://
dx.doi.org/10.1161/CIRCEP.111.966465.

99. Pachon JC, Pachon EI, Cunha Pachon MZ, et al.
Catheter ablation of severe neurally meditated
reflex (neurocardiogenic or vasovagal) syncope:
cardioneuroablation long-term results. Europace
2011;13(9):1231–42.

Syncope in the Older Person

Iain G. Matthews, MBChB, MRCP[a], Isabel A.E. Tresham, MBBS, MRCP[b],
Steve W. Parry, MBBS, MRCP, PhD[a,b,*]

KEYWORDS

- Syncope • Older people • Neurally mediated disorders • Orthostatic hypotension • Falls
- Arrhythmia

KEY POINTS

- Syncope can be a more challenging diagnostic and therapeutic exercise in older patients compared with younger patients.
- Syncope in older patients carries a significantly higher morbidity, mortality, and health economic burden.
- The examining clinician needs to be alert to the protean manifestations of underlying syncope in the older patient, and although the importance of ensuring that cardiac causes are exposed and acted on, neurally mediated disorders and orthostatic hypotension still cause most syncopal episodes in this age group.
- While diagnosing and managing the syncopal event and its adverse health and social consequences, clinicians need to be aware of the management of potential comorbid issues such as osteoporosis and cognitive impairment and if not in a position to act on them, ensure that appropriate specialist help is sought.

INTRODUCTION

Syncope imposes a disproportionately greater health and symptom burden on the older patient. Comorbidity and polypharmacy in tandem with age-related cardiovascular, autonomic, and cerebrovascular physiologic impairment account for this burden. In addition, cognitive decline complicates many aspects of investigation and management. Subsequently, the care of the older patient with syncope requires enhanced and additional skills to those needed to manage the younger patient. This article outlines the nature of those skills, using clinical vignettes to describe investigation and management of the older patient with syncope.

EPIDEMIOLOGY

The most frequently reported incidence of syncope in the literature is derived from the Framingham cohort between 1971 and 1998 of 7814 patients, 822 of whom reported syncope, and stands at 6.2 per 1000 person-years.[1] The most contemporary series documenting the incidence of syncope comes from Denmark between 1997 and 2009, comprising 127,508 patients seen in the emergency department or outpatient clinic or admitted to hospital, and describes a higher incidence of 17.2 per 1000 person-years.[2] Similar contemporary series describe different incidences (**Table 1**).

Thus, there is significant discrepancy between the reported incidences of syncope that is almost certainly related to the different populations studied (primary care vs combined emergency department, outpatient, primary care attendance vs inpatients) and the different parameters used as a measure of syncope (first syncope vs diagnosis of syncope). However, common to all series is the bimodal distribution of syncope and the greater burden of

This article originally appeared in Cardiac Electrophysiology Clinics, Volume 5, Issue 4, December 2013.
[a] Institute for Ageing and Health, Newcastle University, Newcastle upon Tyne NE4 5PL, UK; [b] Falls and Syncope Service, Royal Victoria Infirmary, Newcastle upon Tyne NE1 4LP, UK
* Corresponding author. Institute for Ageing and Health, Newcastle University, Newcastle upon Tyne, UK.
E-mail addresses: steve.parry@nuth.nhs.uk; swparry@hotmail.com

Table 1
Incidence of syncope in largest and most recent series reporting incidence as per 1000 person-years

Series	Population	Number	Incidence per 1000 Person-Years	Mean/Median Age (y)
Soteriades et al,[1] 2002	Framingham cohort First syncope 1971–1988	7814	6.2	Mean 65.9
Alshekhlee et al,[3] 2009	US National Inpatient Sample Diagnosis of syncope 2000–2005	305,932	0.80–0.93	Mean 69 ± 17
Vanbrabant et al,[4] 2011	Belgian primary care cohort First syncope 1994–2008	2785	0.80–2.91	Mean 54.5
Ruwald et al,[2] 2012	Danish National Patient Register Diagnosis of syncope 1997–2009	127,508	17.2	Median 65 (interquartile range 49–81)

syncope shouldered by those of advancing years. With the exception of the Belgian primary care cohort,[4] the mean or median age of presentation with first syncope or diagnosis is 65 years or older (see **Table 1**).

In the Framingham cohort, the incidences in men and women aged 20 to 29 years were 2.6 and 4.7 per 1000 person-years, respectively, compared with 16.9 per 1000 person-years in men and 19.5 per 1000 person-years in women in those older than 80 years.[1] The incidence is relatively static between the ages of 30 and 70 years, before it increases and reaches its peak in those older than 80 years. In a similar vein, in a recent study from Denmark,[2] the incidence in those aged 20 to 29 years is 9.0 per 1000 person-years and there is an increase to 40.2 per 1000 person-years at age 70 years and a peak of 81.2 per 1000 person-years in those older than 80 years. In a study describing a primary-care cohort from Belgium,[4] the incidences in men and women aged 15 to 24 years were 1.3 and 2.4 per 1000 person-years, respectively, compared with 6.1 and 8.7 per 1000 person-years in those older than 75 years.

PATHOPHYSIOLOGY
Cardiac Causes of Syncope

Cardiac causes of syncope are more common in the older patient (**Fig. 1**), reflecting the exponential increase in cardiac conducting tissue disease and structural heart disease with advancing age. Cardiac causes account for around a third of syncopal events in the older patient, with a concomitant increase in morbidity and mortality compared with younger patients.[5] Most are arrhythmic, with bradyarrhythmias

predominating,[5] although valvular disease, particularly aortic stenosis, is not uncommon.[6]

Neurally Mediated Syncope

There is limited evidence regarding the mechanism of syncope in older people, because most studies have looked at younger adults.[7] Typical vasovagal syncope (VVS), mediated by emotional stress such as severe pain or instrumentation, as seen in younger adults, is rarely seen in older adults. Also, VVS in younger adults is not generally associated with other cardiovascular or neurologic disease. In contrast, in older adults, VVS is associated with other comorbidities and medication use.

Often, multiple causes are found of syncope in the elderly, particularly in the neurally mediated disorders (carotid sinus syndrome (CSS), VVS, and situational syncope) and orthostatic hypotension

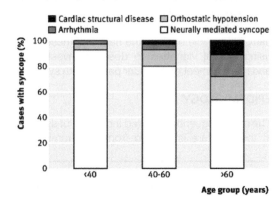

Fig. 1. Causes of syncope in different age groups. (*From* Parry SW, Tan MP. An approach to the evaluation and management of syncope in adults. BMJ 2010;340:c880; with permission.)

(OH).[8,9] The overlap in pathophysiology is further complicated by other age-related factors that contribute to the challenge of diagnosing and managing syncope in the elderly, including multiple comorbidities and polypharmacy. This situation leads to multiple possible attributable or contributory diagnoses, with an overlap not only between syncope type and classification but also between syncope and falls. In the older patient, there is an overlap between syncope and falls, and syncopal events may initially present as falls.[10] Falls and drop attacks may be multifactorial because of problems with gait and balance, visual impairment and cognitive impairment, with amnesia for loss of consciousness[11] and lack of a witness account providing further diagnostic challenges. Up to almost a third of cognitively normal older people with confirmed falls are unable to recall falling 3 months later.[12]

Not only does syncope become more common with increasing age, it is associated with a higher likelihood of an adverse outcome. Related to this worse outcome is the burden of comorbidity and polypharmacy encountered in the older patient. In a study[13] of 242 referrals to a group of syncope centers in Italy, mortality was significantly associated with age and comorbidity (hazard ratio [HR] 1.17, 95% confidence interval [CI] 1.0–1.37 for age and HR 1.39, 95% CI 1.01–1.93 for comorbidity). In the Danish cohort study, 74% to 78% of all those older than 80 years were on cardiovascular medication, whereas compared with age-matched and sex-matched controls, those with syncope were significantly more likely to have a diagnosis of ischemic heart disease, cerebrovascular and peripheral vascular disease, atrial fibrillation, diabetes mellitus, chronic obstructive pulmonary disease, renal failure, liver disease, rheumatologic disease, cancer, and dementia.[2]

There are physiologic changes associated with aging that may help to account for the differences in presentation and cause of syncope in older people. VVS in older adults may be an expression of other underlying pathologic processes, which, although not clearly defined, reflect underlying autonomic disturbances. There is also an increase in positive responses to carotid sinus massage (CSM) with age, and carotid sinus hypersensitivity (CSH) is a cause of syncope almost exclusive to older adults (mean age 70 years).[14] Recent work showing differences in heart rate variability and baroreflex sensitivity[15] and brainstem autonomic nuclei disease[16] in patients with symptomatic CSH suggest a widespread autonomic disorder, although the pathophysiology of CSH remains obscure.[17] There is debate as to whether or not CSH represents a disease state at all. In a randomly

selected sample of 272 individuals older than 65 years from a UK general practice register, CSH was present in 39%. The 95th percentiles response to CSM were 7.3 seconds asystole and 77 mm Hg systolic blood pressure decrease.[18] Coupled with the dearth of randomized controlled trials of pacing therapy in CSS,[19] these findings raise the possibility that CSS may be an age-related epiphenomenon rather than a pathologic entity.[15]

A dysautonomic response to head-up tilt (HUT) testing, with a progressive decrease in blood pressure before a typical vasovagal reaction, tends to be seen in older adults rather than the classic response of blood pressure and heart rate maintenance with sudden hemodynamic collapse seen in the young.[20] This response is also more commonly associated with CSH, suggesting an underlying complex autonomic dysfunction. A similar progressive decrease in blood pressure can also be shown in older adults with orthostatic intolerance, with similar features as seen in a dysautonomic response, but without progression to loss of consciousness within 5 minutes of onset of symptoms of hypotension (eg, light-headedness, sweating, blurring of vision).[21]

Autonomic regulation of heart rate variability differs with age, with reduced heart rate variability in older adults,[22,23] and this is more pronounced in the standing position. This situation may be the result of reduced baroreceptor modulation of heart rate.[24] The pattern of heart rate variability is similar in older and younger patients with VVS, although older patients are more likely to have a predominantly vasodepressor response.[25]

Unlike in younger people, in whom there is a significant increase in plasma renin activity in response to hypotension and postural change induced by tilt table testing, plasma renin activity is not influenced by hypotension or prolonged HUT (120 minutes) in the elderly.[26] This age-related change in plasma renin response to orthostasis suggests sympathetic involvement in the maintenance of blood pressure responses in older adults. Changes in circulating catecholamine concentrations in VVS have been well documented, with a more rapid increase in adrenaline levels found to be associated with VVS than in comparable controls undergoing tilt table testing.[27] However, measurement of arterial catecholamines in older adults (age >65 years) shows a tendency toward higher baseline adrenaline concentration, with less adrenaline surge before onset of syncope compared with younger adults (age <35 years), but with comparable noradrenaline responses.[28] Several other hormonal factors have been hypothesized to play a role in VVS; however, a clear pathophysiologic cause has yet to be shown.[29]

Dynamic cerebral autoregulation is not affected by aging alone[30,31] and is preserved in older people, although disease states which do affect cerebral autoregulation, such as hypertension, are more common in the elderly. It has been suggested that higher baseline blood pressure in older adults provides a blood pressure reserve for maintenance of consciousness compared with younger adults.[32] This theory is supported by older adults (age >60 years) having a significantly higher baseline arterial systolic blood pressure, but with little difference in the lower blood pressure limit to maintain cerebral autoregulation. There is a trend for the blood pressure at syncope induced by tilt table testing to increase with age, but older adults are able to tolerate an upright posture for a longer period before the onset of syncope during HUT. Age and baseline blood pressure has only a minor effect on the lower limit of blood pressure necessary to maintain consciousness.[32] Cerebral autoregulation is also impaired in CSS, with alterations in cerebral blood flow velocities detected by transcranial Doppler during lower body negative pressure–induced hypotension[33] and CSM[34] in patients with CSS versus control individuals. However, the pathophysiologic and potential therapeutic implications of this finding have yet to be elucidated.

The pathophysiology of neurally mediated syncope in older patients is yet to be confirmed but is likely to result from changes in autonomic regulation, in combination with hormonal factors and exacerbated by comorbidity and polypharmacy.

MANAGING SYNCOPE IN THE OLDER PATIENT: A CASE-BASED APPROACH

The older patient is more likely to suffer syncope, more likely to have comorbid conditions, more likely to be taking multiple medications, and more likely to have an adverse outcome. Cardiac causes of syncope are straightforward in terms of treatment; for example, device implantation and antiarrhythmic therapy or surgical and endovascular management of valvular disease are well described elsewhere.[5,35–37] However, even within the bradycardia pacing arena, there are gaps in the evidence base, with consensus on, for example, pacing in bifascicular and trifascicular block challenged by the imminent commencement of a randomized controlled Canadian-led study.[38] However, managing the older patient with less clear-cut syncopal disease requires a broad knowledge base across multiple body systems and of multiple chronic conditions, a solid grounding in clinical pharmacology, and appreciation of the vagaries of presentation. In the neurally mediated disorders, the evidence base in relation to the older patient is even less clear-cut, with randomized controlled trials related to the management of the older syncopal patient being limited to pacing intervention studies in patients with a positive adenosine test,[39,40] CSS associated with unexplained falls,[41–43] and VVS.[19,44] The remainder of this article uses real-life clinical vignettes to describe, explain, and offer practical hints and tips in each of these areas.

Case Vignette 1: When is a Fall Not a Fall?

A 75-year-old man reported 2 episodes of falling whilst walking in the last 2 months. On each occasion, he was suddenly aware of bilateral tinnitus ("loud whooshing in both ears") and fell forward onto the ground. When he was questioned in more detail, his falls were clearly associated with transient loss of consciousness (TLOC), and he had had intermittent postural dizziness, which improved with sitting down, for the previous 7 months. He was immediately orientated, and on 1 occasion suffered a wrist fracture. There was no postural element or any relationship to neck movement. His only medication was bendroflumethiazide for hypertension.

On examination, pulse was 68 beats per minute (bpm) and regular and supine blood pressure was 124/78 mm Hg, with a transient decrease to 88/65 mm Hg on immediate standing, before recovering to 101/72 mm Hg at 3 minutes, with associated mild light-headedness. Cardiovascular, neurologic, and locomotor examinations were normal. Twelve-lead electrocardiography (ECG) showed normal sinus rhythm with left bundle branch block (QRS duration 138 milliseconds). He declined CSM, having been quoted a 1:1000 risk of stroke.

A plan to insert an implantable loop recorder was formulated because the clinical suspicion was of arrhythmic syncope. In the interim, a 48-hour ambulatory ECG was arranged. Approximately 2 hours after having the ambulatory ECG fitted, the patient suffered a syncopal episode in the bathroom. Analysis of the monitor revealed a 19.5-second sinus pause. He was referred for permanent pacing that day.

Discussion

Although neurally mediated syncope still predominates as the leading cause of syncope in the older person (see **Fig. 1**), there is a proportionally greater contribution from structural cardiac disease, OH, and cardiac arrhythmia, with cardiac arrhythmia carrying a significantly higher rate of mortality than other forms.[1,2,13]

Arrhythmic syncope in the older person frequently presents in the classic Stokes-Adams fashion, with sudden unheralded loss of consciousness and prompt, full spontaneous recovery. However, the presentation may be more subtle, as in this case, in the form of drop attacks ("I just went down, didn't trip or slip and didn't lose consciousness") or unexplained falls, particularly with comorbid cognitive impairment or the absence of a witness account. Bradyarrhythmias predominate, with ECG pointers to these being an important component of investigation and management (**Box 1**). As per the ISSUE studies (International Studies of Syncope of Uncertain Etiology)[45] of implantable loop recorder use in unexplained syncope, left or right bundle branch block should prompt further investigation for a potential bradycardic cause, whereas a resting heart rate of less than 50 bpm is strongly suggestive of underlying sinus node dysfunction. In the presence of ischemic heart disease and left ventricular dysfunction, it is important to consider the possibility of ventricular arrhythmia, and clinical examination findings may prompt further echocardiographic or electrophysiologic investigation.

One of the central pillars of diagnosis in arrhythmic syncope is symptom-rhythm correlation, with noninvasive and more invasive monitoring strategies usefully summarized in the UK National Institute of Clinical Excellence (NICE) guidance on TLOC.[46] Up to 48 hours Holter monitoring is suggested in those with TLOC several times per week; with the option to add a patient-activated external event recorder should there be no TLOC in those 48 hours. In those with TLOC every 1 to 2 weeks, an external event recorder should be offered first line, with an implantable loop recorder the next option should there be no TLOC in this time frame. In those with TLOC occurring at a frequency of less than every 2 weeks, then an implantable loop recorder should be offered first line.[46] Patient-activated devices can be problematic in the older patient, although appropriate training[47] and the use of autoactivation mitigate these issues.

Although arrhythmic syncope is more common in the older person, OH is a common problem. This patient had significant OH, and improved symptomatically with substitution of an angiotensin-converting enzyme inhibitor for his thiazide diuretic. Although not the cause of his syncopal event, OH is an independent risk factor for falls in the older patient[48] and caused significant dizziness symptoms. Given the comorbid profile of the aging population, it is not uncommon that both an OH/vasovagal syncope (VVS) overlap and arrhythmic (bradycardic) syncope may coexist, which further complicates matters. It is important to remember osteoporosis in the older patient, as prompted by our case's wrist fracture. Appropriate treatment with bone protection therapy halves the risk of a subsequent fracture over the next 12 months, making assessment using standardized tools like FRAX (fracture risk assessment) vital (http://www.shef.ac.uk/FRAX).

This case is a typical one for a Stokes-Adams–type attack in an older patient, but highlights several important points:

1. The greater preponderance of arrhythmic (particularly bradycardic) syncope in the older person, and the need for greater awareness of soft ECG indicators of these
2. The importance of symptom-rhythm correlation and the optimal strategies for achieving this
3. The presentation of syncope may be with a drop attack or unexplained fall
4. OH or neurally mediated syncope may complicate an apparently simple arrhythmia diagnosis
5. The importance of considering osteoporosis investigation and management.

Case Vignette 2: The Swoon

An 82-year-old woman presented with 4 episodes of collapse in the previous year, with TLOC on 2 occasions. She did not recall any prodromal symptoms, "just going down," and on 3 occasions felt nauseous and very tired after the event. She had injured herself on 1 occasion, with soft tissue injuries to her right upper limb and the right periorbital region. She reported regular transient dizziness on standing from sitting, requiring her to hold on to furniture to maintain balance. Her past history was notable for hypertension, osteoarthritis, type 2 diabetes mellitus, and hypercholesterolemia. She was taking amlodipine, bendroflumethiazide, simvastatin, amitriptyline at night, and bone protection in the form of a bisphosphonate and calcium/vitamin D.

Clinical examination of the cardiovascular and neurologic systems was unremarkable. A 12-lead ECG showed normal sinus rhythm, with no evidence of conducting system disease and a normal

---

Box 1
ECG diagnoses suggestive of arrhythmic (bradycardic) syncope

Left or right bundle branch block

Prolonged first-degree atrioventricular block (PR interval >250 milliseconds)

Asymptomatic inappropriate sinus bradycardia (<50 bpm)

Sinus pauses greater than 3 seconds

Evidence of chronotropic incompetence

corrected QT interval. Her supine blood pressure was 159/72 mm Hg, with an symptomatic immediate dip to 104/68 mm Hg on standing, which corrected after 30 seconds, with no further dropout to 3 minutes. CSM was nondiagnostic. Routine laboratory testing was unremarkable.

The patient went on to have a 20:15 glyceryl trinitrate (GTN) HUT test per the Italian protocol.[49] At 24 minutes, she felt "strange" and hot for 10 to 15 seconds, with a decrease in blood pressure from 123/55 mm Hg to 42/18 mm Hg over a period of 45 seconds, with attendant loss of consciousness and a relative bradycardia of 56 bpm. When the patient was returned supine and with bilateral leg raise, blood pressure and consciousness promptly returned. The patient was transiently disorientated, asking what had happened and where she was, but this settled quickly, and she noted that this was how her collapses had occurred.

A diagnosis of vasodepressor VVS (VASIS [Vasovagal International Study] type 3) was made. Her bendroflumethiazide was discontinued; she was given advice to increase her fluid intake to 1.5 to 2 L of noncaffeinated beverages before midday, be fitted for compression hosiery, and on the importance of immediate abortive action at the onset of the newly identified premonitory symptoms. She was syncope free at 1 year follow-up.

Discussion

The classic vasovagal prodrome of pallor, diaphoresis, light-headedness, dizziness, and nausea is often short or nonexistent in the older patient.[50] Similarly, the classic provoking factors of prolonged standing, posture change, or hot environments are less common.[7] In contrast to younger fainters, the older patient with VVS is less likely to report both total or near loss of consciousness and more likely to present with unexplained falls.[7] The patient in question had no remembered prodrome, but during tilt table testing, clearly identified a short-lived feeling of strangeness and heat of particular import for future abortive maneuvers in real-life fainting. Tilt table testing has been criticized for diagnostic purposes,[46] but its usefulness in showing prodromal symptoms in patients with poorly remembered or unrecognized premonitory symptoms should not be underestimated. Furthermore, tilt table testing is safe and well tolerated in older patients, even in those with cognitive impairment.[7,51,52] Both passive and GTN-provoked protocols have been used extensively, whereas a shorter front-loaded GTN-provoked test may be used in those with mobility issues who might have difficulty standing for long periods.[53]

This elderly woman's diagnosis of VVS was made in the context of a normal surface ECG, no

structural heart disease, and a diagnostic tilt table test, per European Society of Cardiology (ESC) guidelines.[5] Given her cardiovascular risk factors, it would be important to guide further investigations along the cardiac route should further syncope occur despite optimal therapy. Further syncope would have prompted implantable loop recorder use. The presence of multiple comorbid conditions results directly in polypharmacy, with the most culpable in terms of hypotensive disorders being antihypertensives and antianginals. However, more important than the class of agent, is the presence of multiple agents. Polypharmacy is directly linked to an increased rate of VVS in older people.[7] As in the previous case, OH (defined as a sustained 20 mm Hg decrease in systolic blood pressure or 10 mm Hg decrease in diastolic blood pressure associated with typical clinical symptoms of cerebral hypoperfusion on transfer from supine to standing)[54] may be contributory. This symptom can be on either active standing or passive unprovoked tilt testing. It is said to be present in 20% of community-dwelling adults older than 65 years, increasing to 30% in those older than 75 years, and is higher still in institutionalized adults. The mechanism is believed to be failure of the physiologic mechanisms designed to cope with the significantly reduced venous return associated with standing from lying or sitting, as a consequence of the aging process, distinct pathophysiologic entities, and culprit medication. Autonomic neuropathy and Parkinson disease/ Parkinson plus syndrome-related OH are particular issues for the older patient, which warrant further specialist investigation and management.

Treatment in VVS is, as in the younger population, for the most part conservative[55] and has 2 key principals: long-term prevention and mechanisms to abort syncope. Long-term prevention involves ensuring adequate fluid intake, the reduction in dose or cessation of culprit medications, and the wearing of compression hosiery, although these may not be well tolerated by older people. Physical counterpressure maneuvers,[56] lying supine, and elevating the legs are as useful as in younger patients, but physical deconditioning, impaired mobility, and mechanical difficulties from arthritic joints often make these more challenging for the older patient.

There is little evidence for benefit of pharmacologic agents in the older patient. A multicenter randomized controlled study of metoprolol showed no benefit overall, but suggested benefit in patients older than 42 years.[57,58] This theory will be the subject of a further randomized trial of metoprolol in this age group (POST 5 [Prevention of Syncope Trial 5], RS Sheldon, personal communication,

June 2013). Fludrocortisone is commonly used in VVS management, but there have been no published randomized data in adults, although the POST II study[59] in abstract form suggests that there may no benefit at all (http://www.theheart.org/article/1301615.do). Midodrine has been shown to be of benefit in small randomized studies and is the subject of a larger randomized trial.[60] However, our own audit data show that up to 25% of older patients may discontinue midodrine because of its side effect profile (which may include urinary frequency, urgency, piloerection, and worsening of angina).

Pacing therapy in VVS has had a checkered history, with the initial promise of successful observational studies countermanded by blinded, randomized trials that failed to show any benefit.[19] However, the recent ISSUE 3 study[44] showed clear benefit of pacing therapy in patients with neurally mediated syncope and asystole documented on an implantable loop recorder (2-year syncope recurrence rate of 57% in pacemaker-off arm vs 25% in pacemaker-on arm, $P = .039$). The mean age of those paced in ISSUE 3 was 63 ± 14 years, raising the possibility that perhaps latent conducting system disease rather than cardioinhibitory VVS is being identified. Regardless, there is now clear evidence that asystole shown by loop recorder and treated with pacing seems to reduce the syncope burden, although in a highly selected patient group representing less than 10% of VVS cases overall. This evidence, combined with the effectiveness of conservative therapy, means that pacing has only a limited role.

Thus, VVS is the most common diagnosis in the older patient with syncope, in much the same way as it is in the young, with several important riders:

1. It is vital to appreciate the different presentations in the older person, with particular emphasis on the variable reporting of loss of consciousness and the frequent absence of typical vasovagal symptoms
2. Tilt-testing is safe and well tolerated in the older age group and can be important in both accurate diagnosis and the identification of prodromal symptoms
3. Permanent pacing can be a suitable therapy for vasovagal patients with asystole documented by implantable loop recorder
4. Further work is soon to commence on the potential for β-blockers to ameliorate symptoms in VVS in the older patient. In the interim, only midodrine has proven benefit, although it may cause troublesome side effects in this age group
5. Particular care needs to be taken to consider cardiac causes of syncope in the older patient.

Case Vignette 3: Don't Look Now...

An 82-year-old man reported 2 episodes of falling to the ground in the preceding 6 months. On 1 occasion, he was sitting waiting for a bus, and on the other he was crossing the road. There was no prodrome. He denied losing consciousness but suffered soft tissue injuries to his face on both occasions.

His past history was notable for hypertension, hypercholesterolemia, and adenocarcinoma of the prostate on hormonal therapy. His current mediation included aspirin, perindopril, and simvastatin, in addition to the hormonal injections for prostate carcinoma.

On examination, his pulse was 70 bpm and blood pressure 137/64 mm Hg with no evidence of a postural drop. There were no carotid bruits. Examination of the cardiovascular system was normal, and surface ECG was unremarkable. CSM was performed with beat-to-beat blood pressure and continuous ECG monitoring. Supine CSM resulted in asymptomatic slowing of the sinus rate by 10 to 15 bpm, with a concurrent decrease of 15 mm Hg in the systolic blood pressure. Pressure on the right carotid sinus in the upright position resulted in a 7.2-second sinus pause, with loss of consciousness and collapse. The patient recovered quickly, and afterward, he had no awareness of the episode. He was referred for implantation of a dual chamber permanent pacemaker with rate-drop response capability and remained symptom free at 2 years.

Discussion

CSS is a subtype of neurally mediated syncope almost exclusive to the older person, certainly to those older than 40 years.[5] Traditional diagnostic criteria (the method of symptoms[5]) rest on showing CSH (ie, ≥3 seconds of asystole [cardioinhibitory type] or ≥50 mm Hg decrease in systolic blood pressure [vasodepressor type] or both [mixed type] precipitated by CSM in association with reproduction of usual clinical symptoms during 10 seconds of sequential, bilateral CSM in the supine and erect positions). However, more recent guidance[35] suggests that 6 seconds of asystole should be the benchmark for permanent pacing in CSS.

CSS, like VVS and arrhythmic syncope, can have a varied clinical presentation in the older person. Syncope associated with head turning (as in our vignette as the patient crossed the road) or carotid pressure from, for example, shaving[61] is found in only 44% of patients with CSH as an attributable cause of symptoms.[8] Precipitating and premonitory symptoms may be completely absent; in 1 series, 40% of 90 patients with unexplained drop attacks were found to have CSS.[62]

The only treatment modality for CSS investigated in any significant detail is permanent pacing. There are no large, randomized controlled trials of permanent pacing in CSS associated with syncope, but a recent review of the observational evidence[63] suggested a 5-year 75% reduction in syncopal episodes associated with CSS. CSS associated with unexplained falls is less clear-cut. The SAFE PACE study[42] randomized 175 patients presenting with syncope or an unexplained fall who had a positive cardioinhibitory response to CSM to pacing or standard therapy. There was a significant decrease in the mean number of falls/episodes of syncope in the paced group (4.1 [range 0–29] vs 9.3 [range 0–89] odds ratio 0.42, 95% confidence interval [CI] 0.32–0.75). This study was followed by the SAFE PACE 2 study,[43] in which similar numbers were randomized to pacing or implantable loop recorder insertion. This time, the number of falls/syncopal episodes was greater in the paced arm (3.42 vs 2.63, HR 1.38, 95% CI 0.80–2.12). The only placebo-controlled study implanted pacemakers in recurrent unexplained fallers and randomized to pacemaker on or off for 6 months before crossing over to the alternative limb.[41] No effect was associated with pacing on the number of falls, although the trial was underpowered. Thus, the most recent iteration of the ESC syncope guidance[5] guidance gives a class IIa indication for permanent pacing in cardioinhibitory CSS but mentions only syncope as a presenting symptom. On the other hand, the North American equivalent[64] gives pacing a class I recommendation and mentions both syncope and unexplained falls as possible presenting symptoms, as does a recent Cochrane review on falls prevention.[65] The most recent guidance on pacing therapy from the ESC[35] gives a class I recommendation but requires the presence of more than 6 seconds asystole in the presence of syncope reproduction.

RECAPITULATION

1. CSS can be associated with syncope, drop attacks, and unexplained falls, with the propensity for significant injury in many cases.
2. Upright CSM should be performed if supine, bilateral, sequential CSM is unremarkable.[66] Symptoms should be reproduced to confirm a positive diagnosis. In our experience, supine rest for a minimum of 15 minutes after CSM further minimizes the risk of neurologic complications of the test.
3. Permanent pacing is indicated for CSS associated with syncope; in addition, it is our practice to pace patients with unexplained falls and drop attacks and no alternative cause of symptoms if a positive response to CSM is associated with symptoms of collapse or syncope.
4. Criteria for CSS diagnosis are currently debated, and although many laboratories still use the 3-second asystole diagnostic criterion,[66] increasing momentum is gathering to use the 6-second cutoff.[35,67]

SUMMARY

Syncope in the older person can be a more challenging diagnostic and therapeutic exercise compared with the younger patient, and carries a significantly higher morbidity, mortality, and health economic burden. The examining clinician needs to be alert to the protean manifestations of underlying syncope in the older patient, and although the importance of ensuring that cardiac causes are exposed and acted on cannot be overemphasized, neurally mediated disorders and OH still cause most syncopal episodes in this age group. While diagnosing and managing the syncopal event and its adverse health and social consequences, clinicians need to be aware of the management of potential comorbid issues, such as osteoporosis and cognitive impairment, and if not in a position to act on them, ensure that appropriate specialist help is sought. Further work is needed to understand the pathophysiology and hence the management of syncope in the older patient, with ongoing studies helping tease out some of the treatment controversies.

REFERENCES

1. Soteriades ES, Evans JC, Larson MG, et al. Incidence and prognosis of syncope. N Engl J Med 2002;347(12):878–85.
2. Ruwald MH, Hansen ML, Lamberts M, et al. The relation between age, sex, comorbidity, and pharmacotherapy and the risk of syncope: a Danish nationwide study. Europace 2012;14(10):1506–14.
3. Alshekhlee A, Shen WK, Mackall J, et al. Incidence and mortality rates of syncope in the United States. Am J Med 2009;122(2):181–8.
4. Vanbrabant P, Gillet JB, Buntinx F, et al. Incidence and outcome of first syncope in primary care: a retrospective cohort study. BMC Fam Pract 2011; 12(1):102.
5. Task Force for the Diagnosis and Management of Syncope, European Society of Cardiology (ESC), European Heart Rhythm Association (EHRA), et al. Guidelines for the diagnosis and management of syncope (version 2009). Eur Heart J 2009;30(21):2631–71.

6. Aronow WS. Recognition and management of aortic stenosis in the elderly. Geriatrics 2007; 62(12):23–32.

7. Duncan GW, Tan MP, Newton JL, et al. Vasovagal syncope in the older person: differences in presentation between older and younger patients. Age Ageing 2010;39(4):465–70.

8. McIntosh SJ, Lawson J, Kenny RA. Clinical characteristics of vasodepressor, cardioinhibitory, and mixed carotid sinus syndrome in the elderly. Am J Med 1993;95(2):203–8.

9. Tan MP, Newton JL, Chadwick TJ, et al. The relationship between carotid sinus hypersensitivity, orthostatic hypotension, and vasovagal syncope: a case-control study. Europace 2008;10(12): 1400–5.

10. Kenny RA, Bhangu J, King-Kallimanis BL. Epidemiology of syncope/collapse in younger and older Western patient populations. Prog Cardiovasc Dis 2013;55(4):357–63.

11. Parry SW, Steen IN, Baptist M, et al. Amnesia for loss of consciousness in carotid sinus syndrome: implications for presentation with falls. J Am Coll Cardiol 2005;45(11):1840–3.

12. Cummings SR, Nevitt MC, Kidd S. Forgetting falls. The limited accuracy of recall of falls in the elderly. J Am Geriatr Soc 1988;36(7):613–6.

13. Ungar A, Galizia G, Morrione A, et al. Two-year morbidity and mortality in elderly patients with syncope. Age Ageing 2011;40(6):696–702.

14. Alboni P, Brignole M, Menozzi C, et al. Clinical spectrum of neurally mediated reflex syncopes. Europace 2004;6(1):55–62.

15. Tan MP, Kenny RA, Chadwick TJ, et al. Carotid sinus hypersensitivity: disease state or clinical sign of ageing? Insights from a controlled study of autonomic function in symptomatic and asymptomatic subjects. Europace 2010;12(11):1630–6.

16. Miller VM, Kenny RA, Slade JY, et al. Medullary autonomic pathology in carotid sinus hypersensitivity. Neuropathol Appl Neurobiol 2008;34(4): 403–11.

17. Parry SW, Baptist M, Gilroy JJ, et al. Central alpha2 adrenoceptors and the pathogenesis of carotid sinus hypersensitivity. Heart 2004;90(8):935–6.

18. Kerr SR, Pearce MS, Brayne C, et al. Carotid sinus hypersensitivity in asymptomatic older persons: implications for diagnosis of syncope and falls. Arch Intern Med 2006;166(5):515–20.

19. Parry SW, Matthews IG. Update on the role of pacemaker therapy in vasovagal syncope and carotid sinus syndrome. Prog Cardiovasc Dis 2013;55(4):434–42.

20. Sutton R, Brignole M, Menozzi C, et al. Dual-chamber pacing in the treatment of neurally mediated tilt-positive cardioinhibitory syncope: pacemaker versus no therapy: a multicenter randomized study. The Vasovagal Syncope International Study (VASIS) Investigators. Circulation 2000;102(3):294–9.

21. Brignole M, Menozzi C, Del Rosso A, et al. New classification of haemodynamics of vasovagal syncope: beyond the VASIS classification. Analysis of the pre-syncopal phase of the tilt test without and with nitroglycerin challenge. Vasovagal Syncope International Study. Europace 2000;2(1):66–76.

22. Ruiz GA, Madoery C, Arnaldo F, et al. Frequency-domain analysis of heart rate variability during positive and negative head-up tilt test: importance of age. Pacing Clin Electrophysiol 2000;23(3):325–32.

23. Lipsitz LA, Mietus J, Moody GB, et al. Spectral characteristics of heart rate variability before and during postural tilt. Relations to aging and risk of syncope. Circulation 1990;81(6):1803–10.

24. Simpson DM, Wicks R. Spectral analysis of heart rate indicates reduced baroreceptor-related heart rate variability in elderly persons. J Gerontol 1988;43(1):M21–4.

25. Kochiadakis GE, Papadimitriou EA, Marketou ME, et al. Autonomic nervous system changes in vasovagal syncope: is there any difference between young and older patients? Pacing Clin Electrophysiol 2004;27(10):1371–7.

26. Kenny RA, Lyon CC, Bayliss J, et al. Reduced plasma renin activity in elderly subjects in response to vasovagal hypotension and head-up tilt. Age Ageing 1987;16(3):171–7.

27. Benditt DG, Ermis C, Padanilam B, et al. Catecholamine response during haemodynamically stable upright posture in individuals with and without tilt-table induced vasovagal syncope. Europace 2003;5(1):65–70.

28. Ermis C, Samniah N, Sakaguchi S, et al. Comparison of catecholamine response during tilt-table-induced vasovagal syncope in patients <35 to those >65 years of age. Am J Cardiol 2004;93(2): 225–7.

29. Alboni P, Brignole M, Degli Uberti EC. Is vasovagal syncope a disease? Europace 2007;9(2):83–7.

30. Carey BJ, Eames PJ, Blake MJ, et al. Dynamic cerebral autoregulation is unaffected by aging. Stroke 2000;31(12):2895–900.

31. van Beek AH, Claassen JA, Rikkert MG, et al. Cerebral autoregulation: an overview of current concepts and methodology with special focus on the elderly. J Cereb Blood Flow Metab 2008;28(6):1071–85.

32. Giese AE, Li V, McKnite S, et al. Impact of age and blood pressure on the lower arterial pressure limit for maintenance of consciousness during passive upright posture in healthy vasovagal fainters: preliminary observations. Europace 2004;6(5):457–62 [discussion: 63].

33. Parry SW, Steen N, Baptist M, et al. Cerebral autoregulation is impaired in cardioinhibitory carotid sinus syndrome. Heart 2006;92(6):792–7.

34. Leftheriotis G, Rozak P, Dupuis JM, et al. Cerebral hemodynamics during carotid massage in patients with carotid sinus syndrome. Pacing Clin Electrophysiol 1998;21(10):1885–92.

35. Authors/Task Force Members, Brignole M, Auricchio A, et al. 2013 ESC Guidelines on cardiac pacing and cardiac resynchronization therapy: The Task Force on cardiac pacing and resynchronization therapy of the European Society of Cardiology (ESC). Developed in collaboration with the European Heart Rhythm Association (EHRA). Europace 2013;15(8):1070–118.

36. Kappetein AP, Head SJ, Genereux P, et al. Updated standardized endpoint definitions for transcatheter aortic valve implantation: the Valve Academic Research Consortium-2 consensus document. J Thorac Cardiovasc Surg 2013; 145(1):6–23.

37. Bonow RO, Carabello BA, Chatterjee K, et al. 2008 focused update incorporated into the ACC/AHA 2006 guidelines for the management of patients with valvular heart disease: a report of the American College of Cardiology/American Heart Association Task Force on Practice Guidelines (Writing Committee to revise the 1998 guidelines for the management of patients with valvular heart disease). Endorsed by the Society of Cardiovascular Anesthesiologists, Society for Cardiovascular Angiography and Interventions, and Society of Thoracic Surgeons. J Am Coll Cardiol 2008;52(13):e1–142.

38. Krahn AD, Morillo CA, Kus T, et al. Empiric pacemaker compared with a monitoring strategy in patients with syncope and bifascicular conduction block–rationale and design of the Syncope: Pacing or Recording in the Later Years (SPRITELY) study. Europace 2012;14(7):1044–8.

39. Parry SW, Nath S, Bourke JP, et al. Adenosine test in the diagnosis of unexplained syncope: marker of conducting tissue disease or neurally mediated syncope? Eur Heart J 2006;27(12):1396–400.

40. Flammang D, Church TR, De Roy L, et al. Treatment of unexplained syncope: a multicenter, randomized trial of cardiac pacing guided by adenosine 5'-triphosphate testing. Circulation 2012;125(1):31–6.

41. Parry SW, Steen N, Bexton RS, et al. Pacing in elderly recurrent fallers with carotid sinus hypersensitivity: a randomised, double-blind, placebo controlled crossover trial. Heart 2009;95(5):405–9.

42. Kenny RA, Richardson DA, Steen N, et al. Carotid sinus syndrome: a modifiable risk factor for nonaccidental falls in older adults (SAFE PACE). J Am Coll Cardiol 2001;38(5):1491–6.

43. Ryan DJ, Nick S, Colette SM, et al. Carotid sinus syndrome, should we pace? A multicentre, randomised control trial (Safepace 2). Heart 2010; 96(5):347–51.

44. Brignole M, Menozzi C, Moya A, et al. Pacemaker therapy in patients with neurally mediated syncope and documented asystole: Third International Study on Syncope of Uncertain Etiology (ISSUE-3): a randomized trial. Circulation 2012; 125(21):2566–71.

45. Brignole M, Menozzi C, Moya A, et al. Mechanism of syncope in patients with bundle branch block and negative electrophysiological test. Circulation 2001;104(17):2045–50.

46. Westby M, Davis S, Bullock I, et al. Transient loss of consciousness ('blackouts') management in adults and young people. London: National Clinical Guideline Centre for Acute and Chronic Condition, Royal College of Physicians; 2010.

47. Farwell DJ, Freemantle N, Sulke N. The clinical impact of implantable loop recorders in patients with syncope. Eur Heart J 2006;27(3):351–6.

48. Panel on Prevention of Falls in Older Persons, American Geriatrics Society and British Geriatrics Society. Summary of the Updated American Geriatrics Society/British Geriatrics Society clinical practice guideline for prevention of falls in older persons. J Am Geriatr Soc 2011;59(1):148–57.

49. Bartoletti A, Alboni P, Ammirati F, et al. 'The Italian Protocol': a simplified head-up tilt testing potentiated with oral nitroglycerin to assess patients with unexplained syncope. Europace 2000;2(4):339–42.

50. Graham LA, Kenny RA. Clinical characteristics of patients with vasovagal reactions presenting as unexplained syncope. Europace 2001;3(2):141–6.

51. Shaw FE, Bond J, Richardson DA, et al. Multifactorial intervention after a fall in older people with cognitive impairment and dementia presenting to the accident and emergency department: randomised controlled trial. BMJ 2003;326(7380):73.

52. Gieroba ZJ, Newton JL, Parry SW, et al. Unprovoked and glyceryl trinitrate-provoked head-up tilt table test is safe in older people: a review of 10 years' experience. J Am Geriatr Soc 2004;52(11): 1913–5.

53. Parry SW, Gray JC, Newton JL, et al. 'Front-loaded' head-up tilt table testing: validation of a rapid first line nitrate-provoked tilt protocol for the diagnosis of vasovagal syncope. Age Ageing 2008;37(4): 411–5.

54. Freeman R, Wieling W, Axelrod FB, et al. Consensus statement on the definition of orthostatic hypotension, neurally mediated syncope and the postural tachycardia syndrome. Clin Auton Res 2011;21(2): 69–72.

55. Tan MP, Parry SW. Vasovagal syncope in the older patient. J Am Coll Cardiol 2008;51(6):599–606.

56. van Dijk N, Quartieri F, Blanc JJ, et al. Effectiveness of physical counterpressure maneuvers in preventing vasovagal syncope: the Physical Counterpressure

Manoeuvres Trial (PC-Trial). J Am Coll Cardiol 2006; 48(8):1652–7.

57. Sheldon RS, Morillo CA, Klingenheben T, et al. Age-dependent effect of beta-blockers in preventing vasovagal syncope. Circ Arrhythm Electrophysiol 2012;5(5):920–6.

58. Sheldon R, Connolly S, Rose S, et al. Prevention of Syncope Trial (POST): a randomized, placebo-controlled study of metoprolol in the prevention of vasovagal syncope. Circulation 2006;113(9):1164–70.

59. Raj SR, Rose S, Ritchie D, et al. The Second Prevention of Syncope Trial (POST II)–a randomized clinical trial of fludrocortisone for the prevention of neurally mediated syncope: rationale and study design. Am Heart J 2006;151(6):1186.e11–7.

60. Raj SR, Faris PD, McRae M, et al. Rationale for the prevention of syncope trial IV: assessment of midodrine. Clin Auton Res 2012;22(6):275–80.

61. Roskam J. Un syndrome nouveau. Syncopes cardiaques graves et syncope répétées par hyperreflectivité sinocardotidienne. Presse Med 1930;38: 590–1.

62. Parry SW, Kenny RA. Drop attacks in older adults: systematic assessment has a high diagnostic yield. J Am Geriatr Soc 2005;53(1):74–8.

63. Brignole M, Menozzi C. The natural history of carotid sinus syncope and the effect of cardiac pacing. Europace 2011;13(4):462–4.

64. Epstein AE, Dimarco JP, Ellenbogen KA, et al. ACC/AHA/HRS 2008 guidelines for device-based therapy of cardiac rhythm abnormalities: executive summary. Heart Rhythm 2008;5(6):934–55.

65. Gillespie LD, Robertson MC, Gillespie WJ, et al. Interventions for preventing falls in older people living in the community. Cochrane Database Syst Rev 2012;(9):CD007146.

66. Parry SW, Reeve P, Lawson J, et al. The Newcastle protocols 2008: an update on head-up tilt table testing and the management of vasovagal syncope and related disorders. Heart 2009;95(5):416–20.

67. Krediet CT, Parry SW, Jardine DL, et al. The history of diagnosing carotid sinus hypersensitivity: why are the current criteria too sensitive? Europace 2011;13(1):14–22.

Syncope as a Warning Symptom of Sudden Cardiac Death in Athletes

Giulia Vettor, MD[a], Alessandro Zorzi, MD[a], Cristina Basso, MD, PhD[c], Gaetano Thiene, MD[c], Domenico Corrado, MD, PhD[a,b],*

KEYWORDS

- Syncope • Sudden cardiac death • Athletes • Cardiomyopathy

KEY POINTS

- Clinical evaluation of syncope in the athlete remains a challenge.
- Although benign mechanisms predominate, syncope may be arrhythmic and precede SCD.
- Exercise-induced syncope should be regarded as an important alarming symptom of an underlying cardiac disease predisposing to arrhythmic cardiac arrest.
- All athletes with syncope require a focused and detailed workup for underlying cardiac cause, either structural or electrical.
- Major aim is to identify athletes at risk and to protect them from SCD.
- Athletes with potentially life-threatening etiologies of syncope should be restricted from competitive sports.

INTRODUCTION

Syncope is a sudden transient loss of consciousness and postural tone with spontaneous recovery after a brief period, which does not require electrical or medical therapy.[1–9]

Loss of consciousness results from a reduction of blood flow to the reticular activating system located in the brainstem. The metabolism of the brain is strongly dependent on perfusion and, consequently, cessation of cerebral blood flow leads to loss of consciousness within approximately 10 seconds; restoration of appropriate behavior and orientation after a syncopal episode are also immediate.[5]

Syncope is an important health problem because it is common in the general population, is often disabling, may cause injury, and may represent a prelude to SCD.[2,3]

Syncope accounts for 1% of admissions to hospitals and 3% of admissions to emergency departments. In the Framingham study, in a population of 7814 individuals, the incidence of syncope was 3% in men and 3.5% in women during a 26-year follow-up.[3] The prevalence of syncope varies with age, with a peak of first faints in patients aged 10 to 30 years (47% in female patients and 31% in patients at approximately age 15).

Causes of syncope can be classified into vascular, cardiac, neurologic-cerebrovascular, psychogenic, metabolic-miscellaneous, and syncope of unknown origin.[1–5]

This article originally appeared in Cardiac Electrophysiology Clinics, Volume 5, Issue 4, December 2013.
The authors have nothing to disclose.
[a] Department of Cardiac, Thoracic and Vascular Sciences, University of Padova Medical School, Via Giustiniani, 2, Padova 35121, Italy; [b] Arrhythmogenic Inherited Cardiomyopathy Unit, Department of Cardiac, Thoracic and Vascular Sciences, University of Padova Medical School, Via Giustiniani, 2, Padova 35121, Italy; [c] Cardiovascular Pathology, Department of Cardiac, Thoracic and Vascular Sciences, University of Padova, Via A. Gabelli 61, Padova 35121, Italy
* Corresponding author.
E-mail address: domenico.corrado@unipd.it

Athletes with syncope presents a unique challenge for physicians. The causes of syncope in athletes range from benign neurocardiogenic episodes to life-threatening conditions, such as ventricular arrhythmias leading to SCD.

It is mandatory to identify causes and mechanisms of syncope with the aim of excluding the underlying heart disease at risk for arrhythmic cardiac arrest.

The early detection of malignant variants of syncope has important implications for prevention of fatal events during sports. Detection of cardiovascular disorders responsible for syncope has an impact on eligibility for competitive sports activity because of the increased exercise-related risk.[10]

EPIDEMIOLOGY AND CAUSES OF SYNCOPE IN ATHLETES

There are few available data on the epidemiology and causes of syncope in athletes. Colivicchi and colleagues[8] studied a large population of 7568 athletes undergoing preparticipation screening. A syncopal episode was reported in 474 (6.2%) in the previous 5 years. Syncopal episodes were exercise unrelated in 87.7% and exercise related in 13.3%, i.e. postexertional in 12.0% and exertional in 1.3%. Over follow-up, the recurrence rate of syncope was 20 per 1000 subject-years, whereas the rate of new syncopal episodes was 2.2 per 1000 subject-years. Athletes with exercise-unrelated events had a diagnosis of either vasovagal or situational syncope. Unlike postexertional syncope, 50% of syncopal episodes occurring during exertion were "cardiogenic" (2 of 4) and caused by either hypertrophic cardiomyopathy or ventricular tachycardia.[8]

NEURALLY MEDIATED SYNCOPE

In athletes, syncope is most often neurocardiogenic and seems to have a fair prognosis.[6] Specific triggers are blood draws and prolonged standing. Classic prodromal symptoms, such as warmth, nausea, and palpitations, are present in almost cases. Usually the syncopal episodes are brief (5–30 s) and patients awake nauseous. The pathophysiology of neurally mediated syncope is not completely understood.[7]

Experimental studies demonstrated that endurance athletes, having more compliant and distensible ventricles and subject to a chronic volume load during exercise, experience a decrease in their stroke volume during orthostatic position because of a reduction in their filling pressures.

Another hypothesis is that after exertion there is a rapid decrease in venous return, causing vigorous ventricular contraction that activates mechanoreceptors, causing increased afferent neural output.[7]

ORTHOSTATIC HYPOTENSION

Orthostatic hypotension may also cause syncope during sports.[4] It is defined as a 20–mm Hg drop in systolic blood pressure or a 10–mm Hg drop in diastolic blood pressure within 3 minutes of standing and results from a defect in any portion of this blood pressure control system. Orthostatic hypotension can be asymptomatic or associated with symptoms, such as lightheadedness, dizziness, blurred vision, weakness, palpitations, and syncope. These symptoms often arise in the morning or after meals or exercise. Middle-aged and senior athletes are particularly susceptible to hypotension. Orthostatic hypotension is favored by volume depletion and reduced vasomotor tone caused by long periods of training.

CARDIOGENIC SYNCOPE IN THE ATHLETE

Approximately 1% of syncope in athletes is secondary to cardiac disease.[8] Many cardiac causes of syncope are also associated with an increased risk of SCD. In adult ages (>35 years), the most common cause is atherosclerotic coronary artery disease, whereas in younger competitive athletes (≤35 years), many different conditions, such as cardiomyopathies, congenital anomalies of coronary arteries, myocarditis, aortic rupture, valvular disease, preexcitation syndromes, conduction diseases, ion channel diseases, and congenital heart disease may cause cardiogenic syncope. HCM and arrhythmogenic RV cardiomyopathy (ARVC) are leading causes of fatalities in young competitors.[11]

Hypertrophic Cardiomyopathy

HCM is a heart muscle disease, usually genetically transmitted, and characterized by a hypertrophied, nondilated left ventricle (LV) in the absence of another cardiac or systemic disease capable of producing the magnitude of hypertrophy evident.[12,13] Characteristic morphologic and functional cardiac abnormalities include asymmetric LV hypertrophy with disproportionate septal thickening and reduction in LV chamber size with increased myocardial stiffness, which may critically impair diastolic LV and intramural coronary blood filling (**Fig. 1**A). Dynamic LV outflow tract obstruction is also demonstrable at rest or with exercise in a large proportion of patients. The histopathologic hallmark of HCM is myocardial disarray, with widespread, bizarre, and disordered

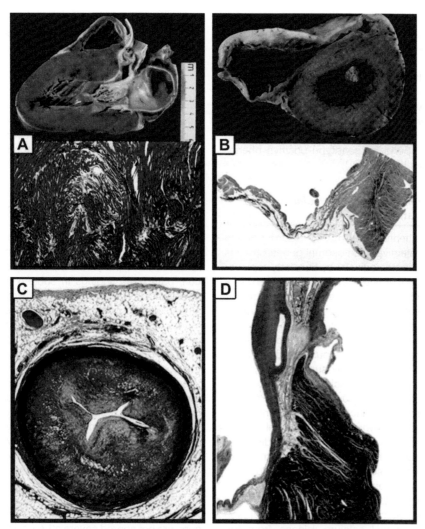

Fig. 1. Leading causes of SCD in young competitive athletes. (*A*) HCM: long-axis cut of the heart specimen showing asymmetric septal hypertrophy with subaortic bulging and septal endocardial fibrous plaque (*top*); histology of the interventricular septum revealing typical myocardial disarray with interstitial fibrosis (*bottom*) (Heidenhain trichrome). (*B*) ARVC: cross-section of the heart specimen with infundibular and inferior subtricuspidal aneurysms (*top*); panoramic histologic view of an aneurysm of the inferior wall showing wall thinning with fibrofatty replacement (*bottom*) (Heidenhain trichrome). (*C*) Premature coronary artery disease: histology of the proximal tract of the left anterior descending coronary artery showing a fibrous plaque causing severe lumen narrowing (Heidenhain trichrome). (*D*) Congenital coronary anomaly: panoramic histologic view showing the intramural aortic course with a slit-like lumen of the anomalous right coronary artery arising from the left aortic sinus of Valsalva and running between the aorta and the pulmonary trunk (Heidenhain trichrome). (*From* Corrado D, Drezner J, Basso C, et al. Strategies for the prevention of sudden cardiac death during sports. Eur J Cardiovasc Prev Rehabil 2011;18:197–208; with permission.)

arrangement of myocytes associated with diffuse interstitial and/or replacement-type fibrosis (see **Fig. 1**A). Myocardial scarring is an acquired phenomenon, in part related to abnormalities of the intramural coronary arteries, which show dysplasia of the tunica media with luminal narrowing (small vessel disease).

Cardiac arrest in affected athletes has been attributed to ventricular arrhythmias, most likely arising from an electrically instable myocardial substrate. The observation of acquired myocardial damage, either acute or in the setting of large septal scars, supports the hypothesis that myocardial ischemia intervenes in the natural history of the disease and contributes to the arrhythmogenicity.[14]

In North America, HCM is the most frequent cause of SCD in young people, including participants in high school and college competitive sports. Athletes affected by HCM are at risk of syncope during exercise by 2 mechanisms: LV outflow tract obstruction and arrhythmias. Based on these observations, it seems prudent to withdraw young people from intense competitive sports when a diagnosis of HCM is made in order to lower the risk. The European Society of Cardiology also recommends restriction from competitive sports for genotype-positive phenotype-negative individuals.[10]

Arrhythmogenic Right Ventricular Cardiomyopathy

ARVC is an inherited heart muscle disorder due to genetically defective desmosomal genes/proteins characterized pathologically by fibrofatty replacement of RV myocardium and clinically by the peculiar RV involvement with electrical ventricular instability leading to SCD, mostly in young people.[15,16]

In patients with ARVC, SCD is frequently preceded by syncope mostly occurring during exercise.[11] The propensity for sudden arrhythmic death during physical exercise is linked to both hemodynamic and neurohumoral factors. Physical exercise may acutely increase RV afterload and cavity enlargement, which, in turn, may elicit ventricular arrhythmias by stretching the diseased RV musculature. Alternatively, the hypothesis of "denervation supersensitivity" of the RV to catecholamines has been advanced. Finally, in a subgroup of patients with ARVC, the cardiac ryanodine receptor 2 (RYR2) missense mutation leading to abnormal calcium release from the sarcoplasmic reticulum during effort has been identified.[15–18]

The heart of young competitive athletes dying suddenly from ARVC demonstrates RV dilatation and massive transmural fibrofatty replacement of the RV musculature, resulting in aneurysmal dilatations of posterobasal, apical, and outflow tract regions, which are potential sources of life-threatening ventricular arrhythmias (see **Fig. 1**B). These pathologic features of the RV allow differential diagnosis with training-induced RV changes (athlete's heart), usually consisting of global RV enlargement without wall motion abnormalities.

Corrado and colleagues[16] reported that among 11 young competitive athletes with ARVC who died suddenly, 5 (45%) had previously experienced at least one syncopal episode as a warning symptom.

In Italy, sudden deaths due to HCM have been largely prevented by identification and disqualification of affected athletes at preparticipation screening.[11,19] Therefore, other cardiovascular conditions, such as ARVC, have come to account for a greater proportion of all sudden death in Italian athletes.

Atherosclerotic Coronary Disease

Atherosclerotic coronary artery disease is the major cause of fatal events in athletes over 35 years of age.[20] Most deaths occur with running, jogging, long-distance racing, and other vigorous sports, such as soccer, tennis, and squash. During exercise, physical and metabolic changes occur, leading to an increased risk of acute coronary complications and life-threatening myocardial ischemia. Even in highly conditioned individuals, sudden coronary death may be precipitated by underlying concealed atherosclerotic plaques. At postmortem examination, pathologic findings in sudden death victims are consistent with an underlying severe and diffuse atherosclerotic coronary artery disease, with 2 or more coronary trunks critically obstructed ($\geq$75% cross-sectional area) and associated with acute coronary thrombosis. In the territory tributary of the culprit coronary artery, the myocardium may show signs of hyperacute myocardial ischemia and/or myocardial scar due to a healed (often previously unrecognized) myocardial infarction. Therefore, the mechanism involved responsible for arrhythmic cardiac arrest consists of VT/ventricular fibrillation related to ventricular scar, acute myocardial ischemia, or both, with sympathetic stimulation during physical exertion favoring the electrical instability.

Highly trained athletes, such as marathon runners, are not spared severe atherosclerotic disease and sudden coronary death.[21] Alarming symptoms suggestive of coronary artery disease and/or coronary risk factors, including smoking, hypertension, hypercholesterolemia, and family history of coronary events before 55 years, have been often recognized in adults who experienced exercise-induced cardiac arrest. It is thus recommended that the presence of risk factors or symptoms of coronary artery disease are investigated in athletes older than 35 years and sports activity undertaken cautiously, particularly in the presence of risk factors. Stress testing may have significant limitations for detecting subjects at risk among the general population, and acute myocardial infarction and sudden coronary death may occur despite a negative exercise testing. Education of athletes should be aimed at increasing awareness of warning symptoms, such as chest pain, palpitations, or syncope, mostly occurring during physical exercise, and at improving lifestyle for prevention of coronary artery disease.

Coronary atherosclerosis is an important substrate for sudden death even in young competitive athletes (≤35 years).[22] Young athletes dying of premature coronary artery disease usually have neither risk factors nor history of angina pectoris and previous myocardial infarction, and sudden death is often the first manifestation of the disease. Exercise testing may fail to show myocardial ischemia or arrhythmias. Fatal coronary atherosclerosis is more often a single-vessel disease that characteristically affects the proximal left anterior descending coronary artery and is often due to fibrocellular plaques (ie, fibrous plaques with intimal smooth muscle cell hyperplasia, so-called accelerated atherosclerosis) and a preserved tunica media in absence of acute thrombosis (**Fig. 1**C).[21] These morphologic features have been suggested as underlying abnormal hypervasoreactivity, possibly culminating on cardiac arrest by vasospastic myocardial ischemia. Because of the scarcity of warning symptoms and the limitation of exercise testing, the identification at preparticipation screening of these young athletes with premature coronary atherosclerosis at risk of ischemic cardiac arrest remains a challenge.

Congenital Coronary Artery Anomaly

Congenital anomalous origin of the coronaries is the second most common cause of syncope and SCD in athletes.[23]

Some studies demonstrated that syncope was the only cardiac symptom present in the history of patients with congenital anomalies of the origin of the coronaries who died suddenly. Anomalous origin of a coronary artery from the wrong coronary sinus is a congenital malformation with a silent clinical course, which may precipitate sudden and unexpected ischemic cardiac arrest in young competitive athletes. The most frequent anatomic findings consist of both left and right coronary arteries arising either from the right or the left coronary sinus. In both conditions, as the anomalous coronary vessel leaves the aorta, it adopts an acute angle with the aortic wall and, thus, traverses between the aorta and the pulmonary trunk, often after an aortic intramural course, with a slit-like lumen (**Fig. 1**D). Fatal myocardial ischemia has been hypothesized as caused by exercise-induced aortic root expansion, which compresses the anomalous vessel against the pulmonary trunk, increasing the acute angulation of the coronary take-off, aggravating the slit-like shape of the lumen of the proximal intramural portion of the aberrant coronary vessel. This mechanism of myocardial ischemia is difficult to reproduce in clinical setting, as shown by the occurrence of negative ECG exercise testing in young athletes who have subsequently died suddenly from the this coronary anomaly.[23]

Ion Channel Diseases

Among the channelopathies group, a major role is played by long QT syndrome (LQTS), Brugada syndrome, and cathecolaminergic polymorphic VT (CPVT).

LQTS is a genetically determined ion-channel disease that may cause life-threatening ventricular arrhythmias, such as torsades de pointes and ventricular fibrillation. The LQTS genes encode ion-channel subunits involved in the repolarization phase of the cardiac action potential. Approximately 90% of genotype-positive patients have a mutation in 3 genes: KCNQ1 (LQT1), KCNH2 (LQT2), and the cardiac Na+ channel gene (SCN5A). Loss-of-function mutations of KCNQ1 (LQT1) and KCNH2 (LQT2) genes are associated with impaired function of cardiac potassium channels regulating outward K+ currents active during late ventricular repolarization. Gain-of-function mutations of SCN5A gene, instead, account for the rare and highly malignant LQT3 variant, which is characterized by impaired function of cardiac Na+ channels with late persistent inward currents delaying ventricular repolarization. Different molecular mechanisms may explain differences seen in clinical manifestations and circumstances of arrhythmic events in patients with different genotypes. LQT1 patients are prone to syncope or cardiac arrest during physical exercise, mostly while swimming. LQT2 subjects are more susceptible during emotional stress and acoustic stimuli. LQT3 patients show a bradycardia-dependent QT prolongation and they usually experience SCD at rest (while sleeping). Molecular screening for gene mutations in patients with LQTS has important prognostic implications, because genotype is an independent predictor of clinical outcome.[24]

Brugada syndrome is a disorder characterized by a typical electrocardiographic pattern. It is a familial disorder transmitted as an autosomal dominant gene and occurs most commonly in young and middle aged males. The syndrome is due to a mutation involving the cardiac Na+ channel gene (SCN5A). In affected patients, many factors are implicated in the onset of fatal arrhythmias as the increased vagal tone during sleep or a hyperthermic state.

It is interesting to note that in the athletes both an increased vagal tone and hyperthermia may play a role: the exercise increases the body temperature and the prolonged training results in a high vagal tone. In the majority of patients with Brugada syndrome the malignant ventricular arrhythmias occur at rest and, in many cases, at night. Syncope and sudden cardiac death are usually the results of an interaction between transient acute abnormalities ('triggers') and underlying heart disease ('substrate'). Acute triggers of sudden death during sports include emotional stress, myocardial ischemia, sympathovagal imbalance, and hemodynamic changes, potentially leading to life threatening ventricular arrhythmias.[25]

Although in the majority of patients with Brugada syndrome malignant ventricular arrhythmias occur at rest, intense exercise may increase the body temperature, and prolonged training may results in a high vagal tone, both factors exacerbating ECG abnormalities of Brugada syndrome and predisposing to SCD. Specifically, the systematic conditioning in athletes with Brugada syndrome may enhance the resting vagal tone and exaggerate the vagal reaction during postexercise recovery period, thus facilitating the occurrence of

syncope at rest or immediately after sports. There is a possibility that an adaptation of the cardiac autonomic nervous system to training, with results in increased vagal activity and/or withdrawal of sympathetic activity, may enhance the propensity of athletes with Brugada syndrome to die suddenly at rest, during sleep, or immediately after exercise (**Fig. 2**).[26]

Another cause of syncope in athletes is CPVT.[17] Mutations in RYR2 (the calcium release channel of the sarcoplasmic reticulum), calsequestrin 2 (CASQ2) (another protein involved in intracellular calcium handling), or the structural protein ankyrin-B (also referred to as LQT4 syndrome) have been defined as the underlying molecular mechanism of arrhythmias typically provoked by exercise or stress. The ECG at baseline is nondiagnostic, but exercise ECG shows multifocal ventricular premature beats or VT with alternating QRS axis (bidirectional VT). They may degenerate

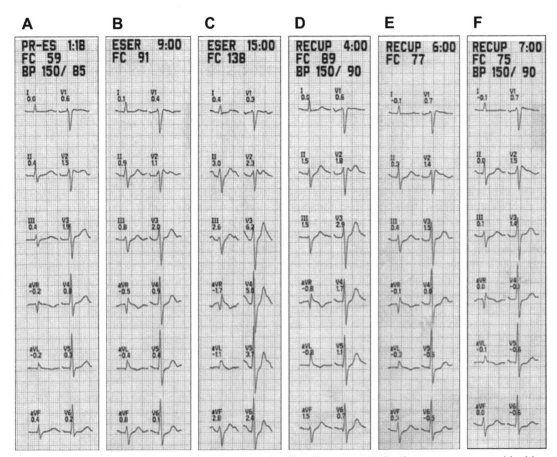

Fig. 2. ECG-recorded pre-exercise (*A*), during exercise (*B, C*), and postexercise (*D–F*) steps in a 31-year-old athlete with Brugada syndrome. Note the distinctive increase of the segment elevation (up to 3.5 mm at the J point in lead V2) during postexercise as a consequence of enhanced vagal rebound. Sympathetic stimulation aggravates the concomitant intraventricular conduction defect as shown by QRS prolongation from 90 to 130 ms and deeper S waves in inferolateral leads during exercise. (*From* Zorzi A, ElMaghawry M, Migliore F, et al. St-segment elevation and sudden death in the athlete. Card Electrophysiol Clin 2013;5:73–84; with permission.)

into polymorphic VT or ventricular fibrillation. Affected subjects have an 80% of risk of syncope and 30% of risk of SCD.

Finally, athletes with corrected congenital heart disease are at high risk for syncope and SCD, particularly after repair of tetralogy of Fallot but also after ventricular septal defect closure.[27]

CLINICAL WORK-UP OF THE ATHLETE WITH SYNCOPE

Evaluation of an athlete with syncope should differentiate true syncope from other conditions causing loss of consciousness (epilepsy, transitory ischemic attack, drop attack, hypoglycemia) and assess the presence of cardiac disease. Initial evaluation includes history (aimed at a clear description of the syncope), physical examination with blood pressure measurement in the orthostatic and standing positions and 12-lead ECG.

First Level Exams

The history in the evaluation of athletes with symptoms of syncope or presyncope is paramount in diagnosis. Syncope or presyncope that occurs during exertion is more likely life threatening than that occurring at rest. Postexertional syncope (such as standing at a foul line or during a time out) is not likely life threatening but is likely to be caused by vasodilatation and corresponding hypotension.[10] In one of the few epidemiologic series of syncope in athletes, Colivicchi and colleagues[8] reported that of 7568 athletes screened, 474 reported syncope in the prior 5 years. Syncope without prodromal symptoms is more troubling than a gradual onset of syncope. Syncope that occurs only with upright posture is less likely to be arrhythmic than that occurring during sitting or lying down. Syncope with a clear and reproducible trigger of stress, excitement, or fear is more likely to be neurocardiogenic than arrhythmic.

A majority of conditions at risk of syncope and sudden death during sports are genetically determined disease with an autosomal dominant pattern of inheritance, hence, the importance of family history in identifying affected athletes. Family history is considered positive when a close relative has experienced a premature heart attack or sudden death (<55 years of age in men and <65 years in women) or in the presence of a family history of cardiomyopathy, Marfan syndrome, LQTS, Brugada syndrome, severe arrhythmias, coronary artery disease, or other disabling cardiovascular diseases.

Positive physical findings include musculoskeletal and ocular features suggestive of Marfan syndrome, diminished and delayed femoral artery pulses, midsystolic or end-systolic clicks, a second heart sound single or widely split and fixed with respiration, marked heart murmurs (any diastolic and systolic grade >2/6), irregular heart rhythm, and brachial blood pressure greater than 140/90 mm Hg.

The hypothesis that many of the undiagnosed and underlying causes of syncope in athletes are suspected in analysis of ECG seems increasingly validated.[28–30] This approach has important implications for the cardiovascular management of athletes, including preparticipation screening, clinical diagnosis, and risk stratification. An Italian study provided the most compelling evidence of efficacy of ECG screening to save lives by identifying and disqualifying athletes with at-risk heart diseases. A time-trend analysis of the incidence of SCD in young competitive athletes in the Veneto region of Italy over 26 years (1979–2004) showed a sharp decline of mortality rates after the introduction of the nationwide screening program; 55 SCDs occurred in screened athletes (1.9 deaths per 100,000 person-years) and 265 deaths in unscreened nonathletes (0.79 deaths per 100,000 person-years). The annual incidence of SCD in athletes decreased by 89%, from 3.6 per 100,000 person-years in the prescreening period to 0.4 per 100,000 person-years in the late-screening period (**Fig. 3**).[11]

Many of the causes of syncope can be suspected on the base of ECG abnormalities at preparticipation screening.

Second- and Third-level Examinations

In cases of positive findings at any of the first-line examinations, an athlete with syncope should be evaluated with other invasive and noninvasive tests, such as a 2-D echo, stress test, Holter monitoring, MRI, coronary angiography, electrophysiological study, and endomyocardial biopsies. The results of these second-level and third-level examinations determine the eligibility of the subject to any sport competition.

Long-term ECG monitoring with Holter monitors can be useful in those patients with frequent or reproducible symptoms. Athletes with intermittent symptoms are best evaluated with a continuous loop monitor. These monitors continuously record a 1- to 3-minute segment of surface ECG and, with activation by a button on the loop monitor, the tape is frozen and the previous few minutes of the event are recorded.[1,4]

Exercise testing should be adapted to the specific type of exercise/sport responsible for the arrhythmic events, because a conventional exercise test may not replicate the specific clinical

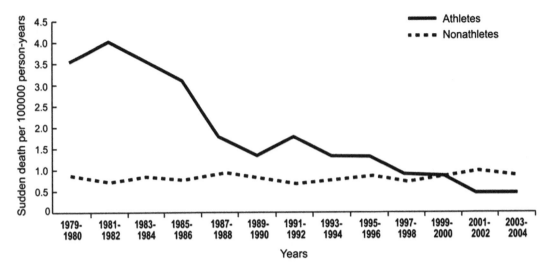

Fig. 3. Annual incidence rates of SCD per 100,000 persons among screened competitive athletes and unscreened nonathletes 12–35 years of age in the Veneto region of Italy, 1979–2004. During the study period (the nationwide preparticipation screening program was launched in 1982), the annual incidence of SCD declined by 89% in screened athletes (*P* for trend <.001). In contrast, the incidence rate of SCD did not demonstrate consistent changes over time in unscreened nonathletes. (*Data from* Corrado D, Basso C, Pavei A, et al. Trends in sudden cardiovascular death in young competitive athletes after implementation of a preparticipation screening program. JAMA 2006;296:1593–601.)

situation and the arrhythmogenic mechanism produced by actively participating in the sport. Increase in the arrhythmia frequency at beginning of exercise, disappearance at peak of exercise, and reappearance during recovery usually suggest the benign nature of the ectopic ventricular rhythm. Triggering or worsening of ventricular arrhythmia during exercise may point to underlying inherited cardiomyopathies or ion channel diseases and may predict malignant arrhythmic events at risk of SD during sports.[10,30–32]

In those athletes who are suspected of having an underlying cardiogenic cause of syncope, a careful echocardiographic evaluation of even subtle morphofunctional ventricular abnormalities is required.[33] Echocardiography is typically normal in CPVT, anomalous coronary arteries, Brugada syndrome, and LQTS.

Echo findings in ARVC include an enlarged hypokinetic RV with a thin RV free wall and heavy RV trabeculations with a hyper-reflective moderator band and occasional sacculations. MRI can also show fatty infiltration and thinning of the RV free wall. In some cases, it can also identify regional or global dilatation of the RV and evaluate for late gadolinium enhancement.[15,16]

Increased LV wall thickness (>13–15 mm with no other cause of hypertrophy), systolic anterior motion of the mitral valve, and LV outflow tract gradients all can be seen in HCM.[12]

MRI is sensitive in detecting increased LV wall thickness in patients with HCM and is particularly useful in detecting apical HCM. Finding a late gadolinium enhancement in the HCM is correlated with a major risk of fatal arrhythmias and SCD.[34]

RV angiography can aid in the diagnosis of ARVC. Dilatation and dysfunction, either global or segmental, of RV are typical findings during cardiac catheterization in patients with ARVC.[15,16]

Cardiac catheterization is also useful in the diagnosis of congenital anomalous coronary arteries and necessary in the diagnosis of atherosclerotic coronary disease.[23]

Management

In athletes with neurocardiogenic syncope, the restriction from sports with intrinsic risk is dictated by the awareness that any transient loss of consciousness will convey adverse effects for the athlete and the people nearby.

In athletes with syncope of arrhythmic origin, with or without an underlying heart disease, recommendation will be granted depending on the type of arrhythmia and/or on the associated abnormal cardiovascular condition.

SUMMARY

Clinical evaluation of syncope in the athlete remains a challenge. Although benign mechanisms predominate, syncope may be arrhythmic and precede SCD. Exercise-induced syncope should be regarded as an important alarming symptom of an underlying cardiac disease predisposing to arrhythmic cardiac arrest. All athletes with syncope require a focused and detailed workup for underlying cardiac cause, either structural or electrical.

Major aim is to identify athletes at risk and to protect them from SCD. Athletes with potentially life-threatening etiologies of syncope should be restricted from competitive sports.

REFERENCES

1. Brignole M, Alboni P, Benditt D, et al. Task force on syncope, european society of cardiology. Part 1. The initial evaluation of patients with syncope. Europace 2001;3:253–60.
2. Moya A, Sutton R, Ammirati F, et al, The Task Force for the Diagnosis and Management of Syncope of the European Society of Cardiology (ESC). Guidelines for the diagnosis and management of syncope (version 2009). Eur Heart J 2009;30:2631–71.
3. Soteriades ES, Evans JC, Larson MG, et al. Incidence and prognosis of syncope. N Engl J Med 2002;347:878–85.
4. Link MS, Estes NA 3rd. How to manage athletes with syncope. Cardiol Clin 2007;25:457–66.
5. Calkins H, Zipes DP. Hypotension and syncope. In: Saunders E, editor. Braunwald's heart disease. Philadelphia: 2005. p. 909–19.
6. Grubb BP. Neurocardiogenic syncope and related disorders of orthostatic intolerance. Circulation 2005;111:2997–3006.
7. Levine BD, Lane LD, Buckey JC, et al. Left ventricular pressure-volume and frank-starling relations in endurance athletes. Implications for orthostatic tolerance and exercise performance. Circulation 1991; 84:1016–23.
8. Colivicchi F, Ammirati F, Santini M. Epidemiology and prognostic implications of syncope in young competing athletes. Eur Heart J 2004;25:1749–53.
9. Gersh BJ, Maron BJ, Bonow RO, et al. 2011 accf/aha guideline for the diagnosis and treatment of hypertrophic cardiomyopathy: a report of the american college of cardiology foundation/american heart association task force on practice guidelines. Circulation 2011;124:e783–831.
10. Pelliccia A, Fagard R, Bjornstad HH, et al. Recommendations for competitive sports participation in athletes with cardiovascular disease: a consensus document from the study group of sports cardiology of the working group of cardiac rehabilitation and exercise physiology and the working group of myocardial and pericardial diseases of the european society of cardiology. Eur Heart J 2005;26: 1422–45.
11. Corrado D, Basso C, Pavei A, et al. Trends in sudden cardiovascular death in young competitive athletesafter implementation of a preparticipation screening program. JAMA 2006;296:1593–601.
12. Maron BJ. Hypertrophic cardiomyopathy: an important global disease. Am J Med 2004;116:63–5.
13. Maron BJ. Sudden death in young athletes. N Engl J Med 2003;349:1064–75.
14. Basso C, Thiene G, Corrado D, et al. Hypertrophic cardiomyopathy and sudden death in the young: pathologic evidence ofmyocardial ischemia. Hum Pathol 2000;31:988–98.
15. Basso C, Corrado D, Marcus FI, et al. Arrhythmogenic right ventricular cardiomyopathy. Lancet 2009;373:1289–300.
16. Corrado D, Basso C, Thiene G. Arrhythmogenic right ventricular cardiomyopathy: an update. Heart 2009;95:766–73.
17. Cerrone M, Napolitano C, Priori SG. Catecholaminergic polymorphic ventricular tachycardia: a paradigm to understand mechanisms of arrhythmias associated to impaired ca(2+) regulation. Heart Rhythm 2009;6:1652–9.
18. Leenhardt A, Lucet V, Denjoy I, et al. Catecholaminergic polymorphic ventricular tachycardia in children. A 7-year follow-up of 21 patients. Circulation 1995;91:1512–9.
19. Corrado D, Basso C, Schiavon M, et al. Screening for hypertrophic cardiomyopathy in young athletes. N Engl J Med 1998;339:364–9.
20. Corrado D, Schmied C, Basso C, et al. Risk of sports: do we need a pre-participation screening for competitive and leisure athletes? Eur Heart J 2011;32:934–44.
21. Corrado D, Thiene G. Sudden cardiac death in marathon runners: can it beprevented? Eur Heart J 2011;32:2591–3.
22. Corrado D, Basso C, Poletti A, et al. Sudden deathin the young. Is acute coronary thrombosis the major precipitating factor? Circulation 1994;90: 2315–23.
23. Basso C, Maron BJ, Corrado D, et al. Clinical profile of congenital coronary artery anomalies with origin from the wrong aortic sinus leading to sudden death in young competitive athletes. J Am Coll Cardiol 2000;35:1493–501.
24. Schwartz PJ, Crotti L, Insolia R. Long-QT syndrome: from genetics to management. Circ Arrhythm Electrophysiol 2012;5:868–77.
25. Antzelevitch C, Brugada P, Borggrefe M, et al. Brugada syndrome: report of the second consensus conference: Endorsed by the heart rhythm society and the european heart rhythm association. Circulation 2005;111:659–70.
26. Zorzi A, ElMaghawry M, Migliore F, et al. St-segment elevation and sudden death in the athlete. Card Electrophysiol Clin 2013;5:73–84.

27. Maron BJ, Thompson PD, Puffer JC, et al. Cardio-vascular preparticipation screening of competitive athletes. A statement for health professionals from the sudden death committee (clinical cardiology) and congenital cardiac defects committee (cardio-vascular disease in the young), american heart association. Circulation 1996;94:850–6.

28. Corrado D, Pelliccia A, Bjornstad HH, et al. Cardiovascular pre-participation screening of young competitive athletes for prevention of sudden death: Proposal for a common european protocol. Consensus statement of the study group of sport car-diology of the working group of cardiac rehabilitation and exercise physiology and the working group of myocardial and pericardial diseases of the European Society of Cardiology. Eur Heart J 2005;26:516–24.

29. Corrado D, Drezner J, Basso C, et al. Strategies for the prevention of sudden cardiac death during sports. Eur J Cardiovasc Prev Rehabil 2011;18: 197–208.

30. Corrado D, Pelliccia A, Heidbuchel H, et al. Rec-ommendations for interpretation of 12-lead elec-trocardiogram in the athlete. Eur Heart J 2010; 31:243–59.

31. Link MS, Estes NA. Athletes and arrhythmias. J Cardiovasc Electrophysiol 2010;21:1184–9.

32. Schmied C, Brunckhorst C, Duru F, et al. Exercise testing for risk stratification of ventricular arrhyth-mias in the athlete. Card Electrophysiol Clin 2013;5:53–64.

33. Steriotis AK, Nava A, Rigato I, et al. Noninvasive cardiac screening in young athletes with ventricular arrhythmias. Am J Cardiol 2013;111:557–62.

34. Uretsky S. Cardiovascular magnetic resonance imaging in hypertrophic cardiomyopathy. Prog Car-diovasc Dis 2012;54:512–6.

Syncope in Hereditary Arrhythmogenic Syndromes

Arnon Adler, MD, Sami Viskin, MD*

KEYWORDS

- Arrhythmogenic syndrome • Syncope • Genotype • Follow-up

KEY POINTS

- Family history of sudden cardiac death in a patient with syncope should always prompt an exhaustive diagnostic workup to exclude a hereditary arrhythmogenic syndrome.
- Symptoms before or after syncope, which are concordant with arrhythmic syncope, should raise the suspicion of an arrhythmic syndrome although symptoms *alone* may be misleading.
- The circumstances of syncope are important as a clue for a hereditary arrhythmogenic syndrome and for directing further diagnostic workup.
- The electrocardiogram is crucial for the diagnosis of a hereditary arrhythmogenic syndrome but a normal electrocardiogram does not exclude these syndromes.

INTRODUCTION

Since the discovery of the first mutation causing long QT syndrome (LQTS) in 1995, the field of hereditary arrhythmogenic syndromes has expanded greatly. Today, these syndromes include LQTS, Brugada syndrome (BrS), catecholaminergic polymorphic ventricular tachycardia (CPVT), and short QT syndrome (SQTS) (**Box 1**). There is also evidence suggesting that the newly described malignant early repolarization syndrome[1,2] also has a genetic cause.[3]

The common characteristic of all hereditary arrhythmogenic syndromes is a genetic mutation influencing the ion flux across the cardiomyocyte's cellular membrane (or inside the cell in the case of CPVT). This pathology creates a substrate for the development of ventricular arrhythmias, primarily polymorphic ventricular tachycardia (VT) or ventricular fibrillation (VF). Importantly, these patients have an otherwise *normal* heart structure. This is in contrast to other genetic syndromes in which the phenotype is principally an *abnormal* heart structure but includes also an increased risk of ventricular arrhythmias (eg, hypertrophic cardiomyopathy, arrhythmogenic right ventricular cardiomyopathy, specific types of dilated cardiomyopathy). The distinction is important because the absence of organic heart disease too often misleads the physician treating a given patient with syncope into leaning to a benign cause once a structurally normal heart is identified.

Syncope is a very common complaint and the most frequent cause is benign reflex syncope, also known as benign vagal (or "vasovagal") syncope.[4] Therefore, the major society guidelines recommend that the preliminary evaluation of syncope include only medical history, physical examination, and an electrocardiogram (ECG).[5,6] Nevertheless, syncope is also the first symptom in many hereditary arrhythmogenic syndrome cases.[7] Because these syndromes involve high risk for fatal arrhythmias, it is crucial that in the haystack of benign syncope these "needles" be

This article originally appeared in Cardiac Electrophysiology Clinics, Volume 5, Issue 4, December 2013.
Conflicts of Interest: None.
Sources of Specific Funding: None.
Sackler School of Medicine, Tel Aviv Medical Center, Tel Aviv University, Israel
* Corresponding author. Department of Cardiology, Tel Aviv Medical Center, Weizman 6, Tel Aviv 64239, Israel.
E-mail address: saviskin@gmail.com

Cardiol Clin 33 (2015) 433–440
http://dx.doi.org/10.1016/j.ccl.2015.04.011
0733-8651/15/$ – see front matter © 2015 Elsevier Inc. All rights reserved.

cardiology.theclinics.com

> **Box 1**
> **Hereditary arrhythmogenic syndromes**
>
> Long QT syndrome (LQTS)
>
> Brugada syndrome (BrS)
>
> Catecholaminergic polymorphic ventricular tachycardia (CPVT)
>
> Short QT syndrome (SQTS)
>
> Malignant early repolarization syndrome

found. In this article, the authors describe what clues in the primary evaluation of a syncopal patient should raise the suspicion of these rare but malignant syndromes.

MEDICAL HISTORY

The importance of the medical history in the evaluation of syncope cannot be overemphasized. The main points that need to be addressed are

- Family history
- Circumstances of syncope
- Symptoms

Family History

Family history of a hereditary arrhythmogenic syndrome or of sudden cardiac death, especially if at a young age, is probably the most important piece of information and should mandate further evaluation. Colman and colleagues[8] examined the yield of history taking in patients with LQTS, those evaluated in the emergency department due to syncope and young (<40 years of age) patients with benign vasovagal syncope (VVS). Family history of sudden cardiac death (SCD) not only was significantly more common in the LQTS patients (as expected) but it actually was one of the strongest differentiators between these groups.

In some cases, a positive family history is the only clue that a patient with syncope has a hereditary arrhythmogenic syndrome. This may be true in cases in which the electrocardiographic manifestation of the arrhythmogenic syndrome is concealed (see later discussion) and the clinical presentation is atypical. The family history is even more crucial in rare cases of familial idiopathic VF (IVF) as in IVF, by definition, causal relationship between the clinical circumstance and the arrhythmia is unidentifiable.[9] It is noteworthy that most cases of IVF are sporadic, yet familiar cases have been identified and in some families links to specific genes have been found.[10] Thus, it is imperative that a patient with syncope and a

strongly positive family history undergoes exhaustive diagnostic workup.

Circumstances of Syncope

The circumstances preceding the syncopal event are also extremely important.[11] As arrhythmias in each one of these syndromes typically occur in specific situations, these "triggers" may aid not only in raising the suspicion of an arrhythmogenic syndrome but also in directing the ensuing workup. In the most prevalent types of LQTS[7] and in CPVT,[12] the typical situational trigger is exercise or emotional stress, whereas arrhythmias related to BrS usually occur during rest or sleep.[13] In SQTS, the circumstances are highly variable with symptoms occurring during exercise, rest, or various other activities.[14] More exact phenotype-genotype correlation may be found in the different subtypes of LQTS. In a study examining different arrhythmogenic triggers in 670 LQTS patients with a known genotype (either LQTS type 1, 2, or 3) 62% of symptomatic patients with LQTS type 1 (LQT1) experienced events during exercise, whereas only 3% experienced events during rest or sleep.[15] This was in stark contrast to the LQT3 group in which 39% of events occurred during sleep or rest and only 13% during exercise. LQT2 patients showed intermediary results. Other studies showed that LQTS patients suffering a cardiac event during swimming had a LQT1 genotype, whereas those who had an acoustic trigger (sudden loud noise) had a LQT2 genotype.[16,17] Considering these data, it is not surprising that syncope during exercise, stress, or while supine was much more common in LQTS (almost entirely LQT1 & 2 in the cohort studied) than in patients with syncope of a different cause.[8]

In the case of CPVT, the circumstances are especially important because the basic ECG is unrevealing (see later discussion). Syncope occurring *during* exercise should always raise the suspicion of CPVT. On the other hand, effort-related benign vagal syncope usually occurs immediately on cessation of strenuous effort (like when standing after a sprint race). Interestingly, we have encountered patients with CPVT who performed strenuous effort for many years in the absence of therapy without ever developing symptoms only to present with cardiac arrest during emotional stress.

Symptoms

The symptoms immediately preceding and following the syncopal event are also of great importance. Thus, it is imperative to personally interview any person who witnessed the event. Arrhythmic syncope is favored by the following: no or little prodrome, associated trauma due to sudden fall, cyanosis, or delay in regaining consciousness even after assuming supine position. On the other hand, prodromal or "warning symptoms," marked pallor during and after the event, nausea, urgent desire to defecate, marked diaphoresis, and prolonged fatigue after the event favor vagal syncope.

The usefulness of symptoms for syncope evaluation has been demonstrated in a recent study that used symptoms to divide 57 BrS patients with syncope to "arrhythmic syncope," "nonarrhythmic syncope," or "doubtful origin."[18] None of the patients presenting with presumed nonarrhythmic or doubtful syncope experienced cardiac arrest during a 65-month follow-up period. In contrast, in the group presenting with suspected arrhythmic syncope (all of which received an implantable cardioverter-defibrillator) 5% subsequently developed spontaneous VF.

On the other hand, the study by Colman and colleagues[8] shows that distinguishing patients with syncope due to LQTS from those with more benign causes based on the clinical characteristics of the event is not always easy. Only palpitations, a relatively common and nonspecific complaint, were reported more frequently by patients with LQTS when compared with syncopal patients in the emergency department. Furthermore, many patients in the LQTS group described symptoms similar to those described by patients with VVS (17% had syncope during micturition, defecation, or coughing). This finding is disconcerting as it implies that we cannot always rely on symptoms as a basis for differentiation between arrhythmic and nonarrhythmic syncope.

It is also important to remember that not all syncopes in patients with a hereditary arrhythmic syndrome are arrhythmia related. VVS is very common in the general population, and there is no reason to believe that it is less common in these patients. Therefore, it is quite likely for a patient to have both.[19] In fact, small studies have shown that patients with LQTS are prone to VVS.[20,21] Furthermore, in all large series reporting on consecutive patients with BrS, the long-term risk for spontaneous VF for patients initially presenting with syncope is intermediate: lower than that for patients presenting with cardiac arrest but significantly higher than that for initially asymptomatic patients.[22,23] This consistent finding suggests that the BrS patient-group presenting with syncope actually includes 2 different patient populations, one presenting with arrhythmic syncope and malignant course during follow-up and one with vagal syncope and benign prognosis. This possibility is supported by the fact that patients with Brugada ECG and syncope who have prodromal "blurred vision" (characteristic of vagal syncope) have a very low risk for spontaneous VF during follow-up.[24] Having said that, it is also important to keep in mind that vagal stimulation may be proarrhythmic in BrS.[25] These confusing points mean that one has to remain mindful of the limitations of symptoms *alone* as a tool for diagnosis of syncope cause.

Some of the hereditary arrhythmogenic syndromes have been associated with atrial fibrillation at a young age. This is especially true for BrS[26,27] and SQTS[28] but has also been described in a minority of LQTS patients.[29–31] Thus, although atrial fibrillation in a patient with otherwise typical vagal syncope usually represents "vagal atrial fibrillation",[32] the presence of such an arrhythmia in a young patient (or family members) being evaluated for syncope should raise the possibility of an arrhythmogenic syndrome.

Finally, one of the toughest tasks is to distinguish malignant arrhythmogenic syncope from epileptic seizures. Although true tonic-clonic seizures occur only in epilepsy, tonic movements occur commonly in syncope.[33] Moreover, the seizures are described by a witness rather than observed by a physician, leading too often to a misdiagnosis. Indeed, many patients with arrhythmic syncope are misdiagnosed at first as having a seizure disorder.[7,34] It is important to remember that generalized tonic-clonic seizures are invariably followed by a postictal phase, during which the patient remains drowsy and confused. Although in some patients with partial seizures originating in the frontal lobe the postictal period may be extremely brief (even seconds), this period usually lasts minutes to hours.[35] Therefore, a patient who becomes fully alert immediately after an episode of "seizures" should be considered to have cardiogenic syncope until proved otherwise.

PHYSICAL EXAMINATION

Almost without exception, the only phenotype of the hereditary arrhythmogenic syndromes is the tendency to develop malignant ventricular arrhythmias and the physical examination is therefore unrevealing. In rare cases of LQTS, there may be other associated conditions such as congenital sensorineural deafness (Jervell and Lange-Nielsen syndrome),[36] the dismorphic features of Andersen-Tawil syndrome (short stature, hypertelorism, broad nose, low-set ears and a hypoplastic mandible),[37] or syndactyly in rare pediatric patients.[38]

Signs of trauma, although not directly implicating an arrhythmogenic syndrome, point to the suddenness of the event, making VVS less likely but still possible. Trauma signs may include bite marks on the anterior part of the tongue caused by hitting the jaw during syncope. Bite marks on the lateral part of the tongue, on the other hand, point to epileptic seizures.

ELECTROCARDIOGRAM

ECG is a crucial part of the initial evaluation of every patient with syncope. Patients with positive findings suggesting a hereditary arrhythmogenic syndrome should undergo further evaluation. Negative findings, although, do not exclude these syndromes and if the medical history is suggestive further evaluation is warranted.

Long QT Syndrome

Population studies[39–41] and studies on patients with LQTS[42] have shown that both groups demonstrate a Gaussian distribution of QTc interval length with a right-shift of the LQTS curve. Thus, the mean QTc of LQTS patients is around 480 msec, whereas the general population's mean QTc is around 400 msec. However, there is an overlapping zone of the QTc interval between healthy subjects and LQTS patients. This overlap creates a "gray zone" in which diagnosis of LQTS gets complicated. For instance, if we use the minimal "positive" QTc intervals in the Schwartz score used for LQTS diagnosis (450 msec for men, 460 msec for women)[43] as a cutoff point, approximately 10% of the healthy population will have a longer QT interval, whereas 10% of LQTS patients will be missed. A cutoff point of 480 msec raises the sensitivity for diagnosis of LQTS to almost 100%[42,44] but with the inevitable price of lowering the specificity. Raising the cutoff point further has mainly prognostic implications with a QTc interval above 500 msec considered a bad prognostic sign.[45]

For practical purposes this means that syncopal patients with a QTc interval longer than 500 msec almost certainly have LQTS. Those with an interval longer than 480 msec should also be heavily suspected. However, the ECG alone can never exclude this diagnosis, and if there are other reasons to suspect LQTS (eg, symptoms concordant with arrhythmic syncope or positive family history) further testing should be performed. Specific attention should be given to those patients with a QTc in the "gray zone" between 450/460 msec (for men/women) and 480 msec. A helpful diagnostic tool in this regard is the Schwartz score mentioned earlier, which estimates the probability of LQTS based mainly on clinical criteria.[43,46]

On top of a long QTc interval, LQTS patients also often exhibit an abnormal T-wave morphology. There are 3 distinct T-wave morphologies typical for each of the 3 most common LQT syndromes (LQT1, LQT2, and LQT3).[47,48] LQT1 patients' T waves are typically broad-based, those with LQT2 often have a "double-humped" T wave, and LQT3 patients usually exhibit a long and flat QT segment with a late-onset T wave. Although an abnormal T-wave morphology may raise the suspicion of LQTS, it is not enough by itself to make the diagnosis.

Whenever a congenital LQTS is suspected in a patient with syncope, the following tests should be considered. (1) Repeated ECG to the index patient and his/her entire family (because there is some variability in day-to-day QT interval duration and because obvious QT prolongation may be easier to identify in additional family members). (2) Holter recordings may unravel pathologic T-wave morphology during bradycardia at night or during post-extrasystolic pauses. (3) Exercise tests may unravel inappropriate QT shortening during exercise or often during the recovery.[44] (4) The bradycardia and reactive tachycardia provoked by adenosine injection during sinus rhythm are very useful for unraveling a LQTS.[49] (5) We recently demonstrated that the instantaneous heart rate acceleration induced by abrupt standing very often leads to diagnostic QT stretching[50] and QT stunning[51] during a simple bed-side test.

Finally, many drugs lead to QT prolongation.[52,53] Syncope in a patient consuming any of these medications should be carefully evaluated because drug-induced LQTS may rarely culminate in fatal arrhythmias.

Brugada Syndrome

The typical ECG in BrS (type 1 BrS ECG) demonstrates a humped ST elevation greater than 2 mm in the right precordial leads (V1-3), usually (but not always) accompanied by an inverted T wave. A saddle-back morphology ST elevation of either greater than 1 mm (type 2) or lower than 1 mm (type 3) are suggestive of BrS but not diagnostic.[54] In fact, it has been lately suggested that type 2 and type 3 be jointly referred to as type 2 for practical reasons.[55] Elevating the precordial leads to the second and third intercostal spaces raises the sensitivity for diagnosis of BrS.[56] It has been suggested that adding another lead on the sternum between the right and left "high leads" raises the sensitivity even further.[57]

It is important to remember, although, that the ECG in BrS is inconsistent. In one large series of patients with type I Brugada pattern who underwent repeated ECG recordings, only one-third of the ECGs were diagnostic and one-third of all ECGs were normal.[58] Clearly, the lack of BrS pattern on the ECG does not exclude BrS.

It is also important to remember that there is a differential diagnosis for BrS pattern, which includes ischemia, post-cardioversion, cocaine or alcohol intoxication, and certain drugs.[54] The latter include sodium channel blockers, calcium channel blockers, beta blockers, antipsychotics, antiepileptic drugs, and others. An updated list may be found in www.brugadadrugs.org.

Catecholaminergic Polymorphic Ventricular Tachycardia

The baseline ECG in CPVT is normal. Therefore, when CPVT is suspected, a maximal (symptom limited) exercise test should be performed. The characteristic response is the appearance of ventricular arrhythmias (and very often atrial arrhythmias as well) that worsen in severity as the exercise intensity increases (from isolated ventricular extrasystoles to repetitive nonsustained VT, bidirectional VT, and rapid polymorphic VT). It should be emphasized that the diagnostic arrhythmias (bidirectional and polymorphic VT) are not always provoked by exercise. In one series,[59] 40% of CPVT mutation carriers had only multiple ventricular extrasystoles (without VT) and 12% had no arrhythmias at all during exercise tests. Recently, an epinephrine challenge test has been proposed to increase sensitivity.[60]

Short QT Syndrome

The lower limit of the QTc interval is less well defined than the upper limit.[61] The first case report of SQTS (only a decade ago) had extremely short QTc interval (<300 msec)[62] but since then more than 100 cases were reported. Almost all of these cases had a QTc less than 360 msec. Population studies have demonstrated that up to 2% of the population has a QTc shorter than this value.[39,40] Taking into account the low prevalence of SQTS leads to the conclusion that most subjects with a QTc less than 360 msec will have a benign course. This finding is also supported by a population study, failing to show an elevated risk for SCD in subjects with a short QTc interval.[63] Therefore, the diagnosis of SQTS should be made with caution.

Further difficulty in the evaluation of the QT interval in SQTS arises from the lack of QT adaptation noticed in these patients.[64] This phenomenon means that in rapid heart rates the QTc interval will be normal (or relatively so) but in slow heart rates the QT will fail to prolong uncovering its true nature. Thus, it is imperative to measure the QT interval during heart rates around 60 bpm (or, at least, <80) in any patient suspected of SQTS. On the other hand, it should be emphasized that the most commonly used formula for correcting the QT for the heart rate (the Bazett formula) overcorrects at slow hearts. In other words, healthy individuals will often have QTc intervals shorter than 360 msec when the calculations are made during sinus bradycardia less than 60/min.[39]

Another electrocardiographic characteristic of SQTS is the noticeable T-wave morphology. The T wave is usually tall and peaked (whether symmetric or not) in the precordial leads and, in SQTS type 1 (SQT1), follows the QRS immediately with no (or almost no) ST segment. In some subsets of SQTS (SQT4-6), the ECG may demonstrate a short QT interval combined with a BrS pattern.[65] In other patients, the ECG may also show signs of early repolarization with J-point elevation in the inferolateral leads.[66]

To aid in the diagnosis a scoring system based on ECG parameters, clinical and familial history and genetic testing have been suggested.[67]

As in other channelopathies, it is important to rule out reversible causes of a short QTc interval. These include hyperkalemia, acidosis, hypercalcaemia, hyperthermia, and digitalis.[14]

SUMMARY

In the primary evaluation of a patient with syncope, any clue suggesting a hereditary arrhythmogenic syndrome should be followed by further appropriate testing. These may include provocative tests (whether exercise test or drug challenge), noninvasive ECG monitoring, electrophysiological studies (in specific situations such as suspected SQTS), and genetic testing. A full discussion of the diagnostic workup is beyond the scope of this article and may be found elsewhere.[68,69]

It is important to remember that some patients with hereditary arrhythmogenic syndromes will have only positive family history or suspicious symptoms with a normal ECG (eg, CPVT or IVF). Others will have symptoms that are typically vasovagal but with an abnormal ECG. Therefore, a high level of suspicion is warranted to diagnose these patients (and family members) before SCD strikes.

REFERENCES

1. Haissaguerre M, Derval N, Sacher F, et al. Sudden cardiac arrest associated with early repolarization. N Engl J Med 2008;358(19):2016–23.
2. Rosso R, Kogan E, Belhassen B, et al. J-point elevation in survivors of primary ventricular

fibrillation and matched control subjects: incidence and clinical significance. J Am Coll Cardiol 2008; 52(15):1231–8.

3. Gourraud JB, Le Scouarnec S, Sacher F, et al. Identification of large families in early repolarization syndrome. J Am Coll Cardiol 2013;61(2):164–72.

4. Ganzeboom KS, Mairuhu G, Reitsma JB, et al. Lifetime cumulative incidence of syncope in the general population: a study of 549 Dutch subjects aged 35-60 years. J Cardiovasc Electrophysiol 2006;17(11):1172–6.

5. Moya A, Sutton R, Ammirati F, et al. Guidelines for the diagnosis and management of syncope (version 2009). Eur Heart J 2009;30(21):2631–71.

6. Strickberger SA, Benson DW, Biaggioni I, et al. AHA/ACCF Scientific Statement on the evaluation of syncope: from the American Heart Association Councils on Clinical Cardiology, Cardiovascular Nursing, Cardiovascular Disease in the Young, and Stroke, and the Quality of Care and Outcomes Research Interdisciplinary Working Group; and the American College of Cardiology Foundation: in collaboration with the Heart Rhythm Society: endorsed by the American Autonomic Society. Circulation 2006;113(2):316–27.

7. Moss AJ, Schwartz PJ, Crampton RS, et al. The long QT syndrome. Prospective longitudinal study of 328 families. Circulation 1991;84(3):1136–44.

8. Colman N, Bakker A, Linzer M, et al. Value of history-taking in syncope patients: in whom to suspect long QT syndrome? Europace 2009;11(7):937–43.

9. Survivors of out-of-hospital cardiac arrest with apparently normal heart. Need for definition and standardized clinical evaluation. Consensus Statement of the Joint Steering Committees of the Unexplained Cardiac Arrest Registry of Europe and of the Idiopathic Ventricular Fibrillation Registry of the United States. Circulation 1997; 95(1):265–72.

10. Postema PG, Christiaans I, Hofman N, et al. Founder mutations in the Netherlands: familial idiopathic ventricular fibrillation and DPP6. Neth Heart J 2011;19(6):290–6.

11. Viskin S, Rosso R, Halkin A. Explaining sudden unexplained death. Circ Arrhythm Electrophysiol 2012;5(5):879–81.

12. Priori SG, Napolitano C, Memmi M, et al. Clinical and molecular characterization of patients with catecholaminergic polymorphic ventricular tachycardia. Circulation 2002;106(1):69–74.

13. Takigawa M, Noda T, Shimizu W, et al. Seasonal and circadian distributions of ventricular fibrillation in patients with Brugada syndrome. Heart Rhythm 2008;5(11):1523–7.

14. Patel C, Yan GX, Antzelevitch C. Short QT syndrome: from bench to bedside. Circ Arrhythm Electrophysiol 2010;3(4):401–8.

15. Schwartz PJ, Priori SG, Spazzolini C, et al. Genotype-phenotype correlation in the long-QT syndrome: gene-specific triggers for life-threatening arrhythmias. Circulation 2001;103(1):89–95.

16. Moss AJ, Robinson JL, Gessman L, et al. Comparison of clinical and genetic variables of cardiac events associated with loud noise versus swimming among subjects with the long QT syndrome. Am J Cardiol 1999;84(8):876–9.

17. Wilde AA, Jongbloed RJ, Doevendans PA, et al. Auditory stimuli as a trigger for arrhythmic events differentiate HERG-related (LQTS2) patients from KVLQT1-related patients (LQTS1). J Am Coll Cardiol 1999;33(2):327–32.

18. Sacher F, Arsac F, Wilton SB, et al. Syncope in Brugada syndrome patients: prevalence, characteristics, and outcome. Heart Rhythm 2012;9(8): 1272–9.

19. Wilde AA, Wieling W. Vasovagal syncope or ventricular fibrillation. Your diagnosis better be accurate. Clin Auton Res 2007;17(4):203–5.

20. Hermosillo AG, Falcon JC, Marquez MF, et al. Positive head-up tilt table test in patients with the long QT syndrome. Europace 1999;1(4):213–7.

21. Toft E, Aaroe J, Jensen BT, et al. Long QT syndrome patients may faint due to neurocardiogenic syncope. Europace 2003;5(4):367–70.

22. Brugada J, Brugada R, Antzelevitch C, et al. Long-term follow-up of individuals with the electrocardiographic pattern of right bundle-branch block and ST-segment elevation in precordial leads V1 to V3. Circulation 2002;105(1):73–8.

23. Probst V, Veltmann C, Eckardt L, et al. Long-term prognosis of patients diagnosed with Brugada syndrome: results from the FINGER Brugada Syndrome Registry. Circulation 2010;121(5):635–43.

24. Take Y, Morita H, Toh N, et al. Identification of high-risk syncope related to ventricular fibrillation in patients with Brugada syndrome. Heart Rhythm 2012; 9(5):752–9.

25. Miyazaki T, Mitamura H, Miyoshi S, et al. Autonomic and antiarrhythmic drug modulation of ST segment elevation in patients with Brugada syndrome. J Am Coll Cardiol 1996;27(5):1061–70.

26. Pappone C, Radinovic A, Manguso F, et al. New-onset atrial fibrillation as first clinical manifestation of latent Brugada syndrome: prevalence and clinical significance. Eur Heart J 2009;30(24): 2985–92.

27. Rodriuez-Manero M, Namdar M, Sarkozy A, et al. Prevalence, clinical characteristics and management of atrial fibrillation in patients with Brugada syndrome. Am J Cardiol 2013;111(3):362–7.

28. Giustetto C, Di Monte F, Wolpert C, et al. Short QT syndrome: clinical findings and diagnostic-therapeutic implications. Eur Heart J 2006;27(20): 2440–7.

29. Olesen MS, Yuan L, Liang B, et al. High prevalence of long QT syndrome-associated SCN5A variants in patients with early-onset lone atrial fibrillation. Circ Cardiovasc Genet 2012;5(4):450–9.

30. Johnson JN, Tester DJ, Perry J, et al. Prevalence of early-onset atrial fibrillation in congenital long QT syndrome. Heart Rhythm 2008;5(5):704–9.

31. Benito B, Brugada R, Perich RM, et al. A mutation in the sodium channel is responsible for the association of long QT syndrome and familial atrial fibrillation. Heart Rhythm 2008;5(10):1434–40.

32. Coumel P, Attuel P, Lavallee J, et al. The atrial arrhythmia syndrome of vagal origin. Arch Mal Coeur Vaiss 1978;71(6):645–56 [in French].

33. Lin JT, Ziegler DK, Lai CW, et al. Convulsive syncope in blood donors. Ann Neurol 1982;11(5):525–8.

34. MacCormick JM, McAlister H, Crawford J, et al. Misdiagnosis of long QT syndrome as epilepsy at first presentation. Ann Emerg Med 2009;54(1):26–32.

35. Theodore WH. The postictal state: effects of age and underlying brain dysfunction. Epilepsy Behav 2010;19(2):118–20.

36. Jervell A, Lange-Nielsen F. Congenital deaf-mutism, functional heart disease with prolongation of the Q-T interval and sudden death. Am Heart J 1957;54(1):59–68.

37. Andersen ED, Krasilnikoff PA, Overvad H. Intermittent muscular weakness, extrasystoles, and multiple developmental anomalies. A new syndrome? Acta Paediatr Scand 1971;60(5):559–64.

38. Marks ML, Whisler SL, Clericuzio C, et al. A new form of long QT syndrome associated with syndactyly. J Am Coll Cardiol 1995;25(1):59–64.

39. Kobza R, Roos M, Niggli B, et al. Prevalence of long and short QT in a young population of 41,767 predominantly male Swiss conscripts. Heart Rhythm 2009;6(5):652–7.

40. Funada A, Hayashi K, Ino H, et al. Assessment of QT intervals and prevalence of short QT syndrome in Japan. Clin Cardiol 2008;31(6):270–4.

41. Gallagher MM, Magliano G, Yap YG, et al. Distribution and prognostic significance of QT intervals in the lowest half centile in 12,012 apparently healthy persons. Am J Cardiol 2006;98(7):933–5.

42. Taggart NW, Haglund CM, Tester DJ, et al. Diagnostic miscues in congenital long-QT syndrome. Circulation 2007;115(20):2613–20.

43. Schwartz PJ, Moss AJ, Vincent GM, et al. Diagnostic criteria for the long QT syndrome. An update. Circulation 1993;88(2):782–4.

44. Sy RW, van der Werf C, Chattha IS, et al. Derivation and validation of a simple exercise-based algorithm for prediction of genetic testing in relatives of LQTS probands. Circulation 2011;124(20):2187–94.

45. Sauer AJ, Moss AJ, McNitt S, et al. Long QT syndrome in adults. J Am Coll Cardiol 2007;49(3):329–37.

46. Schwartz PJ. The congenital long QT syndromes from genotype to phenotype: clinical implications. J Intern Med 2006;259(1):39–47.

47. Moss AJ, Zareba W, Benhorin J, et al. ECG T-wave patterns in genetically distinct forms of the hereditary long QT syndrome. Circulation 1995;92(10):2929–34.

48. Zhang L, Timothy KW, Vincent GM, et al. Spectrum of ST-T-wave patterns and repolarization parameters in congenital long-QT syndrome: ECG findings identify genotypes. Circulation 2000;102(23):2849–55.

49. Viskin S, Rosso R, Rogowski O, et al. Provocation of sudden heart rate oscillation with adenosine exposes abnormal QT responses in patients with long QT syndrome: a bedside test for diagnosing long QT syndrome. Eur Heart J 2006;27(4):469–75.

50. Viskin S, Postema PG, Bhuiyan ZA, et al. The response of the QT interval to the brief tachycardia provoked by standing: a bedside test for diagnosing long QT syndrome. J Am Coll Cardiol 2010;55(18):1955–61.

51. Adler A, van der Werf C, Postema PG, et al. The phenomenon of "QT stunning": the abnormal QT prolongation provoked by standing persists even as the heart rate returns to normal in patients with long QT syndrome. Heart Rhythm 2012;9(6):901–8.

52. Viskin S. Long QT syndromes and torsade de pointes. Lancet 1999;354(9190):1625–33.

53. Available at: www.azcert.rog.

54. Antzelevitch C, Brugada P, Borggrefe M, et al. Brugada syndrome: report of the second consensus conference: endorsed by the Heart Rhythm Society and the European Heart Rhythm Association. Circulation 2005;111(5):659–70.

55. Bayes de Luna A, Brugada J, Baranchuk A, et al. Current electrocardiographic criteria for diagnosis of Brugada pattern: a consensus report. J Electrocardiol 2012;45(5):433–42.

56. Shimizu W, Matsuo K, Takagi M, et al. Body surface distribution and response to drugs of ST segment elevation in Brugada syndrome: clinical implication of eighty-seven-lead body surface potential mapping and its application to twelve-lead electrocardiograms. J Cardiovasc Electrophysiol 2000;11(4):396–404.

57. Veltmann C, Papavassiliu T, Konrad T, et al. Insights into the location of type I ECG in patients with Brugada syndrome: correlation of ECG and cardiovascular magnetic resonance imaging. Heart Rhythm 2012;9(3):414–21.

58. Richter S, Sarkozy A, Veltmann C, et al. Variability of the diagnostic ECG pattern in an ICD patient population with Brugada syndrome. J Cardiovasc Electrophysiol 2009;20(1):69–75.

59. Hayashi M, Denjoy I, Extramiana F, et al. Incidence and risk factors of arrhythmic events in catecholaminergic polymorphic ventricular tachycardia. Circulation 2009;119(18):2426–34.

60. Marjamaa A, Hiippala A, Arrhenius B, et al. Intravenous epinephrine infusion test in diagnosis of catecholaminergic polymorphic ventricular tachycardia. J Cardiovasc Electrophysiol 2012;23(2):194–9.

61. Viskin S. The QT interval: too long, too short or just right. Heart Rhythm 2009;6(5):711–5.

62. Gussak I, Brugada P, Brugada J, et al. Idiopathic short QT interval: a new clinical syndrome? Cardiology 2000;94(2):99–102.

63. Anttonen O, Junttila MJ, Rissanen H, et al. Prevalence and prognostic significance of short QT interval in a middle-aged Finnish population. Circulation 2007;116(7):714–20.

64. Wolpert C, Schimpf R, Giustetto C, et al. Further insights into the effect of quinidine in short QT syndrome caused by a mutation in HERG. J Cardiovasc Electrophysiol 2005;16(1):54–8.

65. Antzelevitch C, Pollevick GD, Cordeiro JM, et al. Loss-of-function mutations in the cardiac calcium channel underlie a new clinical entity characterized by ST-segment elevation, short QT intervals, and sudden cardiac death. Circulation 2007;115(4): 442–9.

66. Watanabe H, Makiyama T, Koyama T, et al. High prevalence of early repolarization in short QT syndrome. Heart Rhythm 2010;7(5):647–52.

67. Gollob MH, Redpath CJ, Roberts JD. The short QT syndrome: proposed diagnostic criteria. J Am Coll Cardiol 2011;57(7):802–12.

68. Obeyesekere MN, Klein GJ, Modi S, et al. How to perform and interpret provocative testing for the diagnosis of Brugada syndrome, long-QT syndrome, and catecholaminergic polymorphic ventricular tachycardia. Circ Arrhythm Electrophysiol 2011;4(6):958–64.

69. Ackerman MJ, Priori SG, Willems S, et al. HRS/EHRA expert consensus statement on the state of genetic testing for the channelopathies and cardiomyopathies: this document was developed as a partnership between the Heart Rhythm Society (HRS) and the European Heart Rhythm Association (EHRA). Europace 2011;13(8):1077–109.

Syncope and Idiopathic (Paroxysmal) AV Block

Michele Brignole, MD, FESC[a],*,
Jean-Claude Deharo, MD, FESC[b], Regis Guieu, MD[c]

KEYWORDS

• Atrioventricular block • Implantable loop recorder • ECG • Syncope

KEY POINTS

• Syncope due to idiopathic AV block is characterized by: 1) ECG documentation (usually by means of prolonged ECG monitoring) of paroxysmal complete AV block with one or multiple consecutive pauses, without P-P cycle lengthening or PR interval prolongation, not triggered by atrial or ventricular premature beats nor by rate variations; 2) long history of recurrent syncope without prodromes; 3) absence of cardiac and ECG abnormalities; 4) absence of progression to persistent forms of AV block; 5) efficacy of cardiac pacing therapy.

• The patients affected by idiopathic AV block have low baseline adenosine plasma level values and show an increased susceptibility to exogenous adenosine. The APL value of the patients with idiopathic AV block is much lower than patients affected by vasovagal syncope who have high adenosine values.

DIAGNOSIS OF IDIOPATHIC AV BLOCK

Syncope due to idiopathic atrioventricular (AV) block (**Box 1**) is a distinct clinical form of syncope characterized by common clinical and electrophysiologic features[1]:

• Electrocardiographic (ECG) documentation (usually by means of prolonged ECG monitoring) of idiopathic paroxysmal complete AV block with one or multiple consecutive pauses; AV block occurs without P-P cycle lengthening or PR interval prolongation and is not triggered by atrial or ventricular premature beats nor by rate variations (**Fig. 1**)

• Long history of recurrent syncope without prodromes

• Absence of cardiac and ECG abnormalities

• Absence of progression to persistent forms of AV block

• Efficacy of cardiac pacing therapy

Patients affected by idiopathic AV block have low baseline adenosine plasma level (APL) values and show an increased susceptibility to exogenous adenosine. In one study,[1] the median baseline APL of these patients was significantly lower than that found in the age-matched and sex-matched population of 81 healthy subjects: 0.33 µM (interquartile range 0.20–0.56) versus 0.49 µM (0.38–0.68) ($P = .017$). APL values of patients with idiopathic AV block are much lower than those of patients affected by typical vasovagal syncope and patients with positive tilt table

This article originally appeared in Cardiac Electrophysiology Clinics, Volume 5, Issue 4, December 2013.
The authors have nothing to disclose.
[a] Department of Cardiology, Arrhythmologic Center, Ospedali del Tigullio, Via Don Bobbio 25, Lavagna 16033, Italy; [b] Department of Cardiology, Timone University Hospital, 264, rue Saint Pierre 13385, Marseille, France; [c] Laboratory of Biochemistry and Molecular Biology, Timone University Hospital, Unité Mixte de Recherche Ministere de la Defense, Aix Marseille Université, Boulevard P Dramard, Marseille 13015, France
* Corresponding author.
E-mail address: mbrignole@ASL4.liguria.it

Cardiol Clin 33 (2015) 441–447
http://dx.doi.org/10.1016/j.ccl.2015.04.012
0733-8651/15/$ – see front matter © 2015 Elsevier Inc. All rights reserved.

testing who have higher APL values than normal subjects (**Fig. 2**).

Other relevant laboratory findings are as follows:

- Most patients with idiopathic AV block show a high susceptibility to the rapid IV injection of 18 mg adenosine or 20 mg adenosine triphosphate (ATP) test (**Fig. 3**). The adenosine/ATP test fairly reproduces spontaneous AV block. The adenosine response is abolished by theophylline, an adenosine antagonist, but not by atropine, a vagal antagonist.[2]
- Tilt table test may be positive, but positivity rate is lower than in patients with vasovagal syncope and is never able to reproduce an AV block. Thus tilt table test response seems to be nonspecific.
- Carotid sinus massage is almost invariably negative.

DIFFERENTIAL DIAGNOSIS FROM OTHER TYPES OF AV BLOCK

Idiopathic paroxysmal AV block has different clinical and electrophysiologic features from those of the 2 other known types of paroxysmal AV block: intrinsic AV block due to AV conduction disease and extrinsic vagal AV block. Well-defined clinical and electrophysiologic features differentiate them.

Intrinsic paroxysmal AV block, which usually occurs in patients with underlying heart disease and/or abnormal standard ECG, is regarded as a manifestation of an intrinsic disease of the AV conduction system (Stokes-Adams attack), which is confirmed by abnormal electrophysiologic findings.[3,4] The AV block is usually initiated by atrial, His, or ventricular premature extrasystole, increased heart rate (tachy-dependent AV block) or decreased heart rate (brady-dependent AV block), all features that support a diagnosis of intrinsic AV block (**Fig. 4**). The outcome is characterized by a rapid progression toward permanent AV block.[3,4]

Extrinsic (vagal) AV block is localized within the AV node and is associated with slowing of the sinus rate. A classic vagal effect on the conduction system includes gradual slowing of the sinus rate (P-P interval) and AV conduction (prolonging PR), which are occasionally followed by sinus arrest or complete AV block. The 2 conditions frequently coexist, indicating a simultaneous vagal action on sinus node and AV node. Even when a more

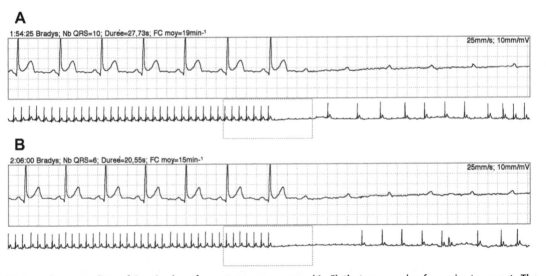

Fig. 1. Holter recording of 2 episodes of spontaneous syncope (*A, B*) that occurred a few minutes apart. The 2 episodes were very similar and were characterized by sudden-onset complete AV block without changes in P-P cycle length, which constantly remained 720 ms (*top, trace*), and long ventricular asystole of 7 and 11 seconds, respectively (*bottom, compressed trace*). (*From* Brignole M, Deharo JC, De Roy L, et al. Syncope due to idiopathic paroxysmal atrioventricular block. Long-term follow-up of a distinct form of atrioventricular block. J Am Coll Cardiol 2011;58:170; with permission.)

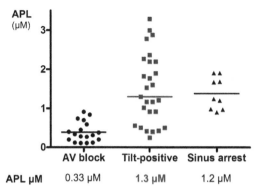

Fig. 2. The individual values of APL in 18 patients with idiopathic AV block patients, 9 patients with typical vasovagal syncope and documentation of sinus arrest during spontaneous syncope, and 27 patients with positive response during tilt table test. The horizontal line shows the median APL value of each group.

prominent AV response occurs, vagally mediated AV block is usually preceded by significant PR prolongation or Wenckebach; P-P interval prolongs markedly also during asystole and there is significant PR prolongation on resumption of AV conduction (**Fig. 5**).[3,5–7] The patients affected by syncope caused by vagal AV block have different

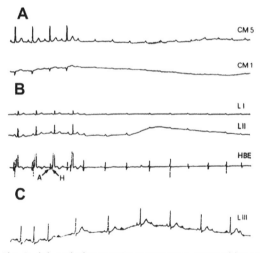

Fig. 3. (A) Ambulatory ECG monitoring. Normal heart rhythm is abruptly interrupted by paroxysmal AV block, which causes syncope. (B) ATP test. An IV bolus of 20 mg ATP reproduces syncope and spontaneous ECG pattern. His-bundle intracavitary recording (HBE) shows that P waves are blocked proximal to His-bundle deflection. (C) During oral theophylline therapy, ATP infusion causes asymptomatic 2:1 AVB without asystolic pauses. (*From* Brignole M, Gaggioli G, Menozzi C, et al. Adenosine-induced atrioventricular block in patients with unexplained syncope: the diagnostic value of ATP testing. Circulation 1997;96:3924; with permission.)

clinical features. Their episodes of syncope have well-identifiable triggers (central, ie, emotional distress, or peripheral, ie, prolonged standing) and are preceded by symptoms of autonomic activation (ie, feeling of warmth, an odd sensation in the abdomen, and lightheadedness or dizziness, nausea, and sweating).[8] In addition, low APL values clearly differentiated idiopathic AV block patients from those with vasovagal syncope. High APL values seem to characterize vasovagal syncope and tilt-positive syncope (see **Fig. 2**). Thus, a different basal APL profile seems to be present in patients with idiopathic AV block and in patients with vasovagal syncope.[9–11] Finally, permanent cardiac pacing is successful in preventing syncopal recurrences during long-term follow-up in idiopathic AV block patients but much less effective in patients affected by reflex cardioinhibitory syncope, even if a spontaneous asystolic reflex has been documented, with syncope recurring in 9% to 45% of patients.[5,12] The cause of persistence of syncopal recurrence in reflex syncope is attributed to the coexistence of a vasodepressor reflex which, to some degree, is present in virtually all patients.

EPIDEMIOLOGY OF SYNCOPE DUE IDIOPATHIC AV BLOCK

Epidemiology of syncope due to idiopathic AV block is largely unknown because its diagnosis requires the (often fortuitous) ECG documentation of AV block at the time of syncope. The first description of adenosine-sensitive paroxysmal AV block was made by Brignole and colleagues[2] in 1997. The authors evaluated 15 syncope patients who had had the fortuitous ECG documentation of paroxysmal AV block. ATP testing showed an abnormal response in 6 of the 7 patients without structural heart disease and negative workup, whereas it was abnormal in only 2 of the 8 patients with associated abnormalities. The ECG of the ATP-sensitive patients showed the same characteristics of idiopathic AV block described above. Similar ECG features have been occasionally described in individual patients in clinical studies[13] and in few case reports.[14–17] The original description[1] included 18 cases.

In the absence of ECG documentation, syncope due to idiopathic AV block is undistinguishable from other forms of syncope without prodromes, which occur in patients with normal heart and normal ECG. Idiopathic AV block might be easily misdiagnosed as an atypical form of neutrally mediated syncope. Therefore, it is likely that its true prevalence is higher than that diagnosed. The prevalence of idiopathic AV block from ISSUE

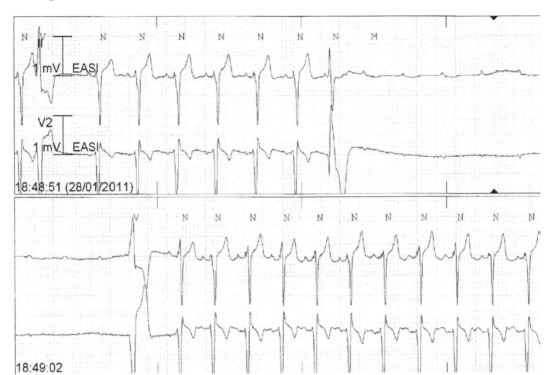

Fig. 4. Intrinsic paroxysmal AV block in a patient with underlying structural heart disease. The AV block was initiated by a ventricular premature extrasystole, and P-P cycle decreased during asytole due to activation of a compensatory reflex. The electrophysiologic study confirmed the site of the block below the His bundle (not shown in the figure).

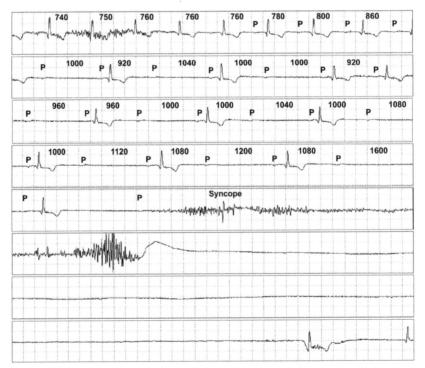

Fig. 5. Extrinsic (vagal) paroxysmal AV block documented by implantable loop recorder. A vagal mechanism is supported by the gradual slowing of the sinus rate (P-P interval) and AV conduction (prolonging PR and 2:1 block). During asystole AV block is replaced by sinus arrest. APL values in this patient were very high (1.9 μM), confirming the reflex nature of the episode.

2 and ISSUE 3 studies can be inferred.[18,19] Type 1C form of the ISSUE classification[6] of asystolic syncopes resembles the ECG features of idiopathic AV block. In ISSUE 2 study,[18] type 1C block was found to be present in 8% of syncope patients with normal ECG and absence of structural heart disease (corresponding to 15% of those who had ECG documentation of syncope). In ISSUE 3 study,[19] type 1C block was found to be present in 22% of those who had a diagnostic asystolic event. It can only be speculated that these figures may represent the prevalence of this new syndrome among patients without structural heart disease who are affected by unexplained syncope. However, a prospective study is needed to confirm this prevalence.

PATHOPHYSIOLOGICAL CONSIDERATIONS: THE PURINERGIC PROFILE AND THE ROLE OF ADENOSINE

The low observed baseline APL value (compared with controls and with patients with reflex asystolic syncope) and the rate of positive ATP test, which was much higher than that found in the literature in normal controls[2] and in patients with unexplained syncope,[2] indicate an increased susceptibility of the AV node to adenosine. These observations led to hypothesize some relationship between the adenosine pathway and the genesis of the AV block.

The effect of adenosine on different structures and organs involves activation of membrane receptor subtypes, named A_1, A_{2A}, A_{2B}, or A_3, depending on their primary sequence and affinity for ligands. The effect of adenosine on the AV node is mainly due to the stimulation of high-affinity A_1 receptors, which are much more numerous in the AV node than in the sinoatrial node.[20–22] Like many other cell surface receptors, the number of cardiac adenosine A_1 receptors undergoes up-regulation and down-regulation when cardiac tissues are chronically exposed to low or elevated concentrations of adenosine receptor agonist (ie, adenosine). A transient release of endogenous adenosine could be sufficient to block conduction in the AV node when a high number of free high-affinity A_1 receptors in the AV node are available (low-APL patients). Conversely, when APL is high, as in patients with vasovagal syncope or positive tilt testing, most A_1 receptors in the AV node are saturated and AV block is unlikely to occur (**Fig. 6**). The cause of the transient release of endogenous adenosine responsible for paroxysmal AV block is unknown. Adenosine is a ubiquitous substance, which is released under several physiologic and pathologic conditions (eg, in

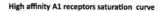

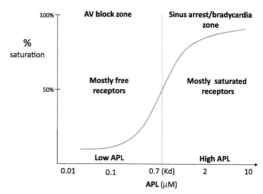

Fig. 6. Schematic description of the adenosine receptor-effector coupling system in the AV node, which is thought to have been responsible for paroxysmal AV block in the patients. The effect of adenosine on the AV node is mainly due to the stimulation of high-affinity adenosine A_1 receptors. Like many other cell surface receptors, the number of cardiac adenosine A_1 receptors undergoes up-regulation and down-regulation when cardiac tissues are chronically exposed to elevated concentrations of adenosine receptor agonist (ie, adenosine). The constant of dissociation (Kd) of A_1 adenosine receptors is 0.7 μM. Around the Kd value, a high number of free high-affinity A_1 receptors in the AV node are available for activation. In this range, even a moderate increase in endogenous APL binds a high number of A_1 receptors, leading to AV block. Conversely, at high APL values, most A_1 receptors in the AV node are already saturated and endogenous adenosine is unlikely to cause AV block.

the case of myocardial hypoxia or during reflex β-adrenergic stimulation).[23,24]

From a wider perspective, central or peripheral baroreceptor reflex abnormalities or alterations in neurohumoral mechanisms could play a pivotal role in the genesis of extrinsic (functional) and reflex syncopes.[25] Despite differences in their receptors, adenosine and the neurotransmitter acetylcholine have remarkably similar effects on cardiac function.[23,24,26,27] A possible explanation is the similarity of their receptor-effector coupling systems. In addition to having direct effects, acetylcholine and adenosine act synergistically against the stimulatory action of the sympathetic neurotransmitters noradrenaline and adrenaline on adenyl cyclase. Thus, excitatory and inhibitory effects of the adrenergic cholinergic and purinergic outflows are integrated at the level of the receptor-effector coupling system, resulting in the final cardiac effect (**Fig. 7**).

In conclusion, even if a role of the adenosine pathway in the genesis of the AV block may be possible, the above data are insufficient to prove

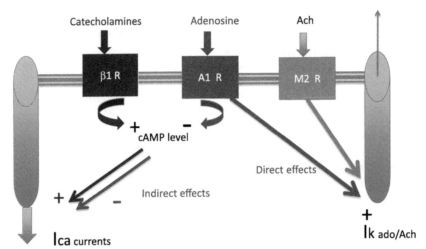

Fig. 7. The final effect of adenosine on heart rate is mediated by direct and indirect mechanisms. The indirect mechanism is the anti-adrenergic action of A1 adenosine receptors by opposing the effect of sympathetic nervous activation and β1 stimulation by lowering intracellular cAMP levels in target cells.[26] The direct mechanism is due to the induction of a potassium current through an inward rectifier potassium channel, which leads to hyperpolarization of sinus node and AV node cells (IK$_{ado}$).[27] This latter effect is very similar to that obtained with acetylcholine (Ach) on muscarinic receptors. β1 R, β1 adrenergic receptor; A1 R, A1 adenosine receptor; IK, inward going rectification; M2R, M2 muscarinic receptor.

a causality relationship. Therefore, the mechanism of the block in the patients remains largely unexplained (idiopathic AV block). The above observations might be of interest for the planning of future studies.

CLINICAL PERSPECTIVES

In clinical practice, patients with syncope who have the ECG documentation of paroxysmal AV block are usually regarded as a manifestation of an intrinsic disease of the AV conduction system and a diagnosis of cardiac syncope (primary arrhythmia) is made. Conversely, in the absence of ECG documentation, patients with unexplained syncope with normal heart would probably be categorized as affected by an atypical form of neurally mediated syncope. Therefore, 2 opposite diagnoses could be made in the same patient, depending on whether or not paroxysmal AV block during a spontaneous attack is documented on ECG.

In patients affected by unexplained syncope without prodromes, normal heart, and normal ECG, the diagnostic strategy usually calls for the early use of the implantable loop recorder (ILR). Most idiopathic AV block cases were identified by means of ILR. However, this strategy implies the implantation of a diagnostic device and the need of waiting until a relapse occurs. Is it possible to identify idiopathic AV block patients based on clinical features? The adenosine/ATP test seemed

to be sensitive enough to identify the patients with idiopathic AV block in this study, but it showed a very low specificity in other studies in which there was a lack of correlation between the responses to the test and the mechanism of spontaneous syncope documented by ILR.[11,12] The ability of APL value to discriminate idiopathic AV block cases from vasovagal syncope patients was evaluated using receiver operating characteristic curve analysis (Deharo JC et al, personal communication, 2013). A cutoff value of APL of ≤0.38 was found to have a sensitivity of 61% and a specificity of 92%. Applying to normal subjects without syncope, 22% of these had an APL value less than the cutoff value. The potential application in clinical practice of this cutoff requires further studies.

REFERENCES

1. Brignole M, Deharo JC, De Roy L, et al. Syncope due to idiopathic paroxysmal atrioventricular block. Long term follow up of a distinct form of atrioventricular block. J Am Coll Cardiol 2011;58:167–73.
2. Brignole M, Gaggioli G, Menozzi C, et al. Adenosine-induced atrioventricular block in patients with unexplained syncope: the diagnostic value of ATP testing. Circulation 1997;96:3921–7.
3. Lee S, Wellens JJ, Josephson M. Paroxysmal atrioventricular block. Heart Rhythm 2009;6:1229–34.
4. El-Sherif N, Jalife J. Paroxysmal atrioventricular block: are phase 3 and phase 4 block mechanisms or misnomers? Heart Rhythm 2009;6:1514–21.

5. Sud S, Klein G, Skanes A, et al. Implications of mechanism of bradycardia on response to pacing in patients with unexplained syncope. Europace 2007;9:312–8.

6. Brignole M, Moya A, Menozzi C, et al. Proposed electrocardiographic classification of spontaneous syncope documented by an implantable loop recorder. Europace 2005;7:14–8.

7. Zyśko D, Gajek J, Koźluk E, et al. Electrocardiographic characteristics of atrioventricular block induced by tilt testing. Europace 2009;11:225–30.

8. Moya A, Sutton R, Ammirati F, et al. Guidelines for the diagnosis and management of syncope (version 2009): the Task Force for the Diagnosis and Management of Syncope of the European Society of Cardiology (ESC). Eur Heart J 2009;30:2631–71.

9. Saadjian A, Lévy S, Franceschi F, et al. Role of endogenous adenosine as a modulator of syncope induced during tilt testing. Circulation 2002;106:569–74.

10. Carrega L, Saadjian AY, Mercier L, et al. Increased expression of adenosine A2A receptors in patients with spontaneous and head-up-tilt-induced syncope. Heart Rhythm 2007;4:870–6.

11. Deharo JC, Mechulan A, Giorgi R, et al. Adenosine plasma level and A2A adenosine receptor expression: correlation with laboratory tests in patients with neurally mediated syncope. Heart 2012;98:855–9.

12. Brignole M, Sutton R, Menozzi C, et al. Early application of an implantable loop recorder allows effective specific therapy in patients with recurrent suspected neurally mediated syncope. Eur Heart J 2006;27:1085–92.

13. Deharo JC, Jego C, Lanteaume A, et al. An implantable loop recorder study of highly symptomatic vasovagal patients. J Am Coll Cardiol 2006;47:587–93.

14. Strasberg B, Lam W, Swiryn S, et al. Symptomatic spontaneous paroxysmal AV nodal block due to localized hyperresponsiveness of the AV node to vagotonic reflexes. Am Heart J 1982;103:795–801.

15. Sra JS, Singh B, Blanck Z, et al. Sinus tachycardia with atrioventricular block: an unusual presentation during neurocardiogenic (vasovagal) syncope. J Cardiovasc Electrophysiol 1998;9:203–7.

16. Mendoza IJ, Castellanos A, Lopera G, et al. Spontaneous paroxysmal atrioventricular block in patients with positive tilt tests and negative electrophysiologic studies. Am J Cardiol 2000;85:893–6.

17. Sanjuán R, Facila L, Blasco ML, et al. Case 13. Neuromediated syncope presenting as high grade AV block. In: Garcia-Civera R, Baron-Esquivias G, Blanc JJ, et al, editors. Syncope cases. Oxford (United Kingdom): Blackwell Futura; 2006. p. 38–40.

18. Brignole M, Sutton R, Menozzi C, et al. Lack of correlation between the responses to tilt testing and adenosine triphosphate test and the mechanism of spontaneous neurally-mediated syncope. Eur Heart J 2006;27:2232–9.

19. Brignole M, Menozzi C, Moya A, et al. Pacemaker therapy in patients with neurally mediated syncope and documented asystole. Third international study on syncope of uncertain etiology (ISSUE-3). A randomized trial. Circulation 2012;125:2566–71.

20. Ralevic V, Burnstock G. Involvement of purinergic signaling in cardiovascular disease. Drug News Perspect 2003;16:133–40.

21. Shryock JC, Belardinelli L. Adenosine and adenosine receptors in the cardiovascular system: biochemistry, physiology and pharmacology. Am J Cardiol 1997;79:2–10.

22. Wu L, Belardinelli L, Zablocki JA, et al. A partial agonist of the A(1)-adenosine receptor selectively slows AV conduction in guinea pig hearts. Am J Physiol Heart Circ Physiol 2001;280:334–43.

23. Lerman B, Belardinelli L. Cardiac electrophysiology of Adenosine. Basic and clinical concepts. Circulation 1991;83:1499–507.

24. Clemo H, Belardinelli L. Effect of adenosine on atrioventricular conduction. I: site and characterization of adenosine action in the guinea pig atrioventricualr node. Circ Res 1986;59:427–36.

25. Mosqueda-Garcia R, Furlan R, Tank J, et al. The elusive pathophysiology of neurally mediated syncope. Circulation 2000;102:2898–906.

26. Olsson RA, Pearson JD. Cardiovascular purinoceptors. Physiol Rev 1990;70:761–845.

27. Koeppen M, Eckle T, Eltzschig HK. Selective deletion of the A1 adenosine receptor abolishes heart-rate slowing effects of intravascular adenosine in vivo. PLoS One 2009;4:e6784.

Syncope in Patients with Organic Heart Disease

Brian Olshansky, MD[a],*, Renee M. Sullivan, MD[b]

KEYWORDS

- Syncope • Organic heart disease • Arrhythmia • Cardiomyopathy

KEY POINTS

- Patients with syncope and organic heart disease remain a small but important subset of those patients who experience transient loss of consciousness.
- Patients with syncope require thoughtful and complete evaluation in an attempt to better understand the mechanism of syncope and its relationship to the underlying disease, and to diagnose and treat both properly.
- The goal is to reduce the risk of further syncope, to improve long-term outcomes with respect to arrhythmic and total mortality, and to improve patients' quality of life.

INTRODUCTION

Syncope, a cause of transient loss of consciousness, is one of the most common conditions clinicians face, and the number of patients with syncope is growing. In 2002, according to the National Hospital Discharge Survey, there were 440,000 inpatients with syncope, based on the ICD-9 code 780.2 (syncope and collapse). Over 1 million office visits occurred in 2001 alone for the same primary diagnosis. Syncope is thought to occur in 3%[1] to 37%[2] of the general population (with women at greatest risk) and has a 6% annual incidence among the elderly.[3] Perhaps 3% of visits to the emergency department and 6% of hospital admissions[4,5] are for syncope, but these numbers underestimate the true prevalence, as syncope may masquerade as falls, collapse, trauma, hip fractures, motor vehicle accidents, or burns.

These statistics do not account for all locations of clinical evaluation or all presentations, may not include patients with syncope that is not documented properly at the time of admission or discharge, and do not take into consideration patients with syncope who fail to be evaluated because of preference or death before evaluation. The wide range in estimates may improve with standardization of data reporting.[6] A recent evaluation of 865 million visits to emergency departments, over a 9-year study period, estimated 6.7 million visits (0.77%) were syncope-related and most frequent among elderly, female, and non-Hispanic patients. The overall admission rate was 32%, with older males and Caucasians most likely to be admitted.[7] In a report from France[8] of 37,475 patients presenting to the emergency department, 454 (1.2%) had syncope, 169 of whom were discharged and 285 admitted. A discharge diagnosis was reported in 76% but was inadequate to explain the cause in 16%. Costs associated with evaluation and treatment of syncope, and related conditions, remain exorbitant.

Despite a meticulous evaluation, the definitive cause of syncope can remain elusive, although it is reassuring that syncope usually carries a benign prognosis. A neurocardiogenic mechanism or

This article originally appeared in Cardiac Electrophysiology Clinics, Volume 5, Issue 4, December 2013.
Disclosures: Dr Olshansky is consultant, honoraria, DSMB - Boston Scientific; Consultant, honoraria - Medtronic; Consultant - Boehringer Ingelheim; Consultant - Biocontrol; DSMB - Amarin; DSMB - Sanofi Aventis. Dr Sullivan has nothing to disclose.
a University of Iowa Hospitals, 200 Hawkins Drive, Iowa City, IA 52242, USA; b University of Missouri, Columbia, MO, USA
* Corresponding author.
E-mail address: brian-olshansky@uiowa.edu

cardiology.theclinics.com

situational trigger, in the absence of apparent structural heart disease, is often causative and self-limited, even if it is recurrent. However, syncope may be due to a myriad of clinical conditions and, when organic heart disease is present, short-term and long-term outcomes may not be so propitious. In this setting, there may be greater risk of early recurrence, and episodes may be more malignant, being linked to injury, hospitalization, imminent and prolonged cardiovascular collapse, sudden death, or total mortality in up to 30% of cases.[9]

Health care providers and casual observers alike corroborate that syncope can appear "the same as sudden death, except in one you wake up."[10,11] Hence, when a patient with organic heart disease passes out, the clinician often has an unparalleled dread leading to expensive and excessive testing, hospitalizing without just cause, and offering treatment before it is necessary.

This article addresses the issue of syncope in the face of organic heart disease, with full recognition that the cause, and therefore management, may be complex and multifaceted. Practical strategies are provided to clarify the underlying mechanism(s) and cause(s) of syncope, and define an approach allowing the clinician to evaluate and manage the individual patient. Because of the complex nature of the conditions addressed, randomized controlled clinical trials and robust data from large studies are generally absent with respect to guiding specific patient management, but guidelines have been published regarding evaluation and management of these patients.[12]

ORGANIC HEART DISEASE: WHAT IT IS AND WHAT IT IS NOT

Although seemingly self-evident, a robust and accepted definition of organic heart disease scarcely exists in the medical literature. However, the definition is crucial because it serves as the basis for the clinical conditions discussed herein and helps to clarify the populations at short-term and long-term risk. Organic heart disease is any condition that alters the structure of the heart (muscle, valves, conduction system, or other cardiovascular structures, including great vessels and conduits to the pulmonary system), either transiently or permanently.

Cardiomyopathy, attributable to a multiplicity of causes, including myocardial infarction, is one form of organic heart disease; various causes of ventricular dilation/hypertrophy/infiltration, or scar that substitutes nonfunctional "substrate" for muscle or damages the conduction system, are other possibilities. Valvular abnormalities can alter the structure of the ventricles and their response to autonomic perturbations and cardiac output. Coronary artery abnormalities (generally atherosclerosis or congenital anomalies) may initiate myocardial ischemia and thus affect ventricular function. Congenital abnormalities can affect filling pressures and cardiac output and lead to ventricular scar formation, especially after repair operations. Furthermore, aortic dissection, pulmonary hypertension, and pulmonary embolism fall under the umbrella of organic heart disease. **Box 1** presents a list of organic heart diseases associated with risk for syncope.

Syncopal arrhythmias are possible in any of the aforementioned conditions. However, the term organic heart disease does not necessarily include arrhythmic conditions such as sick sinus syndrome, atrial fibrillation, or ventricular tachycardia. The presence of organic heart disease can be associated with, exacerbate, or initiate these rhythm disturbances. Channelopathies, such as those present in the Brugada syndrome, the long or short QT syndrome, or catecholaminergic polymorphic ventricular tachycardia, while associated with adverse outcomes in patients with syncope and malignant ventricular arrhythmias, are not necessarily considered organic heart disease.

IS ORGANIC HEART DISEASE COMMON IN THE SYNCOPE PATIENT, AND IS IT REASON FOR CONCERN?

Despite the enormous numbers of individuals who collapse, sufficient epidemiologic data indicating the presence or absence of organic heart disease in these patients is sparse. Schnipper and Kapoor[13] estimated that 3% (range 1%–8%) of syncope is due to organic heart disease, but the accuracy of this estimate is questionable as it is dependent on the overall population considered and the setting of evaluation. Although some retrospective data indicate similar rates of recurrent syncope in patients with and without heart disease, it becomes difficult to factor in the population, the presence and treatment of comorbid conditions, the treatment of syncope, and issues related to outcomes. Syncope seems to have a bimodal distribution that in some ways also reflects its associated risks. For example, younger individuals, often women without heart disease, have isolated episodes of syncope that wane over time, whereas older individuals with new-onset syncope tend to have associated heart disease.[14–17]

An observational study from the Danish National Patient Register of 127,508 patients with a first-time diagnosis of syncope showed 3 age peaks

---

Box 1
Organic heart disease associated with syncope

Coronary Artery Disease

  Ischemia

  Anomalous coronary artery

Valvular Heart Disease

  Stenotic lesions

    Aortic stenosis

    Mitral stenosis

    Tricuspid stenosis

    Pulmonic stenosis

  Regurgitant lesions

    Aortic regurgitation

    Mitral regurgitation

    Tricuspid regurgitation

    Pulmonic regurgitation

Myocardial Disease

  Cardiomyopathy

    Dilated cardiomyopathy

      Ischemic

      Nonischemic

    Infiltrative cardiomyopathy

      Amyloidosis

      Sarcoidosis

      Hemochromatosis

    Noncompaction

  Diastolic dysfunction

  Hypertrophic cardiomyopathy

  Myotonic dystrophy

  Arrhythmogenic right ventricular dysplasia

  Myocarditis

  Pericardial disease

    Pericarditis

    Effusion/tamponade

    Constriction

Congenital Heart Disease

Disease of Cardiac Conduction System

  Kearns-Sayre

  Myotonic dystrophy

  Progressive conduction system disease (Lev, Lenegre)

  Atrioventricular block

Cardiac Tumor (Obstruction)

  Atrial myxoma

  Fibroelastoma

Disease of Great Vessels (Obstruction)

  Aortic dissection

  Subclavian steal

  Carotid disease

Dysautonomia

Disease of Pulmonary System (Dysautonomic)

  Pulmonary hypertension

  Pulmonary embolism

  Cough syncope

(20, 60, and 80 years). Cardiovascular disease and cardiovascular drug therapy was present in 28% and 48% of these patients, respectively; there was greater risk of hospital admission in patients with cardiovascular disease at any age (especially the young).[18] The same group evaluating 37,017 otherwise healthy patients with a first-time diagnosis of syncope and 185,085 control subjects found that 3023 (8.2%) and 14,251 (7.1%) deaths occurred in the syncope and control populations, respectively. There was an increased risk of all-cause mortality (hazard ratio [HR] 1.06, 95% confidence interval [CI] 1.02–1.10), cardiovascular hospitalization (HR 1.74, 95% CI 1.68–1.80), recurrent syncope (45.1/1000 person-years), and stroke rate (6.8/1000 person-years (HR 1.35, 95% CI 1.27–1.44)).[19] Furthermore, diagnostic coding for syncope was found to be reasonably accurate (positive predictive value of 95% and sensitivity of 63%).[20]

Persons with syncope and organic heart disease are at higher risk for death than the general syncope population; this may be based on the underlying heart disease alone rather than the presence of syncope. In the Framingham Study, 822 of 7814 (10.5%) participants had syncope, the suspected cause of which was vasovagal in 21%, cardiac in 9.5%, orthostatic in 9%, and unknown in 37%. Syncope was associated with mortality (multivariable-adjusted HR 1.31, 95% CI 1.14–1.51), especially when due to a cardiac cause (HR 2.01, 95% CI 1.48–2.73), but not if of vasovagal etiology.[17] This study did not investigate the timing between syncope and death; assess if syncope was an independent predictor of death; determine if heart disease, when present, was the proven cause for syncope; or consider how cardiac disease actually caused syncope. Of note, it did not show that syncope increases the risk of death in patients with organic heart disease. In a multivariate analysis, syncope may not be a predictor of poor outcome,[21] but this becomes difficult to reconcile as comorbidities are more common in persons with syncope, especially the elderly.[22]

Syncope represents an adverse prognostic marker in patients with acute myocardial infarction. Data from the MONICA/KORA myocardial infarction registry indicated that patients who have a myocardial infarction associated with syncope are at much greater risk of dying than those with myocardial infarction not associated with syncope (odds ratio [OR] 5.36, 95% CI 2.65–10.85).[23]

In a retrospective and nonrandomized analysis of 88 persons with syncope undergoing electrophysiology testing (75% of whom had heart disease), left ventricular ejection fraction (LVEF) (mean = 0.41 ± 0.20) was the only independent factor associated with sudden death. It was not important if the patients had a cardiac cause for syncope and/or if syncope was related to an arrhythmia. These data highlight the difficulties of assigning risk to patients with syncope and heart disease.[24]

Nevertheless, syncope is associated with adverse outcomes in patients with heart failure. During 1-year follow-up of 491 patients with New York Heart Association (NYHA) Functional Class III or IV heart failure and a mean LVEF of 0.20 ± 0.07, the 60 patients (12%) with syncope had a risk of sudden death far exceeding those without syncope ($P<.00001$) but independent of the purported cause of syncope (cardiac vs noncardiac).[25]

A retrospective analysis from the Sudden Cardiac Death in Heart Failure Trial (SCD-HeFT)[26] supported a high rate of syncope in patients with heart failure. SCD-HeFT included well-treated NYHA Functional Class II to III heart-failure patients with LVEF of 0.35 or less. Of this population, 6% of patients had syncope before randomization, 14% had syncope after randomization, and 2% had syncope before and after randomization. In patients with an implantable cardioverter-defibrillator (ICD), syncope before and after randomization was associated with more appropriate ICD discharges (HR 1.75, 95% CI 1.10–2.80, $P = .019$, and HR 2.91, 95% CI 1.89–4.47, $P = .001$, respectively). Postrandomization syncope predicted total and cardiovascular death (HR 1.41, 95% CI 1.13–1.76, $P = .002$, and HR 1.55, 95% CI 1.19–2.02, $P = .001$, respectively).

However, syncope was associated with increased mortality risk regardless of treatment (placebo, amiodarone, or ICD), indicating that death may be due to causes other than arrhythmia, or be inevitable, especially in the ICD group. The causes of 458 episodes of syncope in 356 patients (16% of the population) were orthostatic hypotension (n = 65), ventricular tachycardia (n = 44), drug-induced hypotension (n = 38), vasomotor (n = 33), cardiac arrest (cardiopulmonary resuscitation given) (n = 24), drug-induced arrhythmia (n = 2), seizures (n = 7), other (n = 159), and unknown (n = 86).

Syncope is not necessarily arrhythmic, life threatening, or recurrent, even in persons with structural heart disease, as shown in a report of 35 individuals with syncope and a negative electrophysiology study. Of these, 6 had recurrent syncope caused by bradycardia with long pauses in 3, sinus tachycardia in 1, and chronic atrial fibrillation in 2. Only 1 patient had sustained ventricular tachycardia with presyncope.[27]

In other reports, those patients with syncope and organic heart disease, impaired LVEF, and other high-risk markers have as high an intermediate-term risk of sudden death as those who have experienced cardiac arrest attributable to sustained ventricular tachycardia or ventricular fibrillation.[28,29] Indeed, syncope may actually represent an aborted cardiac arrest.

SYNCOPE AND DEATH: A TEMPORAL ASSOCIATION

An entire body of literature is devoted to the emergency-room assessment of patients with syncope and obvious organic heart disease. Decision algorithms regarding admission or discharge from the emergency room and observations concerning short-term survival have been developed.[30,31] The presence of organic heart disease alone raises concern that syncope may be due to a potentially life-threatening process, but this concern has not been readily incorporated into guidelines based on good clinical evidence. Nevertheless, a patient with syncope who has organic heart disease, and for whom the cause is not easily determined, must be considered a candidate for hospital admission.

The risk of adverse outcomes in patients with syncope may be short term with some presentations of organic heart disease, particularly if the condition is reversible. For instance, a patient with an acute myocardial infarction may have syncope arising from a variety of mechanisms: transient hypotension, ventricular arrhythmias, or bradycardia. Arrhythmias caused by myocardial ischemia, acute myocardial infarction, or chordal rupture of the mitral valve may resolve with acute treatment. Syncope related to aortic dissection or pulmonary embolism may resolve when the underlying cause is treated.

Recent emergency-room data indicate that heart disease and heart failure in patients with syncope portends a short-term risk of death. A systematic electronic review of the literature from 1990 to 2010 pooled 11 studies of patients evaluated in the emergency department for syncope, of whom 42% were admitted. The risk of death was 4.4%; 1.1% had a cardiovascular cause of death. One-third of patients were discharged without a diagnosis and 10.4% had a diagnosis of heart disease. Palpitations preceding syncope, syncope with exertion, a history consistent with heart failure or ischemic heart disease, and evidence of bleeding were the most powerful predictors of adverse outcomes.[32]

Emergency-room risk-stratification approaches have been attempted[33–38] but have not been fully validated.[39] Any prognostic value may only be short term.[40] In an early report of patients with syncope, multivariate predictors of arrhythmia or 1-year mortality were an abnormal electrocardiogram (ECG) (OR 3.2, 95% CI 1.6–6.4), history of ventricular arrhythmia (OR 4.8, 95% CI 1.7–13.9), and history of congestive heart failure (OR 3.2, 95% CI 1.3–8.1). Outcomes may be related to these factors more than to syncope itself.[38]

The Evaluation of Guidelines in SYncope Study (EGSYS) score[36] has attempted to define who has cardiac syncope using criteria from the European guidelines. The EGSYS Score showed that the presence of palpitations, heart disease, an abnormal ECG, syncope during effort, and syncope when supine were associated with high risk, whereas the presence of precipitating or predisposing factors or an autonomic prodrome were associated with lower risk.[36] Other risk-stratification approaches include: The Osservatorio Epidemiologico sulla Sincope nel Lazio (OESIL and OESIL2) scores; the San Francisco Syncope Rule; the ROSE (Risk Stratification of Syncope in the Emergency Department) study; and the Short Term Prognosis of Syncope (STePS) study.[33–38,41] The OESIL risk score (age >65 years, cardiovascular disease, syncope without prodrome, abnormal ECG) and its validation prospectively in 328 consecutive patients (178 women; average age 57.5 years), indicated a highly significant incremental risk depending on the number of risk factors present, but the score did not determine the cause of syncope.[34,35]

The San Francisco Rule using the CHESS mnemonic (Congestive heart failure, Hematocrit <30%, abnormal ECG, Shortness of breath, Systolic blood pressure <90 mm Hg) showed some promise as a predictor and, although confirmed in validation cohorts, use of this score has not improved outcomes or reduced hospitalization.[42–45] In fact, 48% of patients were considered "high risk," and admission rates increased 9%

when compared with "clinical judgment". Although such "rules" exist, they may not be followed.[46]

In the ROSE Study, brain natriuretic peptide (BNP) and a positive stool guaiac were associated with risk of death, neither of which are necessarily associated with syncope, arrhythmic death, cardiovascular death, or organic heart disease.[47,48]

In a study of 2775 consecutive syncope patients in the STePS study,[41] an abnormal ECG, concomitant trauma, absence of symptoms of impending syncope, and male gender were associated unfavorable outcomes in the short term. Long-term severe outcomes occurring in 9.3% correlated with age older than 65 years, neoplasms, cerebrovascular disease, structural heart disease, and ventricular arrhythmias. One-year mortality was greater in those admitted (14.7%) than in those discharged (1.8%), but it is unclear whether hospital admission has a greater influence than risk stratification alone in patients with syncope.

These data highlight that patients with comorbid conditions and syncope are at greater risk for death, and that syncope alone may have nothing to do with the outcome. After considering the available data, the American College of Emergency Physicians (ACEP) has proposed that emergency-room providers consider the recommendations shown in **Box 2** when evaluating the patient with syncope.

HOW IS SYNCOPE RELATED TO ORGANIC HEART DISEASE? MECHANISMS OF SYNCOPE IN ORGANIC HEART DISEASE

Transient loss of consciousness is caused by paroxysmal, abrupt cessation and usually rapid re-initiation of effective, global cerebral blood flow. Interruption in blood flow may be related directly to an underlying cardiac condition—or not. It is not enough simply to know that an underlying cardiovascular condition exists. Appropriate treatment of the underlying cardiovascular condition may not necessarily address the root cause of syncope, even if syncope is related directly to organic heart disease. Potential mechanism(s) responsible for transient interruption of cerebral blood flow must be considered, and for any given condition or patient several mechanisms may be in play. Such mechanisms include: (1) obstruction to arterial flow; (2) orthostatic or paroxysmal hypotension; (3) a bradyarrhythmia or tachyarrhythmia; (4) a dysautonomic response related directly to the heart condition; (5) an iatrogenic intervention; and (6) an unrelated cause.

Obstruction to blood flow may be due to stenotic valvular lesions (eg, aortic stenosis), cardiac tumors (eg, atrial myxoma) or impaired ventricular dysautonomic condition manifesting as inappropriate peripheral vasodilatation without an adequate compensatory heart rate response, as in amyloidosis or multiple system atrophy) or hemodynamic collapse related to an acute regurgitant valvular lesion (mitral valve chordal rupture). Various tachycardias and bradycardias can cause syncope, and can result from the underlying cardiac condition (progressive conduction system disease leading to heart block, atrial stretch leading to atrial fibrillation, or myocardial scar causing ventricular tachycardia, even if nonsustained). Abrupt changes in rate may be critical to alteration of hemodynamic accommodation, causing transient hypotension and syncope; this is especially true in the elderly and those taking β-blockers and vasodilators, in whom the same rhythm may not cause transient hypotension.

Syncope may be caused by a neurocardiogenic response to the underlying disease (eg, critical aortic stenosis leading to activation of ventricular mechanoreceptors or pulmonary embolus). The Bezold-Jarisch reflex may also occur after inferior wall ischemia. Even syncope in dilated cardiomyopathy may be related to autonomic perturbations with an enhanced neurocardiogenic reflex.[49] Alternatively, a neurocardiogenic response may be independent of the underlying cardiac condition.

In other circumstances, syncope is exacerbated by the underlying condition, but is not related directly. Medications given to treat the underlying heart disease may in fact be responsible in some cases as well. A patient with congestive heart failure and borderline hypotension placed on a diuretic and/or a vasodilator may develop orthostatic hypotension, causing syncope. Antiarrhythmic drugs may have proarrhythmic effects, causing bradycardias or torsades de pointes. Syncope can be completely unrelated to heart disease and may be due to a benign cause such as situational or neurocardiogenic syncope. It is possible, despite multiple explanatory mechanisms (eg, atrial fibrillation with rapid rates in a patient with a cardiomyopathy), that the cause for syncope remains elusive. **Box 3** lists potential mechanisms by which syncope may occur in the presence of organic heart disease.

EVALUATION AND SUBSEQUENT MANAGEMENT OF SYNCOPE IN PATIENTS WITH ORGANIC HEART DISEASE
Clinical Assessment: History and Physical

filling (cardiac tamponade, also triggering an inappropriate dysautonomic mechanism). Transient severe hypotension may be due to an orthostatic mechanism (dehydration, bleeding, or a chronic

The cause for syncope is often inferred and presumptive unless a subsequent episode is provoked or occurs during monitoring. Even then, the mechanism may not be understood fully

---

Box 3
Potential mechanisms responsible for syncope in organic heart disease

Hypotension

    Fluid Shifts

Orthostatic Hypotension

    Dehydration, blood loss

    Dysautonomia

Neurocardiogenic

    Bradycardia

    Hypotension

Arrhythmia (with Abrupt Change in Heart Rate)

    Sinus bradycardia

    Atrioventricular block

    Asystole

    Supraventricular tachycardia including atrial fibrillation

    Ventricular tachycardia

Obstruction to Blood Flow

Iatrogenic

    Medications

    Dehydration

    Vasodilatation

    Bradycardia

    Torsade de pointes

(eg, an asystolic episode may be due to sick sinus syndrome or a neurocardiogenic response). The ascribed cause may be incorrect or go undiagnosed. Triggers may be transient, obscure, or irreproducible. Spontaneous remission is common. Furthermore, the symptom itself may be nonspecific and not easily linked to a cardiac cause[50]; any apparent treatment can be a canard.

Clinically, a sudden otherwise unexplained collapse in a patient with organic heart disease is likely related to the heart disease. The benefits of any subsequent therapy may be misunderstood. This aspect is illustrated in an early report suggesting that tachycardia caused syncope, but the study was marred by the concept that the tachycardia was due to large tonsils and that after tonsillectomy, syncope did not recur.[51] The question remains: which syncope patient requires cardiac evaluation and when is an aggressive management approach justified?

Often the evaluation approach involves inappropriate, unnecessary, and expensive tests such as computed tomography scans of the chest and/or head, carotid dopplers, Holter monitors, cardiac enzymes, d-dimer, BNP, and so forth. This low-yield, high-cost testing approach is still used, although a careful history may be all that is required.[52] An approach to evaluate syncope is described in the European guidelines.[12]

Observational data indicate that patients with long-standing recurrent syncope are more likely to have a benign prognosis, unless the syncope is associated with underlying structural heart disease. The presence of collapse in an older individual with heart disease raises red flags and may be the only premonitory sign of something worse to come. However, syncope alone is not a predictor of outcomes based on age without considering the comorbidities. Careful history taking and uncovering an underlying cardiac cause of syncope may not improve an already poor prognosis.[53]

Alboni and colleagues[54] evaluated 356 patients with syncope prospectively (of whom 337 were assessed); 191 had suspected or certain heart disease and 146 did not. Of those having suspected or certain heart disease, 39% were thought to have a cardiac cause for syncope, 49% were considered to have a neurally mediated cause independent of the heart disease, and 12% had "unexplained" syncope. In those without suspected or diagnosed heart disease, 3% were thought to have a cardiac cause for syncope and 72% were considered to have neurally mediated syncope, whereas 23% were considered to have syncope of an unexplained cause.

From these data, several important points emerge. First, heart disease alone, when present, does not necessarily explain syncope. Second, syncope is often unexplained. Third, many patients with heart disease have syncope unrelated to heart disease. Fourth, the history may be diagnostic.

In another prospective evaluation of 139 syncope patients with organic heart disease, a cardiac cause was identified in 83 patients and a reflex cause was found in 30. In 185 patients without organic heart disease, reflex syncope was diagnosed in 127, cardiac syncope in 30, and vascular syncope in 2.[55]

No prospective study has yet demonstrated a tacit independent relationship between syncope and adverse outcomes, particularly death, in patients with organic heart disease. Such a study would be difficult, if not impossible, to design and conduct, considering the diverse conditions that comprise organic heart disease and the necessity to treat patients based on a presumptive cause.

A stepwise approach advocated by several groups[56–59] can streamline the evaluation process, strip away unnecessary testing, and define a management pathway that will, it is hoped, lead to proper diagnoses, reduce syncopal episodes, lead to fewer hospitalizations, and improve survival. While simple on the surface, in clinical practice every step remains a challenge.[60] **Box 4** presents a list of considerations that must be taken into account when evaluating the patient with syncope and organic heart disease.

Specific clinical features can identify individuals with syncope and a potential underlying cardiac condition. The Calgary Syncope Score, a 118-item questionnaire, was used to determine the etiology of syncope and define the risk for sudden cardiac death in the Cardiac Arrest Survivors with Preserved Ejection Fraction Registry (CAS-PER).[61] The questionnaire predicted those who were tilt-table test positive (n = 21; prolonged sitting or standing, developing presyncope preceded by stress, recurrent headaches, and experiencing fatigue lasting >1 minute after syncope) and those who had spontaneous or inducible ventricular tachycardia (n = 78; male sex, age at onset >35 years); 35 had no cause identified. Using these criteria, 92% were classified correctly (negative predictive value ≥96%), diagnosing ventricular tachycardia with 99% sensitivity and 68% specificity.[62] The 9-year arrhythmia-free and total survival was predicted from the history, but even low risk does not mean no risk.[63]

In another study of 1060 consecutive patients with presumed vasovagal syncope, patients older than 60 years were less likely to give a typical history, more likely to present with unexplained falls, and less likely to have episodes triggered by prolonged standing (OR 0.55, 95% CI 0.40–0.72), posture change (OR 0.61, 95% CI 0.46–0.82), or hot environments (OR 0.57, 95% CI 0.42–0.78).[15] A report of more than 3000 patients showed that younger patients had more vasovagal faints whereas the elderly had more orthostatic hypotension.[14]

Critical and specific to the evaluation of the patient with organic heart disease is consideration of the condition itself, whether or not it has been diagnosed, timing of diagnosis, and any medical therapy prescribed. The circumstances of the event are important to help better determine whether the cause could be arrhythmic, orthostatic, or dysautonomic. Although many conditions may be diagnosed by the history and physical alone, the presumptive cause of syncope may be obscure or difficult to link to the history exactly.

WHAT EVALUATION IS NECESSARY TO RULE OUT A CARDIAC CAUSE FOR HEART DISEASE?

There are no specific guidelines with regard to the proper diagnostic approach to determine the presence or absence of organic heart disease. In some instances, the diagnosis becomes clear based on the history of the patient. In many instances, other clinical circumstances indicate concomitant conditions, such as a myocardial infarction, which, though rare in the syncopal patient, is a marker of high risk.[23] For the patient who presents with syncope and no other cardiac diagnosis (but a suspected cardiac cause), the clinical history, coupled with the ECG and the echocardiogram, which may show structural and functional abnormalities,[64] are a useful beginning before tailoring the approach based on other clinical findings and risk markers manifest in the patient. Cardiac magnetic resonance imaging may be valuable for select patients.

It is important to recognize, however, even if syncope appears to be due to a benign process, that during follow-up evaluation a cardiac cause and/or underlying cardiac diagnosis may become manifest.[54,65] The importance of follow-up evaluation cannot be overstated. When it comes to testing, "caveat emptor" pertains. A test may be positive but have nothing to do with syncope. A test may be negative but not be sensitive enough to detect the abnormality.

Further evaluation, including use of Holter monitors, event monitors, or implantable loop recorders, as well as electrophysiology testing, should not be used indiscriminately but must be

---

Box 4
Considerations when evaluating syncope in patients with heart disease

1. Attempt to define the cause for syncope based on clinical presentation.

2. Identify if organic heart disease is present.

3. Understand the relationship between organic heart disease and syncope. Did organic heart disease cause syncope, and if so, how?

4. Understand if there is a mechanistic relationship between organic heart disease and syncope, and if so, determine if there is a specific risk for arrhythmic and/or sudden cardiac death.

5. If there is not a risk for arrhythmic or sudden death, is there a risk for death otherwise that can be treated?

6. If the episode is acute, consider risks and assess the need for hospital admission.

ordered based on specific clinical features derived from the history and based on the anticipated effect on long-term outcomes for the patient. If testing poses a continued risk for sudden cardiac death, an ICD implant may be prudent. If, on the other hand, the risk of arrhythmic death is high but there are substantial comorbidities and complications, a patient may not be a candidate for ICD implantation. Decisions about ICD or pacemaker implants may be related directly to other clinical indications that supersede issues related to syncope. Such clinical decisions are driven by the best assessment of the data in light of presumed risk and concerns regarding costs, complications, and quality of life.

Long-term and short-term risk assessment must be individualized and take into account the likelihood of survival based on cardiac and noncardiac conditions, risks of arrhythmias, and risk of recurrence. Thus far, no good markers exist to aid in determining how to proceed with the syncope evaluation other than attempting to reproduce the clinical circumstance that may be the cause of syncope (monitoring during an episode, induction of an arrhythmia, tilt-table test, and so forth).

Other noninvasive markers have been evaluated to determine their association with syncope, but none has proved to be reliable or diagnostic as screening tools. These markers include BNP,[66,67] heart-rate variability,[68] spectral turbulence,[69] T-wave alternans,[70,71] baroreflex sensitivity,[72] QT-interval measurements and dispersion,[67,73] and late potentials measured by the signal-averaged ECG.[72,74,75]

Electrophysiology Testing

The electrophysiology study can be used to assess arrhythmic risk and determine the likelihood of freedom from sudden death in patients with organic heart disease.[76–78] If sustained monomorphic ventricular tachycardia is induced with an accepted protocol in a patient with organic heart disease, the long-term risk is poor,[79] but these risks may be predicted by other means including LVEF or NYHA functional class.[80] The predictive accuracy of an electrophysiology test is greatest in patients with coronary artery disease and impaired LVEF. The electrophysiology test is not particularly good at deciphering the risk of bradyarrhythmias. In a study of 21 patients with documented symptoms attributed to sinus pause or atrioventricular (AV) block, the electrophysiology study reproduced findings in 38% with sinus node dysfunction and in 15% with AV block.[81] Though not so accurate for bradyarrhythmias, not all data are consistent.[76]

For those with organic heart disease in whom the electrophysiology study is positive for ventricular tachycardia an ICD may improve outcomes,[29,78,82,83] but syncope may not be related to an induced arrhythmia. In fact, an induced arrhythmia may not reproduce the clinical event (which could be nonsustained ventricular tachycardia), and the relationship between clinical nonsustained ventricular tachycardia and induced, sustained ventricular tachycardia remains uncertain.

Results are disease dependent. An electrophysiology study may not necessarily be predictive in a patient with nonischemic cardiomyopathy, and has limited or unknown value in arrhythmogenic right ventricular cardiomyopathy, hypertrophic cardiomyopathy, sarcoidosis (and other infiltrative conditions), and other conditions such as Kearns-Sayre syndrome.[84,85]

In addition, arrhythmia induction and the potential for life-threatening outcomes is related directly to disease severity. When considering risk stratification, LVEF is a better predictor of outcomes than is an electrophysiology study that is positive for ventricular tachycardia. The electrophysiology test may add diagnostic but not therapeutic value in patients at high risk with low LVEF values, because it is clear that these patients will benefit most from ICD implantation if the risks of other comorbidities are not high. The ability to risk-stratify using electrophysiology testing remains unsettled, especially in patients who do not have ischemic heart disease.[77,86–91] Those who have a positive electrophysiology study and syncope have poor outcomes with an ICD[92] and a high likelihood of appropriate ICD discharges after implantation.[93]

According to American College of Cardiology/American Heart Association/Heart Rhythm Society (ACC/AHA/HRS) guidelines,[94] an ICD is indicated for patients with syncope who have an electrophysiology study that is positive for ventricular tachyarrhythmia when drug therapy is ineffective, not tolerated, or not preferred; however, an ICD is not indicated for patients with syncope, ventricular tachycardia, but no structural heart disease (idiopathic ventricular tachycardia).

Implantable Loop Recorders

Emerging data have defined a specific and important role for the implantable loop recorder (ILR) in the management of syncope in patients who otherwise have no diagnosis despite the history, physical, ECG, tilt-table test, or electrophysiology study.[95–97] Using an ILR, compared with a conventional approach the time to diagnosis is much shorter[98] and the method is cost effective.[99] It would seem that the ILR should be considered earlier in the evaluation of syncope,[100,101] especially if syncope is recurrent, such that unnecessary and nondiagnostic tests can be avoided.[102] Furthermore, if syncope continues after ILR implantation, a negative result can exclude an arrhythmic cause such that other mechanisms can be investigated further,[103] including seizure disorder.[104] In a tertiary referral center in Poland, it was estimated that approximately 6% of syncope patients (including those with organic heart disease) had an indication for an ILR.[105] It appears that many individuals may be candidates for the ILR based on the European guidelines, but actually do not receive it.[106] Acceptable indications include otherwise undiagnosed syncope whereby recording an episode would provide the best diagnostic yield and yet not place an individual at undue risk for sudden cardiac death. As such, the patients at highest risk and lowest risk would be excluded.

APPROACH TO THE SYNCOPE PATIENT WITH ORGANIC HEART DISEASE IN WHOM THE EVALUATION IS NEGATIVE

After a tailored evaluation based on the clinical diagnoses and use of appropriate risk-stratification tools, a contemplative review of the risks based on standard criteria independent of syncope (ie, LVEF, arrhythmia monitor findings, NYHA classification) must occur. Based on an understanding of the magnitude and profundity of the event, coupled with risk criteria, an educated approach must be undertaken to formulate the best plan of care.

In a patient with left ventricular dysfunction who otherwise fits the criteria for an ICD implant, independent of electrophysiology study results, an ICD may be appropriate. In some instances, the patient does not meet established criteria for ICD implantation but still remains at risk; such an individual may be early post myocardial infarction or post coronary artery revascularization, or have newly diagnosed congestive heart failure or left ventricular dysfunction. In these cases, with a negative evaluation otherwise, it would be appropriate to consider that the high risk will be difficult to define completely, and that a negative evaluation including electrophysiology testing or monitoring may be misleading and only provide false optimism. However, before ICD implantation, consideration must include an understanding of the potential mechanisms involved in the syncope. In the case of a patient with aortic valve stenosis, syncope may, for example, be due to a ventricular arrhythmia, but also may be due to paroxysmal AV

block, a neurocardiogenic response, or some other mechanism. In this setting, treating the aortic stenosis may negate the need for an ICD implant.

Patients with nonischemic cardiomyopathy can be at risk for sudden cardiac death even if an electrophysiology test is negative. However, these patients are also at higher risk of total mortality compared with those without syncope.[24,25,28,107] In a prospective study of patients with nonischemic cardiomyopathy, unexplained syncope, and a negative electrophysiology test, 14 underwent ICD implant. Compared with 19 nonischemic cardiomyopathy patients who had a cardiac arrest and were treated with an ICD, 7 of the 14 syncope patients versus 8 of 19 with cardiac arrest received appropriate ICD shocks. All recurrent syncope was associated with ventricular tachyarrhythmias.[107]

In a report concerning patients with nonischemic cardiomyopathy referred for heart transplantation, 147 (of 639) had syncope but no documented sustained arrhythmia. Actuarial survival at 2 years was 85% with ICD therapy and 67% without an ICD ($P = .04$).[108] In a blinded, matched, case-controlled analysis of patients with cardiomyopathy, a negative electrophysiology study, and unexplained syncope, the risk of death and cardiac arrest was lower in those undergoing an ICD implant than in those who did not (HR 0.18, 95% CI 0.04–0.85; $P = .04$).[109] Thus, patients who have idiopathic dilated cardiomyopathy, a negative electrophysiology test, and syncope unexplained by any other mechanism should be considered for an ICD implant (as recommended in the ACC/AHA/HRS guidelines[94]).

Similarly, if syncope occurs and is otherwise unexplained when organic heart disease is diagnosed, an ICD should be contemplated if a ventricular arrhythmia is suspected. However, there are few compelling data to support this approach, and syncope can be due to other causes, as has been shown in patients with arrhythmogenic right ventricular dysplasia, for example.[110,111]

Several mechanisms can explain syncope in hypertrophic cardiomyopathy, including ventricular or supraventricular arrhythmias, AV block, outflow tract obstruction, or a neurocardiogenic response, among others.[112–115] It can even be neurally mediated.[112] Nevertheless, if syncope is unexplained, and especially if there are markers indicating high risk of sudden cardiac death, an ICD should be considered.[116] These data are supported by a multicenter registry of 506 patients followed for a mean of 3.7 ± 2.8 years.[117]

An ICD should be considered for patients with unexplained syncope who have: repaired or unrepaired congenital heart disease[118]; left ventricular noncompaction[119]; valvular heart disease associated with impaired ventricular function (not mitral valve prolapse, not necessarily critical aortic stenosis, and not when an obstructive lesion caused the collapse); and sarcoidosis and other conditions, presuming the cause for syncope is not otherwise found.

A patient who has syncope before a pacemaker or an ICD may continue to pass out from causes unrelated to the implant (undiagnosed syncope not related to arrhythmia), from device malfunction, or ineffective programming. Most ICDs now can record episodes of tachyarrhythmias that can serve as a guide for device programming.

THE FUTURE OF EVALUATING PATIENTS WITH SYNCOPE

A directed, organized, and stepwise approach to syncope may provide higher diagnostic yield, lower costs and hospitalization rates, and improved outcomes for patients.[58,59] Despite attempts to develop a more disciplined diagnostic approach, inappropriate use of tests continues, as many clinicians are not particularly facile in the evaluation of syncope. Syncope clinics are beginning to develop, leading to the multidisciplinary evaluation of patients.[120] It is hoped that a more organized approach to the management of syncope will lead to improved long-term outcomes. The recent European guidelines serve as an exquisite resource regarding syncope evaluation and management in this regard.[12]

SUMMARY

Patients with syncope and organic heart disease remain a small but important subset of those patients who experience transient loss of consciousness. These patients require thoughtful and complete evaluation in an attempt to better understand the mechanism of syncope and its relationship to the underlying disease, and to diagnose and treat both properly. In so doing, the goal is to reduce the risk of further syncope, to improve long-term outcomes with respect to arrhythmic and total mortality, and to improve the quality of life of patients.

REFERENCES

1. Savage DD, Corwin L, McGee DL, et al. Epidemiologic features of isolated syncope: the Framingham Study. Stroke 1985;16:626–9.
2. Dermksian G, Lamb LE. Syncope in a population of healthy young adults; incidence, mechanisms, and significance. J Am Med Assoc 1958;168:1200–7.
3. Lipsitz LA, Wei JY, Rowe JW. Syncope in an elderly, institutionalised population: prevalence, incidence, and associated risk. Q J Med 1985;55:45–54.
4. Kapoor WN. Evaluation and management of syncope. Contemp Intern Med 1994;6:29–32, 35–9.
5. Kapoor WN. Workup and management of patients with syncope. Med Clin North Am 1995; 79:1153–70.
6. Sun BC, Thiruganasambandamoorthy V, Cruz JD, Consortium to Standardize EDSRSR. Standardized reporting guidelines for emergency department syncope risk-stratification research. Acad Emerg Med 2012;19:694–702.
7. Sun BC, Emond JA, Camargo CA Jr. Characteristics and admission patterns of patients presenting with syncope to U.S. emergency departments, 1992-2000. Acad Emerg Med 2004;11:1029–34.
8. Blanc JJ, L'Her C, Touiza A, et al. Prospective evaluation and outcome of patients admitted for syncope over a 1 year period. Eur Heart J 2002;23: 815–20.
9. Kapoor WN, Karpf M, Wieand S, et al. A prospective evaluation and follow-up of patients with syncope. N Engl J Med 1983;309:197–204.
10. Olshansky B. For whom does the bell toll? J Cardiovasc Electrophysiol 2001;12:1002–3.
11. Olshansky B. Is syncope the same thing as sudden death except that you wake up? J Cardiovasc Electrophysiol 1997;8:1098–101.
12. Task Force for the Diagnosis and Management of Syncope, European Society of Cardiology (ESC), European Heart Rhythm Association (EHRA), et al. Guidelines for the diagnosis and management of syncope (version 2009). Eur Heart J 2009;30:2631–71.
13. Schnipper JL, Kapoor WN. Diagnostic evaluation and management of patients with syncope. Med Clin North Am 2001;85:423–56, xi.
14. Cooke J, Carew S, Costelloe A, et al. The changing face of orthostatic and neurocardiogenic syncope with age. QJM 2011;104:689–95.
15. Duncan GW, Tan MP, Newton JL, et al. Vasovagal syncope in the older person: differences in presentation between older and younger patients. Age Ageing 2010;39:465–70.
16. Colman N, Nahm K, Ganzeboom KS, et al. Epidemiology of reflex syncope. Clin Auton Res 2004; 14(Suppl 1):9–17.
17. Soteriades ES, Evans JC, Larson MG, et al. Incidence and prognosis of syncope. N Engl J Med 2002;347:878–85.
18. Ruwald MH, Hansen ML, Lamberts M, et al. The relation between age, sex, comorbidity, and pharmacotherapy and the risk of syncope: a Danish nationwide study. Europace 2012;14:1506–14.
19. Ruwald MH, Hansen ML, Lamberts M, et al. Prognosis among healthy individuals discharged with

a primary diagnosis of syncope. J Am Coll Cardiol 2013;61(3):325–32.

20. Ruwald MH, Hansen ML, Lamberts M, et al. Accuracy of the ICD-10 discharge diagnosis for syncope. Europace 2013;15(4):595–600.

21. Kapoor WN, Hanusa BH. Is syncope a risk factor for poor outcomes? Comparison of patients with and without syncope. Am J Med 1996;100:646–55.

22. Lipsitz LA, Pluchino FC, Wei JY, et al. Syncope in institutionalized elderly: the impact of multiple pathological conditions and situational stress. J Chronic Dis 1986;39:619–30.

23. Kirchberger I, Heier M, Kuch B, et al. Presenting symptoms of myocardial infarction predict short- and long-term mortality: the MONICA/KORA Myocardial Infarction Registry. Am Heart J 2012;164:856–61.

24. Middlekauff HR, Stevenson WG, Saxon LA. Prognosis after syncope: impact of left ventricular function. Am Heart J 1993;125:121–7.

25. Middlekauff HR, Stevenson WG, Stevenson LW, et al. Syncope in advanced heart failure: high risk of sudden death regardless of origin of syncope. J Am Coll Cardiol 1993;21:110–6.

26. Olshansky B, Poole JE, Johnson G, et al. Syncope predicts the outcome of cardiomyopathy patients: analysis of the SCD-HeFT study. J Am Coll Cardiol 2008;51:1277–82.

27. Menozzi C, Brignole M, Garcia-Civera R, et al, International Study on Syncope of Uncertain Etiology Investigators. Mechanism of syncope in patients with heart disease and negative electrophysiologic test. Circulation 2002;105:2741–5.

28. Olshansky B, Hahn EA, Hartz VL, et al. Clinical significance of syncope in the electrophysiologic study versus electrocardiographic monitoring (ESVEM) trial. The ESVEM Investigators. Am Heart J 1999;137:878–86.

29. Steinberg JS, Beckman K, Greene HL, et al. Follow-up of patients with unexplained syncope and inducible ventricular tachyarrhythmias: analysis of the AVID registry and an AVID substudy. Antiarrhythmics versus implantable defibrillators. J Cardiovasc Electrophysiol 2001;12:996–1001.

30. Grossman SA, Fischer C, Lipsitz LA, et al. Predicting adverse outcomes in syncope. J Emerg Med 2007;33:233–9.

31. Baron-Esquivias G, Moreno SG, Martinez A, et al. Cost of diagnosis and treatment of syncope in patients admitted to a cardiology unit. Europace 2006;8:122–7.

32. D'Ascenzo F, Biondi-Zoccai G, Reed MJ, et al. Incidence, etiology and predictors of adverse outcomes in 43,315 patients presenting to the Emergency Department with syncope: an international meta-analysis. Int J Cardiol 2013;167(1):57–62.

33. Quinn J, McDermott D, Stiell I, et al. Prospective validation of the San Francisco Syncope Rule to predict patients with serious outcomes. Ann Emerg Med 2006;47:448–54.

34. Colivicchi F, Ammirati F, Melina D, et al. Development and prospective validation of a risk stratification system for patients with syncope in the emergency department: the OESIL risk score. Eur Heart J 2003;24:811–9.

35. Ammirati F, Colivicchi F, Minardi G, et al. The management of syncope in the hospital: the OESIL Study (Osservatorio Epidemiologico della Sincope nel Lazio). G Ital Cardiol 1999;29:533–9 [in Italian].

36. Del Rosso A, Ungar A, Maggi R, et al. Clinical predictors of cardiac syncope at initial evaluation in patients referred urgently to a general hospital: the EGSYS score. Heart 2008;94:1620–6.

37. Reed MJ, Newby DE, Coull AJ, et al. The Risk stratification of Syncope in the Emergency department (ROSE) pilot study: a comparison of existing syncope guidelines. Emerg Med J 2007;24:270–5.

38. Martin TP, Hanusa BH, Kapoor WN. Risk stratification of patients with syncope. Ann Emerg Med 1997;29:459–66.

39. Birnbaum A, Esses D, Bijur P, et al. Failure to validate the San Francisco Syncope Rule in an independent emergency department population. Ann Emerg Med 2008;52:151–9.

40. Reed MJ, Henderson SS, Newby DE, et al. One-year prognosis after syncope and the failure of the ROSE decision instrument to predict one-year adverse events. Ann Emerg Med 2011;58:250–6.

41. Costantino G, Perego F, Dipaola F, et al. Short- and long-term prognosis of syncope, risk factors, and role of hospital admission: results from the STePS (Short-Term Prognosis of Syncope) study. J Am Coll Cardiol 2008;51:276–83.

42. Quinn J, McDermott D. External validation of the San Francisco Syncope Rule. Ann Emerg Med 2007;50:742–3 [author reply: 743–4].

43. Quinn JV, Stiell IG, McDermott DA, et al. The San Francisco Syncope Rule vs physician judgment and decision making. Am J Emerg Med 2005;23:782–6.

44. Sun BC, Mangione CM, Merchant G, et al. External validation of the San Francisco Syncope Rule. Ann Emerg Med 2007;49:420–7, 427.e1–4.

45. Cosgriff TM, Kelly AM, Kerr D. External validation of the San Francisco Syncope Rule in the Australian context. CJEM 2007;9:157–61.

46. McCarthy F, McMahon CG, Geary U, et al. Management of syncope in the Emergency Department: a single hospital observational case series based on the application of European Society of Cardiology guidelines. Europace 2009;11:216–24.

47. Reed MJ, Newby DE, Coull AJ, et al. The ROSE (risk stratification of syncope in the emergency department) study. J Am Coll Cardiol 2010;55:713–21.

48. Huff JS, Decker WW, Quinn JV, et al. Clinical policy: critical issues in the evaluation and management of adult patients presenting to the emergency department with syncope. J Emerg Nurs 2007;33:e1–17.

49. Livanis EG, Kostopoulou A, Theodorakis GN, et al. Neurocardiogenic mechanisms of unexplained syncope in idiopathic dilated cardiomyopathy. Am J Cardiol 2007;99:558–62.

50. Oh JH, Hanusa BH, Kapoor WN. Do symptoms predict cardiac arrhythmias and mortality in patients with syncope? Arch Intern Med 1999;159: 375–80.

51. Barnes A. Cerebral manifestations of paroxysmal tachycardia. Am J Med Sci 1926;171:489–95.

52. Olshansky B. A Pepsi challenge. N Engl J Med 1999;340:2006.

53. Reed MJ, Gray A. Collapse query cause: the management of adult syncope in the emergency department. Emerg Med J 2006;23:589–94.

54. Alboni P, Brignole M, Menozzi C, et al. Diagnostic value of history in patients with syncope with or without heart disease. J Am Coll Cardiol 2001;37: 1921–8.

55. Mitro P, Kirsch P, Valocik G, et al. A prospective study of the standardized diagnostic evaluation of syncope. Europace 2011;13:566–71.

56. Iglesias JF, Graf D, Forclaz A, et al. Stepwise evaluation of unexplained syncope in a large ambulatory population. Pacing Clin Electrophysiol 2009; 32(Suppl 1):S202–6.

57. Sarasin FP, Pruvot E, Louis-Simonet M, et al. Stepwise evaluation of syncope: a prospective population-based controlled study. Int J Cardiol 2008;127:103–11.

58. Brignole M, Ungar A, Casagranda I, et al, Syncope Unit Project Investigators. Prospective multicentre systematic guideline-based management of patients referred to the syncope units of general hospitals. Europace 2010;12:109–18.

59. Brignole M, Ungar A, Bartoletti A, et al. Standardized-care pathway vs usual management of syncope patients presenting as emergencies at general hospitals. Europace 2006;8:644–50.

60. Sheldon RS, Morillo CA, Krahn AD, et al. Standardized approaches to the investigation of syncope: Canadian Cardiovascular Society position paper. Can J Cardiol 2011;27:246–53.

61. Krahn AD, Healey JS, Simpson CS, et al. Sentinel symptoms in patients with unexplained cardiac arrest: from the Cardiac Arrest Survivors with Preserved Ejection fraction Registry (CASPER). J Cardiovasc Electrophysiol 2012;23:60–6.

62. Sheldon R, Hersi A, Ritchie D, et al. Syncope and structural heart disease: historical criteria for vasovagal syncope and ventricular tachycardia. J Cardiovasc Electrophysiol 2010;21:1358–64.

63. Sheldon R. Syncope outcomes in a national health database: low risk is not no risk. J Am Coll Cardiol 2013;61:333–4.

64. Sarasin FP, Junod AF, Carballo D, et al. Role of echocardiography in the evaluation of syncope: a prospective study. Heart 2002;88:363–7.

65. Gatzoulis K, Sideris S, Theopistou A, et al. Long-term outcome of patients with recurrent syncope of unknown cause in the absence of organic heart disease and relation to results of baseline tilt table testing. Am J Cardiol 2003;92:876–9.

66. Harrison A, Morrison LK, Krishnaswamy P, et al. B-type natriuretic peptide predicts future cardiac events in patients presenting to the emergency department with dyspnea. Ann Emerg Med 2002; 39:131–8.

67. Vrtovec B, Delgado R, Zewail A, et al. Prolonged QTc interval and high B-type natriuretic peptide levels together predict mortality in patients with advanced heart failure. Circulation 2003;107: 1764–9.

68. Grimm W, Herzum I, Muller HH, et al. Value of heart rate variability to predict ventricular arrhythmias in recipients of prophylactic defibrillators with idiopathic dilated cardiomyopathy. Pacing Clin Electrophysiol 2003;26:411–5.

69. Bauer A, Schmidt G. Heart rate turbulence. J Electrocardiol 2003;36(Suppl):89–93.

70. Hohnloser SH, Ikeda T, Bloomfield DM, et al. T-wave alternans negative coronary patients with low ejection and benefit from defibrillator implantation. Lancet 2003;362:125–6.

71. Cohen RJ. Enhancing specificity without sacrificing sensitivity: potential benefits of using microvolt T-wave alternans testing to risk stratify the MADIT-II population. Card Electrophysiol Rev 2003;7:438–42.

72. Koutalas E, Kanoupakis E, Vardas P. Sudden cardiac death in non-ischemic dilated cardiomyopathy: a critical appraisal of existing and potential risk stratification tools. Int J Cardiol 2013;167(2): 335–41.

73. Priori SG, Napolitano C, Diehl L, et al. Dispersion of the QT interval. A marker of therapeutic efficacy in the idiopathic long QT syndrome. Circulation 1994; 89:1681–9.

74. Berbari EJ, Lazzara R. The significance of electrocardiographic late potentials: predictors of ventricular tachycardia. Annu Rev Med 1992;43:157–69.

75. Kuchar DL, Thorburn CW, Sammel NL. The role of signal averaged electrocardiography in the investigation of unselected patients with syncope. Aust N Z J Med 1985;15:697–703.

76. Gatzoulis KA, Karystinos G, Gialernios T, et al. Correlation of noninvasive electrocardiography with invasive electrophysiology in syncope of unknown origin: implications from a large syncope database. Ann Noninvasive Electrocardiol 2009;14:119–27.

77. Olshansky B, Mazuz M, Martins JB. Significance of inducible tachycardia in patients with syncope of unknown origin: a long-term follow-up. J Am Coll Cardiol 1985;5:216–23.

78. Andrews NP, Fogel RI, Pelargonio G, et al. Implantable defibrillator event rates in patients with unexplained syncope and inducible sustained ventricular tachyarrhythmias: a comparison with patients known to have sustained ventricular tachycardia. J Am Coll Cardiol 1999;34:2023–30.

79. Bass EB, Elson JJ, Fogoros RN, et al. Long-term prognosis of patients undergoing electrophysiologic studies for syncope of unknown origin. Am J Cardiol 1988;62:1186–91.

80. Krol RB, Morady F, Flaker GC, et al. Electrophysiologic testing in patients with unexplained syncope: clinical and noninvasive predictors of outcome. J Am Coll Cardiol 1987;10:358–63.

81. Fujimura O, Yee R, Klein GJ, et al. The diagnostic sensitivity of electrophysiologic testing in patients with syncope caused by transient bradycardia. N Engl J Med 1989;321:1703–7.

82. Pezawas T, Stix G, Kastner J, et al. Unexplained syncope in patients with structural heart disease and no documented ventricular arrhythmias: value of electrophysiologically guided implantable cardioverter defibrillator therapy. Europace 2003;5:305–12.

83. Militianu A, Salacata A, Seibert K, et al. Implantable cardioverter defibrillator utilization among device recipients presenting exclusively with syncope or near-syncope. J Cardiovasc Electrophysiol 1997;8:1087–97.

84. Oginosawa Y, Abe H, Nagatomo T, et al. Sustained polymorphic ventricular tachycardia unassociated with QT prolongation or bradycardia in the Kearns-Sayre syndrome. Pacing Clin Electrophysiol 2003;26:1911–2.

85. Rashid A, Kim MH. Kearns-Sayre syndrome: association with long QT syndrome? J Cardiovasc Electrophysiol 2002;13:184–5.

86. Kapoor WN, Hammill SC, Gersh BJ. Diagnosis and natural history of syncope and the role of invasive electrophysiologic testing. Am J Cardiol 1989;63:730–4.

87. Klein GJ, Gersh BJ, Yee R. Electrophysiological testing. The final court of appeal for diagnosis of syncope? Circulation 1995;92:1332–5.

88. Linzer M, Prystowsky EN, Divine GW, et al. Predicting the outcomes of electrophysiologic studies of patients with unexplained syncope: preliminary validation of a derived model. J Gen Intern Med 1991;6:113–20.

89. Rahimtoola SH, Zipes DP, Akhtar M, et al. Consensus statement of the Conference on the State of the Art of Electrophysiologic Testing in the Diagnosis and Treatment of Patients with Cardiac Arrhythmias. Circulation 1987;75:III3–11.

90. Teichman SL, Felder SD, Matos JA, et al. The value of electrophysiologic studies in syncope of undetermined origin: report of 150 cases. Am Heart J 1985;110:469–79.

91. Linzer M, Yang EH, Estes NA 3rd, et al. Diagnosing syncope. Part 2: unexplained syncope. Clinical Efficacy Assessment Project of the American College of Physicians. Ann Intern Med 1997;127:76–86.

92. Bachinsky WB, Linzer M, Weld L, et al. Usefulness of clinical characteristics in predicting the outcome of electrophysiologic studies in unexplained syncope. Am J Cardiol 1992;69:1044–9.

93. Link MS, Costeas XF, Griffith JL, et al. High incidence of appropriate implantable cardioverter-defibrillator therapy in patients with syncope of unknown etiology and inducible ventricular arrhythmias. J Am Coll Cardiol 1997;29:370–5.

94. Epstein AE, DiMarco JP, Ellenbogen KA, et al. ACC/AHA/HRS 2008 guidelines for device-based therapy of cardiac rhythm abnormalities: a report of the American College of Cardiology/American Heart Association Task Force on Practice Guidelines (writing committee to revise the ACC/AHA/NASPE 2002 guideline update for implantation of cardiac pacemakers and antiarrhythmia devices) developed in collaboration with the American Association for Thoracic Surgery and Society of Thoracic Surgeons. J Am Coll Cardiol 2008;51:e1–62.

95. Krahn AD, Klein GJ, Yee R, et al. Use of an extended monitoring strategy in patients with problematic syncope. Reveal Investigators. Circulation 1999;99:406–10.

96. Krahn AD, Klein GJ, Yee R, et al. The use of monitoring strategies in patients with unexplained syncope–role of the external and implantable loop recorder. Clin Auton Res 2004;14(Suppl 1):55–61.

97. Krahn AD, Klein GJ, Yee R, et al. The high cost of syncope: cost implications of a new insertable loop recorder in the investigation of recurrent syncope. Am Heart J 1999;137:870–7.

98. Farwell DJ, Freemantle N, Sulke N. The clinical impact of implantable loop recorders in patients with syncope. Eur Heart J 2006;27:351–6.

99. Davis S, Westby M, Pitcher D, et al. Implantable loop recorders are cost-effective when used to investigate transient loss of consciousness which is either suspected to be arrhythmic or remains unexplained. Europace 2012;14:402–9.

100. Shanmugam N, Liew R. The implantable loop recorder-an important addition to the armamentarium in the management of unexplained syncope. Ann Acad Med Singapore 2012;41:115–24.

101. Krahn AD, Klein GJ, Yee R, et al. Randomized assessment of syncope trial: conventional

diagnostic testing versus a prolonged monitoring strategy. Circulation 2001;104:46–51.

102. Edvardsson N, Frykman V, van Mechelen R, et al. Use of an implantable loop recorder to increase the diagnostic yield in unexplained syncope: results from the PICTURE registry. Europace 2011; 13:262–9.

103. Kabra R, Gopinathannair R, Sandesara C, et al. The dual role of implantable loop recorder in patients with potentially arrhythmic symptoms: a retrospective single-center study. Pacing Clin Electrophysiol 2009;32:908–12.

104. Petkar S, Hamid T, Iddon P, et al. Prolonged implantable electrocardiographic monitoring indicates a high rate of misdiagnosis of epilepsy—REVISE study. Europace 2012;14:1653–60.

105. Kulakowski P, Lelonek M, Krynski T, et al. Prospective evaluation of diagnostic work-up in syncope patients: results of the PL-US registry. Europace 2010;12:230–9.

106. Vitale E, Ungar A, Maggi R, et al. Discrepancy between clinical practice and standardized indications for an implantable loop recorder in patients with unexplained syncope. Europace 2010;12:1475–9.

107. Knight BP, Goyal R, Pelosi F, et al. Outcome of patients with nonischemic dilated cardiomyopathy and unexplained syncope treated with an implantable defibrillator. J Am Coll Cardiol 1999; 33:1964–70.

108. Fonarow GC, Feliciano Z, Boyle NG, et al. Improved survival in patients with nonischemic advanced heart failure and syncope treated with an implantable cardioverter-defibrillator. Am J Cardiol 2000;85:981–5.

109. Sanchez JM, Katsiyiannis WT, Gage BF, et al. Implantable cardioverter-defibrillator therapy improves long-term survival in patients with unexplained syncope, cardiomyopathy, and a negative electrophysiologic study. Heart Rhythm 2005;2: 367–73.

110. Peters S. Long-term follow-up and risk assessment of arrhythmogenic right ventricular dysplasia/cardiomyopathy: personal experience from different primary and tertiary centres. J Cardiovasc Med (Hagerstown) 2007;8:521–6.

111. Peters S, Trummel M, Koehler B, et al. Mechanisms of syncopes in arrhythmogenic right ventricular dysplasia-cardiomyopathy beyond monomorphic ventricular tachycardia. Int J Cardiol 2006;106: 52–4.

112. Spirito P, Autore C, Rapezzi C, et al. Syncope and risk of sudden death in hypertrophic cardiomyopathy. Circulation 2009;119:1703–10.

113. Khair GZ, Bamrah VS. Syncope in hypertrophic cardiomyopathy. I. Association with atrioventricular block. Am Heart J 1985;110:1081–3.

114. Khair GZ, Soni JS, Bamrah VS. Syncope in hypertrophic cardiomyopathy. II. Coexistence of atrioventricular block and Wolff-Parkinson-White syndrome. Am Heart J 1985;110:1083–6.

115. Nienaber CA, Hiller S, Spielmann RP, et al. Syncope in hypertrophic cardiomyopathy: multivariate analysis of prognostic determinants. J Am Coll Cardiol 1990;15:948–55.

116. Maron BJ, Shen WK, Link MS, et al. Efficacy of implantable cardioverter-defibrillators for the prevention of sudden death in patients with hypertrophic cardiomyopathy. N Engl J Med 2000;342: 365–73.

117. Maron BJ, Spirito P, Shen WK, et al. Implantable cardioverter-defibrillators and prevention of sudden cardiac death in hypertrophic cardiomyopathy. JAMA 2007;298:405–12.

118. Alexander ME, Cecchin F, Walsh EP, et al. Implications of implantable cardioverter defibrillator therapy in congenital heart disease and pediatrics. J Cardiovasc Electrophysiol 2004;15:72–6.

119. Jacob JC, Wang DH. Cardiac noncompaction: a rare cause of exertional syncope in an athlete. Curr Sports Med Rep 2012;11:64–9.

120. Shen WK, Decker WW, Smars PA, et al. Syncope Evaluation in the Emergency Department Study (SEEDS): a multidisciplinary approach to syncope management. Circulation 2004;110:3636–45.

Syncope and Driving

Juan C. Guzman, MD, MSc, FRCPC[a],
Carlos A. Morillo, MD, FRCPC, FESC, FHRS[b],*

KEYWORDS

- Syncope • Automobile driving • Cardiac arrhythmias • Sudden cardiac death • Guidelines
- Prognosis

KEY POINTS

- Syncope occurring while driving, and its recurrence, has obvious implications for personal and public safety.
- Vasovagal syncope is the most common type of syncope during driving, and patients with structural heart disease are potentially at high risk; most guidelines enforce restricting driving privileges under these circumstances, although the evidence that this action in fact reduces traffic accidents is limited.
- The current guidelines seem to be restrictive, given the lack of evidence that patients with syncope have a higher risk of vehicle accidents in comparison with the general population.
- The social, financial, and personal grief created by the current guidelines seems disproportionate to the overall risk. Future guidelines will certainly take this lack of evidence into account to further protect the rights of patients with syncope.

INTRODUCTION

Syncope, defined as a transient loss of consciousness (TLOC), is estimated to account for 1% to 3% of emergency department (ED) annual visits, and up to 6% of hospital admissions in North America[1] and around the world.[2] Although most potential causes of syncope are benign and self-limited, some are associated with significant morbidity and mortality, including life-threatening cardiac arrhythmias and structural heart disease.[3] Recurrence is highly variable and is related to the underlying etiology, and such recurrences can be extremely unpredictable.[4] Syncope while driving, as well as postsyncope recurrence, has obvious implications for personal and public safety. Thus consideration of restriction of privileges is intuitive, so as to protect both the patient and the public. However, restricting driving privileges leads to strained physician-patient

relationships, as most patients do not want to give up the independence offered by driving. However, this must be balanced with public safety.[5] This article reviews the current evidence related to syncope and driving, and the current recommendations pertaining to fitness to drive.

FITNESS TO DRIVE

Physicians are regularly called upon to evaluate medical fitness to drive. However, driving is an essential and daily activity, and the potential effects of a medical condition on driving capability should be a considered once a patient is referred for assessment of syncope.[6] When examining a patient to determine fitness to drive, both the patient's rights and the welfare of the community that will be exposed if the patient will drive should be taken into consideration. Physicians should be aware of

This article originally appeared in Cardiac Electrophysiology Clinics, Volume 5, Issue 4, December 2013.
The authors have nothing to disclose.
a Syncope & Autonomic Disorders Unit, Department of Medicine, Hamilton General Hospital, McMaster University, McMaster Wing Room 601, 237 Barton Street East, Hamilton, Ontario L8L 2X2, Canada; b Syncope & Autonomic Disorder Unit, Cardiology Division, Department of Medicine, McMaster University, David Braley CVSRI, Room C-3-120, 237 Barton Street East, Hamilton, Ontario L8L 2X2, Canada
* Corresponding author.
E-mail addresses: morillo@hhsc.ca; Carlos.Morillo@phri.ca

their responsibility or legislated requirement to report patients with medical conditions that make it unsafe for them to drive, according to the jurisdiction in which they practice.[6] Physicians should also be aware of the circumstances under which patients are likely to function. For example, the extreme demands related to operating emergency vehicles and commercial transportation vehicles suggest that drivers of these vehicles should be cautioned that even relatively minor functional defects may make it unsafe for them to drive.[6] Redelmeier and colleagues[7] recently reported that physicians' warnings to patients who are potentially unfit to drive may contribute to a decrease in subsequent trauma from road crashes, yet they may also exacerbate mood disorders and compromise the doctor-patient relationship.

The rights of individuals, including acceptance of personal risk, compete with society's right to legislate the level of risk it considers acceptable for performance of certain activities by individuals who may potentially cause harm to others. Any such policy must be fair to all persons, recognizing that restrictions may limit personal freedoms, job security, and feelings of well-being.[8]

PATHOPHYSIOLOGIC FEATURES OF SYNCOPE AND DRIVING

The final pathophysiologic pathway leading to syncope is sudden transient global cerebral hypoperfusion. Thus, conditions that reduce cardiac output (CO) and cause excessive vasodilatation can cause syncope. The pathophysiologic classification of the principal causes of syncope is detailed elsewhere in this issue in the article by Jean-Jacques Blanc.

Studies from selected and unselected populations have consistently demonstrated that neurally mediated syncope (NMS) is the most common form of syncope.[9–11] Orthostatic stress is recognized as a common trigger of NMS.[2] As a result, NMS theoretically would be uncommon in the seated position; therefore, a cardiac (as opposed to neurocardiogenic) cause of syncope is often suspected when syncope occurs while driving. In a small case-series study, Li and colleagues[12] reported that among 23 patients undergoing tilt-table testing for syncope while driving, 19 patients had a positive tilt-table response consistent with a neurally mediated origin. Using a case-control design, Sorajja and colleagues[13] studied consecutive patients evaluated for syncope from 1996 through 1998 at the Mayo Clinic. Of 3877 patients identified, 381 (9.8%) had syncope while driving (driving group). Compared with the 3496 patients (90.2%) who did not have syncope while driving,

the driving group was younger (P<.01), and had a higher percentage of male patients (P<.001), patients with a history of any cardiovascular disease, (P<.01) and patients with a history of stroke (P<.02). Syncope while driving was commonly caused by NMS (37.3%) and cardiac arrhythmias (11.8%). Overall, NMS also was the most common type of syncope while driving. The high prevalence of NMS occurring in the seated position during driving suggests that impaired neurally mediated reflexes may still trigger syncope in a significant proportion of patients driving.[13] Several mechanisms that may trigger NMS are plausible in the passively seated position without muscle tension or venous pooling, especially in the setting of pre-existing dehydration or intravascular depletion.[2] The warm environment in a car may lead to a level of cutaneous vasodilatation capable of triggering NMS while driving.[14] Strong emotional stimulation while driving is another potential trigger of syncope in the sitting position.[15] The observation that NMS is common while driving is hypothesis generating, including the possibility that driving may act as a trigger. There may be a role for patient education with respect to minimizing both the risk of recurrent syncope and harm to the individual and others. By encouraging frequent breaks while driving and optimal hydration, and, most importantly, by having patients recognize prodromal symptoms promptly, it may be possible to reduce the incidence of recurrent syncope.[4] However, this is clearly speculative and is based on common sense, as there is insufficient evidence to support this recommendation.

Of note, the etiology and recurrence rate of syncope does not differ whether or not the index episode occurred while driving.[13] Thus, the clinical approach to syncope evaluation and recommendations for driving should not differ with regard to the time or activity related with the presentation of the syncopal episode.[4] A patient with structural heart disease (reduced ejection fraction, previous myocardial infarction, significant congenital heart disease) is potentially at high risk, and should have driving privileges revoked pending clarification of the extent of underlying heart disease and cause of syncope. It is well known that syncope, a previous aborted cardiac arrest, 1 or more episodes of sustained ventricular tachycardia (VT), and a history of sudden death in young family members are strong indicators of a high risk of sudden cardiac death (SCD).[6] Overall, SCD while performing dangerous activities is either rare or underreported, and seldom results in injury to others. Risk depends somewhat on specific underlying cardiac arrhythmias.[8] Moreover, the TOVA trial[16] examined the risk of implantable cardioverter-defibrillator (ICD) shocks for VT or ventricular fibrillation (VF) associated with driving. Although the risk of ICD shock for VT/VF was transiently increased in the 30-minute period after driving, the risk was not elevated during driving and the absolute risk was low. These data provide reassurance that driving by ICD patients should not translate into an important rate of personal or public injury.

PREVALENCE, RECURRENCE, AND PROGNOSIS

In a survey conducted among 104 patients, 3% reported syncope occurring while driving, of which only 1% crashed their vehicles.[17] Among those advised not to drive, only 9% followed this advice. Patients with life-threatening ventricular arrhythmias enrolled in the AVID trial had a significantly higher incidence of symptoms suggestive of tachyarrhythmia while driving, although these episodes were unlikely to lead to motor vehicle accidents (0.4% per patient-year).[18] The probability of an accident was lower than the annual accident rate in the general population, and was independent of the duration of abstinence from driving.

In the study reported by Sorajja and colleagues,[13] the actuarial 12-month syncope-recurrence rate was 14.1% in those who had initial syncope while driving, which was not significantly different from the recurrence rate in patients without initial syncope while driving. The 12-month recurrence rate of syncope while driving was 1.1%, with a 7% cumulative probability over the duration of the 8-year follow-up. A 6-month driving restriction may be supported for patients with initial syncope while driving. Unfortunately, 70% of patients who had a repeated episode of syncope while driving had their follow-up episode more than 1 year after the index syncopal event. Thus, any mandatory postsyncopal driving restriction for a period of 3 to 6 months may not accomplish the goal of public safety.[5] Similarly, it can be argued that the overall burden of syncope while driving within the context of other major traffic accidents that lead to death and significant injury is exceedingly low, potentially not supporting these current recommendations. Finally, the long-term survival in the driving group was comparable with that of an age-matched and sex-matched cohort from the Minnesota population. Among the driving group, syncope recurred in 72 patients, 35 of whom (48.6%) had recurrence more than 6 months after the initial evaluation.[13] The presence of underlying cardiac disease increases the risk of recurrence, and the following markers have been identified as predictive of reduced survival of patients with syncope while

driving[13]: VT (hazard ratio [HR] 5.12), atrioventricular block (HR 4.46), coronary artery disease (HR 2.63), history of myocardial infarction (HR 2.35), any cardiovascular disease (HR 2.28), and advanced age (HR 1.07).

CANADIAN CARDIOVASCULAR SOCIETY RISK OF HARM FORMULA

The Canadian Cardiovascular Society (CCS) sponsored a Consensus Conference at which a formula to calculate risk of harm from driving was developed.[19] The risk of harm (RH) to other road users posed by the driver with heart disease is assumed to be directly proportional to the following: (1) time spent behind the wheel or distance driven in a given time period (TD): 0.04 [16,000 km/y] for the average car driver, 0.25 [138,000 km/y] for the average commercial driver; (2) type of vehicle driven (V): 1.0 for a commercial heavy truck and 0.28 for a standard-size passenger car; (3) risk of sudden cardiac incapacitation (SCI); and (4) the probability that such an event will result in a fatal or injury-producing accident (Ac): 0.02. This statement is expressed by the formula: $RH = TD \times V \times SCI \times Ac$. Based on the above calculations, an acceptable RH was considered to be 1/20,000 or 0.00005. Of note, this equation includes the time spent driving and the special risk of a trucking accident given the size of the vehicle. With the use of this formula and the data reported by Sorajja and colleagues,[13] which showed the actuarial recurrence of syncope over the first 12 months to be 14.1%, the RH for syncope is equal to $0.04 \times 0.28 \times 0.141 \times 0.02 = 0.00003$ (in other words, an acceptable risk according to the formula).[4] For public safety, the risk of syncope-mediated driving accidents (0.8% per year) appeared to be substantially less than in young (16–24 years) and elderly drivers (high-risk accident groups).[2]

COMMERCIAL DRIVING

A unique population of patients whose driving is required for their livelihood is those with commercial driver's licenses.[4] Although a private and a commercial driver may have an identical risk of syncope as a consequence of their particular disease state, the risks of driving over time are very different. Commercial drivers spend more time behind the wheel, their vehicles are larger (and in the event of an accident may lead to more collateral damage than would a car), and the type of driving (local or highway at high speed) may have different attendant risks. As such, from a public safety perspective the risks of loss of consciousness at the wheel are different for private and commercial drivers. Thus, the restrictions for driving for those who operate commercial vehicles are much more stringent than for private driving, often involving permanent prohibition of operating commercial vehicles.[8,20] However, there does not appear to be any hard evidence for an increased overall incidence of fatal traffic accidents in this population.

Table 1
Canadian Medical Association recommendations for nontachyarrhythmic syncope

	Private Driving	Commercial Driving
Single episode of typical VVS[a]	No restriction	
Diagnosed and treated cause (eg, PPM for bradycardia, valvular heart disease, hypertrophic cardiomyopathy)	Wait 1 wk	Wait 1 mo
Reversible cause (eg, hemorrhage, dehydration)	Successful treatment of underlying condition	
Situational syncope with avoidable trigger (eg, micturition/ defecation)	Wait 1 wk	
Single episode of unexplained syncope Recurrent vasovagal syncope (with in 12 mo)	Wait 1 wk	Wait 12 mo
Recurrent episodes of unexplained syncope (within 12 mo)	Wait 3 mo	Wait 12 mo

Abbreviations: PPM, permanent pacemaker; VVS, vasovagal syncope.
[a] No restriction is recommended unless the syncope occurs in the sitting position, or if it is determined that there may be an insufficient prodrome to pilot the vehicle to the roadside to a stop before losing consciousness. If vasovagal syncope is atypical, the restrictions for "unexplained" syncope apply.
Data from Canadian Medical Association. CMA driver's guide: determining medical fitness to operate motor vehicle. 8th edition. Ottawa: CMA; 2012. Available at: http://www.cma.ca/driversguide

ETHICS BEHIND REGULATIONS AND GUIDELINES

Medical ethics examines the rightness and wrongness of human acts, the logic used in ethical arguments, and the assumptions on which ethical decisions are based in the context of the individual health and physicians' medical practice. Owing to the tremendous impact of regulation of activities on individuals, attention is given here to ethical issues related to regulation of patients with arrhythmias and syncope. In principle, most individuals are virtuous and do not want to harm another. Thus, if a person has a medical condition that could cause unconsciousness at any time, and if this risk cannot be controlled or eliminated by medical treatment, it is not unethical to enact guidelines or regulations preventing that person from engaging in certain activities.[8]

Knowledge of a patient's condition is held in confidence in the doctor-patient relationship. Medical information may be released to a third party only when the patient has authorized it. If an employer/government regulatory agency

Table 2
Canadian Medical Association recommendations for tachyarrhythmic syncope

	Private Driving	Commercial Driving
VF (nonreversible cause)	6 mo after event	Disqualified
Hemodynamically unstable VT	6 mo after event	Disqualified
VT or VF due to reversible cause[a]	No driving until/unless successful treatment of underlying condition	
Paroxysmal SVT	Satisfactory control	Satisfactory control
AF or atrial flutter[b]	Satisfactory control	Satisfactory control

Abbreviations: AF, atrial fibrillation; SVT, supraventricular tachycardia; VF, ventricular fibrillation; VT, ventricular tachycardia.
[a] Examples include, but are not limited to: VF within 24 hours of myocardial infarction, VF during coronary angiography, VF with electrocution, VF secondary to drug toxicity. Reversible-cause VF recommendations overrule the VF recommendations if the reversible cause is treated successfully and the VF does not recur.
[b] Drivers should receive chronic anticoagulation if clinically indicated (ie, in presence of AF or atrial flutter).
Data from Canadian Medical Association. CMA driver's guide: determining medical fitness to operate motor vehicle. 8th edition. Ottawa: CMA; 2012. Available at: http://www.cma.ca/driversguide

does not use its own medical staff to evaluate an employee's fitness for certain activities, the physician may release information only with the permission of the patient. However, if the patient wishes to withhold medical information from his or her employer/government regulatory agency to avoid losing his or her job, the physician who knows the patient's condition, the responsibilities of the patient's job, and danger to other parties if the patient remains on the job may not ethically withhold this information. The physician must try to persuade the patient to give permission to release such information, but if the patient does not, it is ethical for the physician to break the rule of confidentiality if he or she knows that grave harm could result from his or her silence. The ethical principles of beneficence and no maleficence outweigh the principle of confidentiality in such a situation. The responsible medical ethical action for the physician is to release the information to the proper authority with full disclosure to the patient.[8]

CURRENT GUIDELINES AND RECOMMENDATIONS
Canadian Medical Association Driver's Guide: Determining the Medical Fitness to Operate a Motor Vehicle

The Canadian Medical Association (CMA) guide on the evaluation of fitness to drive[6] has gained a global reputation since it was first published in 1974. This guide provides physicians and medical practitioners with current, practical information regarding counseling patients on the effects of their state of health on their fitness to drive (**Tables 1** and **2**). According to the CMA guidelines most episodes of syncope are due to NMS, which can usually be diagnosed by history and does not warrant further investigation. If syncope remains unexplained after initial assessment, further testing is recommended to reach a diagnosis and to direct possible therapy.

Table 3
American Heart Association and Heart Rhythm Society recommendations for neurally mediated syncope

	Private Driving	Commercial Driving
NMS mild	No restriction	Wait 1 wk
NMS severe treated	Wait 3 wk	Wait 6 wk
NMS severe untreated	Total restriction	
CSS mild	No restriction	
CSS severe treated with control	Wait 1 wk	Wait 1 wk
CSS severe treated with uncertain control	Wait 3 wk	Wait 6 wk
CCS severe untreated	Total restriction	

Abbreviations: CSS, carotid sinus hypersensitivity syndrome; NMS, neurally mediated syncope.

From Epstein AE, Miles WM, Benditt DG, et al. Personal and public safety issues related to arrhythmias that may affect consciousness: implications for regulation and physician recommendations. A medical/scientific statement from the American Heart Association and the North American Society of Pacing and Electrophysiology. Circulation 1996;94(5):1161; with permission.

Table 4
American Heart Association and Heart Rhythm Society recommendations for syncope and associated arrhythmias before specific treatment

	Private Driving	Commercial Driving
Bradycardia without PPM	Total restriction	
Bradycardia with PPM nondependent	No restriction	
Bradycardia with PPM dependent	Wait for 1 wk	Wait for 4 wk
Nonsustained VT	3 mo free interval	6 mo free nterval
Sustained VT	6 mo free interval	Total restriction
VF	Total restriction	
SVT	Restrictions until after initiation of therapy that eliminates symptoms	
SVT with uncontrolled symptoms	Total restriction	

Abbreviations: PPM, permanent pacemaker; SVT, supraventricular tachycardia; VF, ventricular fibrillation; VT, ventricular tachycardia.

From Epstein AE, Miles WM, Benditt DG, et al. Personal and public safety issues related to arrhythmias that may affect consciousness: implications for regulation and physician recommendations. A medical/scientific statement from the American Heart Association and the North American Society of Pacing and Electrophysiology. Circulation 1996;94(5):1160; with permission.

Table 5
Recommendations concerning patients with syncope who drive

	Group 1: Private Driving	Group 2: Professional Driving
NMS single/mild	No restrictions	No restriction unless it occurred during high-risk activity[a]
Recurrent syncope	After symptoms are controlled	Permanent restriction unless effective treatment has been established
Unexplained syncope	No restriction unless absence of prodrome, occurrence during driving, or presence of severe structural heart disease	After diagnosis and appropriate therapy is established
Cardiac arrhythmia with medical treatment	After successful treatment is established	After successful treatment is established
Pacemaker implant	After 1 wk	After appropriate function is established
Successful catheter ablation	After successful treatment is established	After long-term successful treatment is established

Group 1: private drivers of motorcycles, cars, and other small vehicles with and without a trailer; Group 2: professional drivers of vehicles over 3.5 tons or passenger-carrying vehicles exceeding 8 seats excluding the driver. Drivers of taxicabs, small ambulances, and other vehicles form an intermediate category between the ordinary private driver and the vocational driver, and should follow local legislation.

[a] Neurally mediated syncope (NMS) is defined as severe if it is very frequent, or occurring during the prosecution of a high-risk activity, or recurrent or unpredictable in high-risk patients.

From Moya A, Sutton R, Ammirati F, et al. Guidelines for the diagnosis and management of syncope (version 2009). Eur Heart J 2009;30(21):2664; with permission.

American Heart Association and the Heart Rhythm Society: Personal and Public Safety Issues Related to Arrhythmias that May Affect Consciousness

The American Heart Association (AHA) and the Hearth Rhythm Society (HRS) have formulated several recommendations (**Tables 3** and **4**).[8,21] These guidelines are not applicable to every patient in every situation, and physicians are encouraged to use their own judgment in making a recommendation for any given patient. It must be emphasized that many of the recommendations are based on limited data.

According to the AHA/HRS, the decision to allow a patient to resume driving should be based on the severity and nature of the presenting event. Mild NMS or carotid sinus hypersensitivity (CSS) is characterized by mild symptoms, occurs with warning and usually only with standing, has clear precipitating causes, and is infrequent. By distinction, severe NMS or CSS is characterized by severe symptoms (usually syncope), occurs without warning and in any position, has no clear precipitating causes, and/or occurs frequently.

Guidelines for the Diagnosis and Management of Syncope (Version 2009): The Task Force for the Diagnosis and Management of Syncope of the European Society of Cardiology

The 2009 European Society of Cardiology (ESC) guidelines on syncope made recommendations on driving and syncope. According to the ESC, data suggest that the risk of vehicle accidents in patients with a history of syncope is not different from that of the general population of drivers without syncope.[2] ESC recommendations are shown in **Table 5**.

SUMMARY

Syncope occurring while driving, as well as its recurrence, has obvious implications for personal and public safety. Vasovagal syncope is the most common type of syncope while driving. Patients with structural heart disease are potentially at high risk, and most guidelines enforce restriction of driving privileges under these circumstances, although the evidence that this action in fact reduces traffic accidents is limited. The current guidelines seem to be somewhat restrictive, given the lack of evidence that patients with syncope have a higher risk of vehicle accidents in comparison with the general population. The social, financial, and personal grief created by the current guidelines seems disproportionate to the overall risk. Future guidelines will certainly take this lack of evidence into account to further protect the rights of patients with syncope.

REFERENCES

1. ACEP. Clinical policy: critical issues in the evaluation and management of patients presenting with syncope. Ann Emerg Med 2001;37(6):771–6.

2. Moya A, Sutton R, Ammirati F, et al. Guidelines for the diagnosis and management of syncope (version 2009). Eur Heart J 2009;30(21):2631–71.

3. Kapoor WN, Karpf M, Wieand S, et al. A prospective evaluation and follow-up of patients with syncope. N Engl J Med 1983;309(4):197–204.

4. Curtis AB, Epstein AE. Syncope while driving: how safe is safe? Circulation 2009;120(11):921–3.

5. Raj SR. Driving restrictions in patients following syncope is difficult for physicians. Auton Neurosci 2009; 151(2):71–3.

6. CMA. CMA driver's guide: determining medical fitness to operate motor vehicle. In: CMA, editor. 8th edition. CMA; 2012. Available at: http://www.cma.ca/driversguide. Accessed 2012.

7. Redelmeier DA, Yarnell CJ, Thiruchelvam D, et al. Physicians' warnings for unfit drivers and the risk of trauma from road crashes. N Engl J Med 2012; 367(13):1228–36.

8. Epstein AE, Miles WM, Benditt DG, et al. Personal and public safety issues related to arrhythmias that may affect consciousness: implications for regulation and physician recommendations. A medical/scientific statement from the American Heart Association and the North American Society of Pacing and Electrophysiology. Circulation 1996;94(5):1147–66.

9. Soteriades ES, Evans JC, Larson MG, et al. Incidence and prognosis of syncope. N Engl J Med 2002;347(12):878–85.

10. Blitzer ML, Saliba BC, Ghantous AE, et al. Causes of impaired consciousness while driving a motorized vehicle. Am J Cardiol 2003;91(11):1373–4.

11. Ammirati F, Colivicchi F, Santini M. Diagnosing syncope in clinical practice. Implementation of a simplified diagnostic algorithm in a multicentre prospective trial—the OESIL 2 study (Osservatorio Epidemiologico della Sincope nel Lazio). Eur Heart J 2000;21(11):935–40.

12. Li H, Weitzel M, Easley A, et al. Potential risk of vasovagal syncope for motor vehicle driving. Am J Cardiol 2000;85(2):184–6.

13. Sorajja D, Nesbitt GC, Hodge DO, et al. Syncope while driving: clinical characteristics, causes, and prognosis. Circulation 2009;120(11):928–34.

14. Hainsworth R. Pathophysiology of syncope. Clin Auton Res 2004;14(Suppl 1):18–24.

15. Mosqueda-Garcia R, Furlan R, Tank J, et al. The elusive pathophysiology of neurally mediated syncope. Circulation 2000;102(23):2898–906.

16. Albert CM, Rosenthal L, Calkins H, et al. Driving and implantable cardioverter-defibrillator shocks for ventricular arrhythmias: results from the TOVA study. J Am Coll Cardiol 2007;50(23):2233–40.

17. Maas R, Ventura R, Kretzschmar C, et al. Syncope, driving recommendations, and clinical reality: survey of patients. BMJ 2003;326(7379):21.

18. Akiyama T, Powell JL, Mitchell LB, et al. Resumption of driving after life-threatening ventricular tachyarrhythmia. N Engl J Med 2001;345(6):391–7.

19. Simpson C, Dorian P, Gupta A, et al. Assessment of the cardiac patient for fitness to drive: drive subgroup executive summary. Can J Cardiol 2004; 20(13):1314–20.

20. Blumenthal R, Braunstein J, Connolly H, et al. Cardiovascular Advisory Panel guidelines for the medical examination of commercial motor vehicle drivers. 2009. Available at: http://www.fmcsa.dot.gov/documents/cardio.pdf. Accessed 2009.

21. Epstein AE, Baessler CA, Curtis AB, et al. Addendum to "Personal and public safety issues related to arrhythmias that may affect consciousness: implications for regulation and physician recommendations. A medical/scientific statement from the American Heart Association and the North American Society of Pacing and Electrophysiology". Public safety issues in patients with implantable defibrillators. A scientific statement from the American Heart Association and the Heart Rhythm Society. Heart Rhythm 2007; 4(3):386–93.

Therapy for Syncope

Angel Moya, MD, PhD

KEYWORDS

- Syncope • Reflex syncope • Counterpressure maneuvers • Cardiac syncope
- Syncope secondary to orthostatic hypotension • Pacemaker therapy • Bundle branch block

KEY POINTS

- The treatment of patients with syncope depends on the cause and final mechanism of syncopal episodes.
- Reflex syncope is a benign condition, with a good prognosis in terms of survival and only patients with recurrent and severe episodes need specific treatment.
- The initial measures for treating patients with reflex syncope are nonpharmacologic: provide information about the benign status of their condition, help in identifying and avoiding triggers, water ingestion, counterpressure maneuvers in those patients with prodromal symptoms, and tilt training in selected and motivated patients who are unresponsiveness to other treatments.
- Drug therapy has generally not showed any beneficial effect in patients with reflex syncope, with the possible exception of β-blockers in patients older than 42 years.
- In patients with syncope secondary to orthostatic hypotension, a multifactorial approach, including good hydration, reducing hypotensive drugs, compressive stockings, elevation of the head of the bed, and eventually fludrocortisone, can be helpful.
- In patients with suspected cardiac syncope and a high-risk profile for cardiac events or sudden death, an implantable cardioverter defibrillator must be considered irrespective of the final mechanism of syncope.
- In all patients with syncope of unknown origin, bundle branch block, and preserved left ventricular ejection fraction, 2 different strategies are proposed: a sequential strategy consisting of an electrophysiologic study, and if it is not diagnostic, implanting an implantable loop recorder or to implant a pacemaker without any additional test.

INTRODUCTION

In the therapeutic approach of any cardiovascular disease, 2 different objectives must be taken into consideration: relieving symptoms and improving the prognosis.

In syncope, relieving symptoms involves avoiding syncopal recurrences or, if this is not possible, at least reducing the number of syncopal recurrences. In some patients, another goal can be to convert recurrent sudden unexpected syncope leading to trauma to a syncope preceded by prodromal symptoms, allowing the patients to avoid injury.

The prognosis of patients with syncope depends on the cause (**Table 1**).[1–6] Patients with reflex syncope in general have a good prognosis in terms of survival[7] and, consequently, these patients should only be treated if they have frequent and disabling symptoms. In contrast, most patients with cardiac syncope have a poor prognosis in terms of survival, mainly related to the type and severity of the underlying heart disease and, consequently, in those patients, the treatment should be aimed at not only preventing syncopal recurrences but also decreasing the risk of cardiovascular events or sudden cardiac death.

This article originally appeared in Cardiac Electrophysiology Clinics, Volume 5, Issue 4, December 2013.
Conflict of Interest: Dr A. Moya received some modest fees for lectures from Medtronic, St Jude Medical and Boston Scientific.
Arrhythmia Unit, Cardiology Department, Vall d'Hebron Hospital, Autonoma University Barcelona, P. Vall d'Hebrón 119 – 129, 08035 Barcelona, Spain
E-mail address: amoyamitjans@gmail.com

Table 1	
Etiologic classification of syncope	
Reflex syncope (neurally mediated)	Vasovagal Situational Carotid sinus syncope Atypical forms
Orthostatic hypotension	Primary autonomic failure Secondary autonomic failure Drug-induced Volume depletion
Cardiac	Arrhythmia • Bradycardia • Tachycardia Structural heart disease

Accordingly, the first point in the management of patients with syncope is to establish the cause and risk stratification.[1] The diagnostic process in patients with syncope is not always easy and includes a detailed clinical history, physical examination and baseline electrocardiogram; according to the results of these initial approaches, some additional tests must be performed. Using this strategy, the cause of syncope is diagnosed in 60% to 80% of patients; in the remaining patients, risk stratification can be established to identify those patients at risk of having cardiac events or death at midterm follow-up.

This article reviews the treatment of patients with syncope according to the different causes.

REFLEX SYNCOPE

Reflex syncope (RS) traditionally refers to a heterogeneous group of conditions in which cardiovascular reflexes that are normally useful in controlling the circulation become intermittently inappropriate in response to a trigger, resulting in vasodilatation and/or bradycardia and thereby in a decrease in arterial blood pressure and global cerebral perfusion.[1] The timing, contribution, and magnitude of these 2 components, hypotension and bradycardia, vary from one patient to another, and sometimes from one episode to another in the same patient (**Fig. 1**).

A reflex mechanism is the most common cause of syncope in the general population with a high incidence in the young population.[8,9] Most patients with RS have occasional episodes, usually triggered by some recognizable circumstances, and preceded by prodromal symptoms; however, some patients have frequent recurrences, sometimes without previous prodromal symptoms, which can lead to injury and severe impairment of their quality of life.

In patients with RS, the therapeutic strategy ranges from counseling, only to the possibility of implanting a pacemaker (**Table 2**). Most patients with RS are young without any other comorbidity[8,9] and syncope episodes tend to occur in clusters with several recurrences during a period of time followed by long asymptomatic periods or event complete remission; consequently, caution is advised before implementing aggressive treatments.[10]

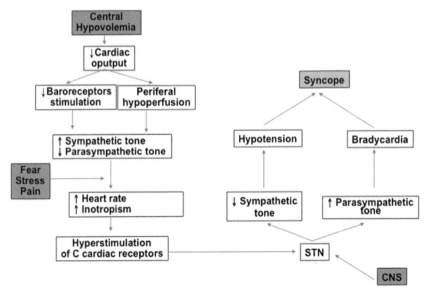

Fig. 1. Syncope pathophysiology. CNS, central nervous system; STN, solitary tract nucleus.

Table 2
Therapeutic strategies for treating patients with reflex syncope

Strategy	Patient Population
Explanation of the diagnosis, provision of reassurance, and explanation of risk of recurrence	In every patient
Increase in ingestion of salt and water	In every patient
Isometric physical counterpressure maneuvers	In patients with prodromal symptoms
Tilt training	In selected and motivated patients with recurrent episodes refractory to other measures
Drugs	No evidence of effectiveness with possible exception of β-blockers in patients older than 42 y
Cardiac pacing	In patients older than 40 y, with recurrent unexpected syncope in whom an asystole is documented during spontaneous syncope or elicited by adenosine 5′-triphosphate

General Measures

Patients with RS should be informed that their condition is benign and usually self-limited, which helps to reduce anxiety.

Some patients recognize the triggers, whereas others are not aware of their presence. A detailed history can be helpful not only in identifying some triggers but also in helping the patient to identify and avoid them.

Water Ingestion

Several studies performed during tilt testing have shown that acute water ingestion (approximately 500 mL) increases peripheral resistance, increasing arterial blood pressure and increasing tolerance to tilt testing.[11–14] Although these studies have been confined to tilt testing and there are no data on their impact in the follow-up of these patients, this measure can be recommended in most patients because it is not harmful and does not incur additional costs.

Physical Counterpressure Maneuvers

In 2001, 2 different studies showed that performing some muscle tensing maneuvers, either with arm tensing[15] or with leg crossing (**Fig. 2**),[16] during the initial phase of the reflex response during tilt testing, abolished or at least delayed the development of induced syncope.

These preliminary data led to a multicenter controlled study of 223 patients with recurrent RS and recognizable prodromal symptoms.[17] Patients were randomized to perform counterpressure maneuvers (arm tensing or leg crossing) when they had prodromal symptoms versus conventional treatment. Over a mean follow-up of 14 months, there was a significant reduction in syncopal recurrences in the group of patients allocated to counterpressure maneuvers compared with the control group.

According to this study, counterpressure maneuvers should be implemented in those patients with RS and prodromal symptoms.

Tilt Training

In 1998, Ector and colleagues[18] published some observational studies in which they showed that in patients with recurrent syncope and a positive tilt testing response, in-hospital sequential tilt testing until they became negative, followed by a similar maneuver daily at home, was effective in reducing syncopal recurrences.

In recent years, several investigators have performed randomized nonblinded trials with conflicting results.[19–21] One of the problems in interpreting the results of these trials was that there was low compliance in the group of patients allocated to tilt training. More recently, Tan and colleagues[22] published a blinded study of 22 patients in which the control group performed a sham maneuver, and those patients allocated to tilt training had fewer recurrences than those in the control group.

Thus, although the data supporting that tilt training is an effective treatment in all patients with recurrent syncope are limited, it can be recommended in selected and well-motivated patients with recurrent syncope who are not responding to other treatments.

Drug Therapy

Based on the pathophysiologic mechanism of RS, several drugs have been proposed and tested for treating patients with RS (**Box 1**).

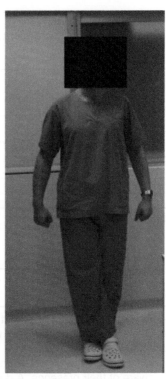

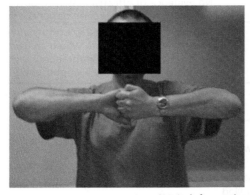

Fig. 2. Counterpressure maneuvers: arm tensing in left panel and leg crossing in right panel.

Scopolamine,[23] dysopiramide,[24] and clonidine[25] were tested in observational trials and none proved to be effective.

Fludrocortisone was tested in a small, randomized, double-blind trial in children, and showed no benefits.[26] Currently, there is an ongoing multicenter randomized trial with fludrocortisone versus placebo in patients with RS, but the final results have not yet been published.[27]

Several studies have analyzed the role of β-blockers (metoprolol,[28–30] propranolol,[28,31] nadolol,[31] and atenolol[32]) in patients with recurrent RS, and overall they did not show beneficial effects in patients with recurrent RS. A recent study including 2 different populations, one an observational cohort and the other patients from a randomized study (POST trial),[29] suggested that β-blockers may be beneficial in patients with RS aged 42 years or older.[33]

Etilefrine has been studied in several randomized studies, both in tilt testing[34] and in clinical follow-up,[35] and there was no benefit compared with placebo.

Initial uncontrolled studies suggested that midodrine was useful in preventing syncope recurrences in patients with RS.[36–38] Two controlled studies, one in an adult population[39] and the other in a pediatric population,[40] showed that midodrine used as a first-line therapy was effective in reducing syncope recurrences. However, most recently, Romme and colleagues[41] performed a randomized crossover study, in which they compared midodrine versus placebo in patients in whom nonpharmacologic therapy failed to prevent syncope recurrences; midodrine was not

> **Box 1**
> **Drugs for treating patients with reflex syncope that have been assessed in controlled trials**
>
> β-Blockers
>
> - Propranolol
> - Nadolol
> - Metoprolol
> - Atenolol
>
> Dysopiramide
>
> Clonidine
>
> Serotonin reuptake inhibitors
>
> Scopolamine
>
> Fludrocortisone
>
> α-Adrenergic
>
> - Etilefrine
> - Midrodine

superior to placebo in preventing syncope recurrences in this population.

Two different controlled trials analyzed the role of serotonin reuptake inhibitors in patients with RS with conflicting results.[42,43] There is not yet enough evidence of the beneficial effect of serotonin reuptake inhibitors in preventing syncope recurrence.

In summary, there is not yet enough evidence favoring the use of drugs for preventing syncope recurrences in patients with RS.[44] Recent data suggest that the use of β-blockers in patients older than 42 years can be effective, but these data need to be confirmed in a specific controlled trial focused on this population.[33]

Cardiac Pacing

RS has 2 components, the cardioinhibitory and vasodepressor, that are always present, therefore several investigators have analyzed the possible role of pacemaker implantation (PI) in patients with recurrent reflex cardioinhibitory syncope.

The first controlled studies were published between 1999 and 2003 (**Table 3**). Two of them compared PI versus conventional treatment[45,46] and the third compared PI with β-blockers,[47] which at the time was considered an effective treatment. In all these studies, patients were included if they had recurrent syncope and a positive cardioinhibitory response to tilt testing. In all 3 trials, patients allocated to PI, had a significant reduction in the rate of syncope recurrence compared with controls. To eliminate a possible

placebo effect of PI,[48] new trials were designed with similar selection criteria but PI was performed in all eligible patients. Once a pacemaker had been implanted, patients were randomized to pacemaker ON versus pacemaker OFF. In 2 of these studies, the syncopal recurrence rate at follow-up was the same in both groups.[49,50] In a third study, which used a pacemaker with a closed-loop stimulation algorithm, showed a reduction of syncopal recurrence in paced patients.[51] However, this study had methodological problems linked to randomization. However, in all these studies, the response to tilt testing was used to identify patients eligible for PI. In recent years, it has been demonstrated that there is poor correlation between the response observed during tilt testing and spontaneous episodes mainly in terms of heart rate pattern, suggesting that the response to tilt testing may not be the best tool for identifying those patients who might benefit from PI.[52–54]

Two more recent controlled blinded trials that also compared pacemaker ON and OFF in patients with syncope and asystole, either triggered with intravenous administration of adenosine 5′-triphosphate[55] or documented by an implantable loop recorder (ILR) during spontaneous syncope,[56] have shown that those patients with the pacemaker ON had a significant reduction in syncope recurrences.

In summary, it seems that in a selected population of adult patients (usually older than 40 years), with recurrent RS in whom an asystole longer the 3 seconds is documented during spontaneous

Table 3
Trials that have assessed the role of pacing in reflex syncope

Trial	Inclusion Criteria	Design
VPS[45]	Positive TT with HR <60, 70, 80 bpm	PI vs conventional treatment
VASIS[46]	Positive TT with HR <40 bpm or asystole >3 s	PI vs conventional treatment
SYDIT[47]	Positive TT with HR <40 bpm or asystole >3 s	PI vs atenolol
VPSII[49]	Positive TT with BP × HR <6000	PI with randomization DDD vs ODO
SYNPACE[50]	Positive TT with HR <40 bpm or asystole >3 s	PI with randomization DDD vs ODO
INVASY[51]	Positive TT with cardioinhibitory or mixed response	PI with randomization DDD-CLS vs DDI
Flamang et al,[55] 2012	Asystole >10 s after intravenous ATP administration	PI with randomization DDD vs AAI
ISSUE 3[56]	Syncope with documented asystole >3 s or asymptomatic spontaneous asystole >6 s (usually documented by ILR)	PI with randomization DDD vs VVI 40 bpm

Abbreviations: ATP, adenosine 5′-triphosphate; BP, blood pressure; bpm, beats per minute; HR, heart rhythm; ILR, implantable loop recorder; PI, pacemaker implantation; TT, tilt testing.

syncope or eventually after adenosine 5'-triphosphate, the implantation of a dual-chamber pacemaker can be useful in decreasing syncopal recurrences.

SYNCOPE SECONDARY TO ORTHOSTATIC HYPOTENSION

Syncope secondary to orthostatic hypotension is more common in the older population and it can be potentiated by the use of antihypertensive drugs, such as vasodilators or diuretics.

In these patients, adequate hydration is crucial.[12] In addition, antihypertensive treatment should be reevaluated. Fludrocortisone administration can be useful. Other nonpharmacologic treatments include application of compression stockings[57] and sleeping with the head of the bed elevated up to 10°.[58,59]

CARDIAC SYNCOPE

There some preliminary considerations with regard to cardiac syncope. The first is that, although there is an apparent cardiac mechanism that can trigger syncope in many cases, there can be some competitive additional mechanisms that can play a role in the development of syncope. This is the case, for example, with syncope occurring at the beginning of paroxysmal supraventricular or ventricular tachycardia. In those cases, in addition to the low cardiac output that can happen at the beginning of the arrhythmia, a reflex mechanism with inappropriate vasodilatation contributes to the transient decrease in cerebral hypoperfusion. The other consideration is that in some patients at risk of presenting ventricular arrhythmias (eg, those with depressed left ventricular ejection fraction or with some channelopathies), even though an arrhythmic origin of syncope has not been documented, an implantable cardioverter defibrillator (ICD) must be implanted to prevent sudden cardiac death irrespective of the cause of syncope.

In any case in which a cardiac cause of syncope is identified, treatment should be directed to the specific mechanism. Those patients in whom syncope can be clearly attributed to a primary bradycardia should receive a pacemaker. In those in whom syncope is clearly related to a supraventricular or ventricular arrhythmia, the arrhythmia should be treated, usually with catheter ablation or drugs.

SYNCOPE AND BIFASCICULAR BLOCK

It is known that the most common cause of syncope in patients with bifascicular block is atrioventricular block.[60] However, other mechanisms can be the cause of syncope in these patients; in particular tachyarrhythmias (ventricular or supraventricular) or RS may be responsible.[61,62]

Some of these patients, by virtue of severe underlying structural heart disease, are at risk of sudden death. It is well known that syncope is associated with increased mortality and appropriate ICD discharges in patients with structural heart disease and impaired left ventricular function.[62] Therefore, it is essential to assess the risk of sudden death and determine whether the implantation of an ICD is indicated. In scenarios in which severe structural disease is not present, treatment is controversial.

An observational study of 323 patients with syncope, bundle branch block, and normal left ventricular function used a 3-phase diagnostic strategy (initial evaluation, electrophysiologic study, and insertion of an ILR). In this series, the cause of syncope could be diagnosed in 267 (82.7%) patients. Although in most cases (202 patients), the cause of the syncope was a bradyarrhythmia, in some cases, other causes, such as ventricular tachycardia or RS, were diagnosed leading to specific treatment, including implantation of an ICD in 19 (5.8%).[63] Thus, in this specific population, current guidelines on cardiac pacing suggest that a strategy consisting of carotid sinus massage and an electrophysiologic study should be followed, and if they are diagnostic, the patient should be treated according to the findings; if those tests are negative, insertion of an ILR is recommended to follow up the patient.[64] However, these guidelines also recommend class IIb PI in selected cases. Recently, Santini and colleagues[65] published the results of a controlled trial in patients with syncope of unknown origin and bundle branch block, in which a pacemaker was implanted in all patients who were randomized to DDD at 60 bpm versus DDI at 30 bpm with a significant decrease in the syncope recurrence rate in those programmed at DDD 60 bpm. Currently, there is an ongoing randomized trial of patients with normal ventricular function that will assess the optimal management strategy for this subset of patients: an empirical permanent pacemaker or prolonged monitoring with an ILR.[66]

REFERENCES

1. Moya A, Sutton R, Ammirati F, et al. Guidelines for the diagnosis and management of syncope (version 2009). Eur Heart J 2009;30:2631–71.
2. Martin TP, Hanusa BH, Kapoor WN. Risk stratification of patients with syncope. Ann Emerg Med 1997;29:459–66.

3. Colivicchi F, Ammirati F, Melina D, et al, OESIL (Osservatorio Epidemiologico sulla Sincope nel Lazio) Study Investigators. Development and prospective validation of a risk stratification system for patients with syncope in the emergency department: the OESIL risk score. Eur Heart J 2003;24:811–9.

4. Del Rosso A, Ungar A, Maggi R, et al. Clinical predictors of cardiac syncope at initial evaluation in patients referred urgently to a general hospital: the EGSYS score. Heart 2008;94:1620–6.

5. Sarasin FP, Hanusa BH, Perneger T, et al. A risk score to predict arrhythmias in patients with unexplained syncope. Acad Emerg Med 2003;10: 1312–7.

6. Quinn J, McDermott D, Stiell I, et al. Prospective validation of the San Francisco Syncope Rule to predict patients with serious outcomes. Ann Emerg Med 2006;47:448–54.

7. Soteriades ES, Evans JC, Larson MG, et al. Incidence and prognosis of syncope. N Engl J Med 2002;347:878–85.

8. Wieling W, Ganzeboom KS, Saul JP. Reflex syncope in children and adolescents. Heart 2004;90: 1094–100.

9. Ganzeboom KS, Colman N, Reitsma JB, et al. Prevalence and triggers of syncope in medical students. Am J Cardiol 2003;91:1006–8.

10. Natale A, Geiger MJ, Maglio C, et al. Recurrence of neurocardiogenic syncope without pharmacologic interventions. Am J Cardiol 1996;77:1001–3.

11. May M, Jordan J. The osmopressor response to water drinking. Am J Physiol Regul Integr Comp Physiol 2011;300:R40–6.

12. Schroeder C, Bush VE, Norcliffe LJ, et al. Water drinking acutely improves orthostatic tolerance in healthy subjects. Circulation 2002;106:2806–11.

13. Wieling W, Colman N, Krediet CT, et al. Nonpharmacological treatment of reflex syncope. Clin Auton Res 2004;14(Suppl 1):62–70.

14. Flevari P, Fountoulaki K, Leftheriotis D, et al. Vasodilation in vasovagal syncope and the effect of water ingestion. Am J Cardiol 2008;102:1060–3.

15. Brignole M, Croci F, Menozzi C, et al. Isometric arm counter-pressure maneuvers to abort impending vasovagal syncope. J Am Coll Cardiol 2002;40: 2053–9.

16. Krediet CT, van Dijk N, Linzer M, et al. Management of vasovagal syncope: controlling or aborting faints by leg crossing and muscle tensing. Circulation 2002;106:1684–9.

17. van Dijk N, Quartieri F, Blanc JJ, et al. Effectiveness of physical counterpressure maneuvers in preventing vasovagal syncope: the Physical Counterpressure Manoeuvres Trial (PC-Trial). J Am Coll Cardiol 2006;48:1652–7.

18. Ector H, Reybrouck T, Heidbüchel H, et al. Tilt training: a new treatment for recurrent neurocardiogenic syncope and severe orthostatic intolerance. Pacing Clin Electrophysiol 1998;2: 193–6.

19. Foglia-Manzillo G, Giada F, Gaggioli G, et al. Efficacy of tilt training in the treatment of neurally mediated syncope. A randomized study. Europace 2004;6:199–204.

20. On YK, Park J, Huh J, et al. Is home orthostatic self-training effective in preventing neurocardiogenic syncope? A prospective and randomized study. Pacing Clin Electrophysiol 2007;30:638–43.

21. Gurevitz O, Barsheshet A, Bar-Lev D, et al. Tilt training: does it have a role in preventing vasovagal syncope? Pacing Clin Electrophysiol 2007;30: 1499–505.

22. Tan MP, Newton JL, Chadwick TJ, et al. Home orthostatic training in vasovagal syncope modifies autonomic tone: results of a randomized, placebo-controlled pilot study. Europace 2010;12: 240–6.

23. Lee TM, Su SF, Chen MF, et al. Usefulness of transdermal scopolamine for vasovagal syncope. Am J Cardiol 1996;78:480–2.

24. Morillo CA, Leitch JW, Yee R, et al. A placebo-controlled trial of intravenous and oral disopyramide for prevention of neurally mediated syncope induced by head-up tilt. J Am Coll Cardiol 1993; 22:1843–8.

25. Biffi M, Boriani G, Sabbatani P, et al. Malignant vasovagal syncope: a randomised trial of metoprolol and clonidine. Heart 1997;77:268–72.

26. Salim MA, Di Sessa TG. Effectiveness of fludrocortisone and salt in preventing syncope recurrence in children: a double-blind, placebo-controlled, randomized trial. J Am Coll Cardiol 2005;45:484–8.

27. Raj SR, Rose S, Ritchie D, et al. The Second Prevention of Syncope Trial (POST II)–a randomized clinical trial of fludrocortisone for the prevention of neurally mediated syncope: rationale and study design. Am Heart J 2006;151:1186.e11–7.

28. Ventura R, Maas R, Zeidler D, et al. A randomized and controlled pilot trial of beta-blockers for the treatment of recurrent syncope in patients with a positive or negative response to head-up tilt test. Pacing Clin Electrophysiol 2002;25:816–21.

29. Sheldon R, Connolly S, Rose S, et al. Prevention of Syncope Trial (POST): a randomized, placebo-controlled study of metoprolol in the prevention of vasovagal syncope. Circulation 2006;113: 1164–70.

30. Sheldon RS, Amuah JE, Connolly SJ, et al. Effect of metoprolol on quality of life in the Prevention of Syncope Trial. J Cardiovasc Electrophysiol 2009; 20:1083–8.

31. Flevari P, Livanis EG, Theodorakis GN, et al. Vasovagal syncope: a prospective, randomized, crossover evaluation of the effect of propranolol, nadolol

and placebo on syncope recurrence and patients well-being. J Am Coll Cardiol 2002;40:499–504.

32. Madrid AH, Ortega J, Rebollo JG, et al. Lack of efficacy of atenolol for the prevention of neurally mediated syncope in a highly symptomatic population: a prospective, double-blind, randomized and placebo-controlled study. J Am Coll Cardiol 2001; 37:554–9.

33. Sheldon R, Morillo CA, Klingenheben T, et al. Age dependent effects of beta-blockers in preventing vasovagal syncope. Circ Arrhythm Electrophysiol 2012;5:920–6.

34. Moya A, Permanyer-Miralda G, Sagrista-Sauleda J, et al. Limitations of head-up tilt test for evaluating the efficacy of therapeutic interventions in patients with vasovagal syncope: results of a controlled study of etilefrine versus placebo. J Am Coll Cardiol 1995;25:65–9.

35. Raviele A, Brignole M, Sutton R, et al. Effect of etilefrine in preventing syncopal recurrence in patients with vasovagal syncope: a double-blind, randomized, placebo-controlled trial. The Vasovagal Syncope International Study. Circulation 1999;99:1452–7.

36. Grubb BP, Karas B, Kosinski D, et al. Preliminary observations on the use of midodrine hydrochloride in the treatment of refractory neurocardiogenic syncope. J Interv Card Electrophysiol 1999;3:139–43.

37. Mitro P, Trajbal D, Rybar AR. Midodrine hydrochloride in the treatment of vasovagal syncope. Pacing Clin Electrophysiol 1999;22:1620–4.

38. Samniah N, Sakaguchi S, Lurie KG, et al. Efficacy and safety of midodrine hydrochloride in patients with refractory vasovagal syncope. Am J Cardiol 2001;88:A7, 80–3.

39. Perez-Lugones A, Schweikert R, Pavia S, et al. Usefulness of midodrine in patients with severely symptomatic neurocardiogenic syncope: a randomized control study. J Cardiovasc Electrophysiol 2001;12:935–8.

40. Qingyou Z, Junbao D, Chaoshu T, et al. The efficacy of midodrine hydrochloride in the treatment of children with vasovagal syncope. J Pediatr 2006;149:777–80.

41. Romme JJ, van Dijk N, Go-Schön IK, et al. Effectiveness of midodrine treatment in patients with recurrent vasovagal syncope not responding to non-pharmacological treatment (STAND-trial). Europace 2011;13:1639–47.

42. Di Girolamo E, Di Iorio C, Sabatini P, et al. Effects of paroxetine hydrochloride, a selective serotonin reuptake inhibitor, on refractory vasovagal syncope: a randomized, double-blind, placebo-controlled study. J Am Coll Cardiol 1999;33:1227–30.

43. Theodorakis GN, Leftheriotis D, Livanis EG, et al. Fluoxetine vs. propranolol in the treatment of

vasovagal syncope: a prospective, randomized, placebo-controlled study. Europace 2006;8:193–8.

44. Romme JJ, Reitsma JB, Black CN, et al. Drugs and pacemakers for vasovagal, carotid sinus and situational syncope. Cochrane Database Syst Rev 2011;(10):CD004194.

45. Connolly SJ, Sheldon R, Roberts RS, et al. The North American Vasovagal Pacemaker Study (VPS). A randomized trial of permanent cardiac pacing for the prevention of vasovagal syncope. J Am Coll Cardiol 1999;33:16–20.

46. Sutton R, Brignole M, Menozzi C, et al. Dual-chamber pacing in the treatment of neurally mediated tilt-positive cardioinhibitory syncope: pacemaker versus no therapy: a multicenter randomized study. The Vasovagal Syncope International Study (VASIS) Investigators. Circulation 2000;102:294–9.

47. Ammirati F, Colivicchi F, Santini M, et al, Syncope Diagnosis and Treatment Study Investigators. Permanent cardiac pacing versus medical treatment for the prevention of recurrent vasovagal syncope: a multicenter, randomized, controlled trial. Circulation 2001;104:52–5.

48. Sud S, Massel D, Klein GJ, et al. The expectation effect and cardiac pacing for refractory vasovagal syncope. Am J Med 2007;120:54–62.

49. Connolly SJ, Sheldon R, Thorpe KE, et al. Pacemaker therapy for prevention of syncope in patients with recurrent severe vasovagal syncope: Second Vasovagal Pacemaker Study (VPS II): a randomized trial. JAMA 2003;289:2224–9.

50. Raviele A, Giada F, Menozzi C, et al. A randomized, double-blind, placebo-controlled study of permanent cardiac pacing for the treatment of recurrent tilt-induced vasovagal syncope. The vasovagal syncope and pacing trial (SYNPACE). Eur Heart J 2004;25:1741–8.

51. Occhetta E, Bortnik M, Audoglio R, et al. Closed loop stimulation in prevention of vasovagal syncope. Inotropy Controlled Pacing in Vasovagal Syncope (INVASY): a multicentre randomized, single blind, controlled study. Europace 2004;6: 538–47.

52. Brignole M, Sutton R, Menozzi C, et al, International Study on Syncope of Uncertain Etiology 2 (ISSUE 2) Group. Lack of correlation between the responses to tilt testing and adenosine triphosphate test and the mechanism of spontaneous neurally mediated syncope. Eur Heart J 2006;27:2232–9.

53. Moya A, Brignole M, Menozzi C, et al, International Study on Syncope of Uncertain Etiology (ISSUE) Investigators. Mechanism of syncope in patients with isolated syncope and in patients with tilt-positive syncope. Circulation 2001;104:1261–7.

54. Deharo JC, Jego C, Lanteaume A, et al. An implantable loop recorder study of highly symptomatic vasovagal patients: the heart rhythm

observed during a spontaneous syncope is identical to the recurrent syncope but not correlated with the head-up tilt test or adenosine triphosphate test. J Am Coll Cardiol 2006;47:587–93.

55. Flammang D, Church TR, De Roy L, et al. Treatment of unexplained syncope: a multicenter, randomized trial of cardiac pacing guided by adenosine 5′-triphosphate testing. Circulation 2012;125:31–6.

56. Brignole M, Menozzi C, Moya A, et al. Pacemaker therapy in patients with neurally mediated syncope and documented asystole: Third International Study on Syncope of Uncertain Etiology (ISSUE-3): a randomized trial. Circulation 2012;125:2566–71.

57. Podoleanu C, Maggi R, Brignole M, et al. Lower limb and abdominal compression bandages prevent progressive orthostatic hypotension in elderly persons: a randomized single-blind controlled study. J Am Coll Cardiol 2006;48:1425–32.

58. Carasca E. Lower limb and abdominal compression bandages prevent progressive orthostatic hypotension in the elderly. A randomized placebo-controlled study. J Am Coll Cardiol 2006;48:1425–32.

59. Ten Harkel AD, Van Lieshout JJ, Wieling W. Treatment of orthostatic hypotension with sleeping in the head-up tilt position, alone and in combination with fludrocortisone. J Intern Med 1992;232:139–45.

60. McAnulty JH, Rahimtoola SH, Murphy E, et al. Natural history of high risk bundle branch block: final report of a prospective study. N Engl J Med 1982;307:137–43.

61. Brignole M, Menozzi C, Moya A, et al. Mechanism of syncope in patients with bundle branch block and negative electrophysiological test. Circulation 2001;104:2045–50.

62. Olshansky B, Poole JE, Johnson G, et al. Syncope predicts the outcome of cardiomyopathy patients: analysis of the SCD-HeFT study. J Am Coll Cardiol 2008;51:1277–82.

63. Moya A, García-Civera R, Croci F, et al. Diagnosis, management, and outcomes of patients with syncope and bundle branch block on behalf of the Bradycardia detection in Bundle Branch Block (B4) study. Eur Heart J 2011;32:1535–41.

64. Brignole M, Auricchio A, Baron-Esquivias G, et al. 2013 ESC Guidelines on cardiac pacing and cardiac resynchronization therapy: the task force on cardiac pacing and resynchronization therapy of the European Society of Cardiology (ESC). Developed in collaboration with the European Heart Rhythm Association (EHRA). Europace 2013;15:1070–118.

65. Santini M, Castro A, Giada F, et al. Prevention of syncope through permanent cardiac pacing in patients with bifascicular block and syncope of unexplained origin: the PRESS study. Circ Arrhythm Electrophysiol 2013;6:101–7.

66. Krahn AD, Morillo CA, Kus T, et al. Empiric pacemaker compared with a monitoring strategy in patients with syncope and bifascicular conduction block–rationale and design of the Syncope: Pacing or Recording in ThE Later Years (SPRITELY) study. Europace 2012;14:1044–8.

The Role of the Syncope Management Unit

Rose Anne Kenny, MD, FRCPI, FRCP, FRCPE, FTCD*,
Ciara Rice, RGN, BNS, Grad Dip Crit Care,
Lisa Byrne, RGN, Postgrad Dip Crit Care

KEYWORDS

- Syncope • Syncope management unit • Cost

KEY POINTS

- Syncope (fainting) is a common and costly health care issue.
- Patients who are managed by a syncope management unit (SMU) have better outcomes, shorter hospital stays, and incur lower health care costs.
- The skill mix of SMU staff includes training in common disorders that cause syncope: cardiovascular, neurologic, geriatric and psychiatric.
- The model of SMU can vary according to the best fit for current practice.

GENERAL FEATURES OF THE SYNCOPE CARE DELIVERY ORGANIZATION

There is no single syncope care delivery model suitable for all environments. The following offers a list of some of the most important features to consider when establishing such an organization:

- The model of care delivery should be appropriate to existing practice and maximize resources and local expertise while ensuring implementation of published practice guidelines.
- Models of care delivery vary from a single one site–one stop syncope facility to a wider multifaceted practice in which several specialists are involved in syncope management. The management strategy should be agreed on and practiced by all practitioners (encompassing a range of specialties) involved in syncope management.
- The age range and symptom characteristics of patients appropriate for syncope investigation should be determined in advance. Some facilities are prepared to evaluate both pediatric and adult patients with syncope, whereas others limit practice to adult or pediatric cases.

- Potential referral sources should be taken into consideration. Referral can be directly from family practitioners, from the accident and emergency department (ED), from hospital admissions, and from patients in institutional settings. The scope of referral source has implications for resources and skill mix.
- In a single dedicated facility the skill mix depends on the specialty designated to take a lead in the development of the facility. There are existing models in which cardiologists (commonly with an interest in cardiac pacing and electrophysiology), neurologists (commonly with an interest in autonomic disorders and/or epilepsy), general physicians, and geriatricians (with an interest in age-related cardiology or falls) each lead syncope facilities. There is no evidence for the superiority of any model.
- The skill mix (ie, the types of professionals/expertise required to staff the facility) required depends on the extent to which screening of referrals occurs before presentation at the facility. If referrals hail directly from the community and/or from the ED, a broader skill mix than just cardiology is required. Under these

This article originally appeared in Cardiac Electrophysiology Clinics, Volume 5, Issue 4, December 2013.
Conflict of Interest: The author has no conflict of interest.
School of Medicine, Trinity College Dublin, Health Sciences Institute, St James's Hospital, Dublin 8, Ireland
* Corresponding author.
E-mail address: rkenny@tcd.ie

circumstances, other differential diagnoses such as epilepsy, neurodegenerative disorders, metabolic disorders, and falls are more likely to be referred.

- It is essential to establish a mechanism through which regular communication can be established with all stakeholders (ie, patients, referring physicians, hospital/clinic management, consultant physicians, nurses, and other allied medical professionals) in order to ensure an ongoing consensus for and understanding of proposed management strategies. This mechanism includes the implications of and implementation of published guidelines. Among the medical profession stakeholders it is important to consider staff members in the ED, neurology department, general medicine service, orthopedic surgery, geriatric medicine, psychiatry, and ear, nose, and throat (ENT) departments.

RATIONALE FOR A SYNCOPE MANAGEMENT UNIT
Syncope: the Challenge

Syncope is a transient self-limiting event characterized by loss of consciousness caused by global cerebral hypoperfusion. Because the onset is rapid, or in some instances sudden, and because the event is of short duration with spontaneous recovery, the diagnosis is challenging and depends on reproduction of symptoms during testing or the ability to capture events during long-term monitoring.

Several characteristics of syncope make it challenging:

- Patients with syncope present to many different specialties: family practitioners, general physicians, cardiologists, geriatricians, neurologists, ED physicians, and ENT specialists.[1]
- Syncope is common, and the lifetime prevalence is high.[2,3]
- Syncopal episodes can be periodic, often with long time intervals between episodes during which no abnormality is noted.
- The differential diagnosis is extensive.
- Although life-threatening causes of syncope are rare, the fear of missing such a diagnosis can lead to long, unnecessary work-ups.[4]
- Despite the ever-increasing diagnostic tools (**Table 1**), the diagnosis may be elusive.
- For most causes of syncope, there is no single test that leads to an incontrovertible diagnosis.
- There is wide variation in practice. In one review of practices in 28 Italian hospitals,

application of carotid sinus massage varied from 0% to 58%, and diagnoses of reflex syncope and cardiac pacing for cardioinhibitory carotid sinus syndrome from 10% to 79% and 1% to 25% respectively, showing wide variation in practice and diagnoses.[5] Therefore a systematic approach, by a dedicated service equipped to evaluate and manage syncope, is recommended. This system can be virtual (an ambulatory a team) or based in a fixed setting, for example in the ED, or a combination of both approaches.[6–8]

Syncope: a Common Problem

Syncope is a common problem that can be debilitating and associated with high health care costs; its incidence is difficult to estimate because of variation in definition, differences in population prevalence, and under-reporting in the general population. The median peak of first syncope is around 15 years with a sharp increase after 70 years. Vasovagal syncope is the commonest cause of syncope for all age groups, but cardiac causes become more common with advancing age. The cumulative incidence of syncope ranges from 5% in women aged 20 to 29 years, up to 50% in women aged 80 years and older. One-third of medical students report at least one syncopal episode in their lifetime. The lifetime cumulative incidence of syncope in women is almost twice that of men. Syncope accounts for up to 1% to 3% of hospital admissions and emergency room (ER) visits and in these settings is associated with cardiovascular comorbidity and cardiovascular pharmacotherapy. In older adults, syncope is a major cause of morbidity and mortality with serious personal and wider health economic costs. Prevalence and incidence figures for syncope in older adults are confounded by an overlap with presentations classified as falls. In addition to injury and increasing dependency, quality-of-life studies consistently show that functional impairment in persons with recurrent syncope is similar to other chronic diseases.[1,9,10]

Only a small fraction of patients with syncope in the general population present to a clinical setting. The prevalence of syncope is 18.1 to 39.7 per 1000 patient years in the general population, of whom 9.3 attend their general practice because of the event and 0.7 present to the ER.[11] General practitioners in the Netherlands refer only 10% of patients with reflex syncope to specialists for further evaluation. In most cases, referrals are made to a neurologist or to a cardiologist.[12] These data may explain the discrepancies in diagnostic rates from history and initial physical

Table 1
Tests and assessments used in diagnosis of syncope

Initial Assessment	Blood Tests	Provocative Tests	Monitoring	Video Recording of Events	Autonomic Function Tests	Tests for Exclusion of Other Diagnoses
History Physical examination, Medications review	Electrolytes Hemoglobin	Exercise stress test Carotid sinus massage	Inpatient telemetry Ambulatory monitoring:	Smart phone	Ewing battery Sweat tests	EEG CT brain
12-lead ECG	White cell count	Tilt-table test: Unprovoked GTN provocation With simultaneous EEG Lower body negative pressure	Holter	—	Heart rate variability: spectral analysis and time domain	MRI brain
Lying and standing BP	Troponin	ATP test	External loop recorder	—	—	—
—	BNP	Drug challenge	Implantable loop recorder	—	—	—
—	HbA1c/glucose Cortisol	Electrophysiology —	Smart phone apps for heart rate and rhythm monitoring	— —	— —	—
—	Autoantibody screen for autonomic neuropathy	—	24 hour (BP) monitoring	—	—	—

Abbreviations: BNP, brain natriuretic peptide; BP, blood pressure; GTN, glyceryl trinitrate; HbA1c, hemoglobin A1c.
Adapted from Krahn A, Andrade JG, Deyell MW. Selective appropriate diagnostic tools for evaluating the patient with syncope/collapse. Prog Cardiovasc Dis 2013;55(4):402–9.

evaluation; the results depend on how typical the history of an episode is, how many practitioners have seen the patient before index presentation, and to which setting the patient presents. In most hospitals without a syncope management unit (SMU), activity for syncope and collapse is based on inpatient rather than elective activity (**Table 2**).[7]

Syncope is Costly

The annual health care cost of syncopal episodes in the United States was estimated in 2005 as $2.4 billion per year for patients who were hospitalized,[8] an amount that equated to 0.1% of the US Federal Government budget for that year, which compares with the treatment of asthma at $2.8 billion, human immunodeficiency virus at $2.1 billion, and chronic obstructive pulmonary disease at $1.9 billion per year.[8,13,14]

In noneconomic terms, syncope is a debilitating symptom. There are at present no financial estimates available, but Linzer and colleagues[9] showed that quality of life is seriously and adversely affected by syncope and, for those of working age, it is frequently associated with loss of employment. Data from the Netherlands concur with this view.[10]

The high cost of syncope evaluation has been documented by several studies during the past 3 decades.[13–28] Because the cause of a given episode of syncope may initially be unclear and because syncope can on occasion be caused by a life-threatening problem such as ventricular arrhythmias, physicians may have a tendency to err on the side of caution by hospitalizing a large proportion of patients with syncope. Between 2000 and 2010, the number of patients hospitalized with a diagnosis of syncope in the United States (ICD-9780.2) increased by 30% from to 462,000 to 602,000.[15] Enhancing the ability of

physicians to identify patients who can safely undergo evaluation of syncope on a less costly outpatient basis may substantially reduce the cost of syncope care.

A targeted approach to the investigation of syncope increases the overall diagnostic yield, thereby improving patient care with the initiation of cause-specific treatment. A targeted approach also reduces unnecessary and expensive hospital admissions (see **Table 2**). Unknown or incorrect diagnoses can lead to unnecessary life-altering consequences, such as loss of personal freedom from the inability to drive a vehicle, or the loss of employment or inappropriate medications (eg, epileptic drug therapy). In an effort to determine the cause of syncope, overuse of diagnostic tools, which consume a significant amount of health care resources, is common.[7,8]

STAKEHOLDERS

Education of all stakeholders about the scope of the SMU and appropriate referral pathways is important. The initial evaluation, if correctly applied, can be delivered by the first professional to come into contact with the patient. Adherence to protocols thereafter ensures correct further assessment by a specialist SMU team. Other disciplines involved in assessment may include cardiology, geriatric medicine, neurology, psychiatry, psychology, and ENT. Services that use systematic application of algorithms may be nurse led with syncope consultant specialist backup.[17,29]

SETTINGS
Syncope Management in the ED

The prevalence of syncope referrals to EDs range from 0.9% to 3.4%, and syncope is the sixth most common cause of hospital admission in adults more than 65 years of age.[7,30–32] Reflex

Table 2
Activities for ICD codes for syncope and collapse in 4 UK inner city teaching hospitals

Activity Data in a Single Year (1999)	Hospital 4 No SMU	Hospital 8 No SMU	Hospital 13 No SMU	Hospital 1 SMU
Number of episodes	837	1099	1249	1150
Mean inpatient length of stay (d)	7.9	17.0	5.2	2.7
Percentage of activity that was emergency	97	97	99	38
Percentage of activity that was elective	3	3	1	62
Percentage of elective activity delivered as outpatient	8	38	0	98

Hospital 1 was the only hospital with an SMU. Emergency and elective episodes represent percentage of activity for syncope and collapse in 1 year.
Adapted from Kenny RA, O'Shea D, Walker HF. Impact of a dedicated syncope and falls facility for older adults on emergency beds. Age Aging 2002;31(4):272–5.

syncope is the most common cause (up to 40%), orthostatic hypotension occurs in 6% to 24%, cardiac syncope 10% to 20%, and psychogenic syncope 1% to 5%. Cardiac causes and orthostatic hypotension are most common in elderly patients.[30,33]

ED physicians evaluating syncope often face the challenge of selecting who requires immediate admission and who can be safely discharged and evaluated as an outpatient. In 2 validation studies[34,35] investigators sought to define the application of ESC guidelines to hospital admission or discharge in the ED and suggested that a significantly higher number of hospital admissions occurred in clinical practice despite many patients not meeting admission criteria. The overuse of hospital admissions could be caused by insufficient training or lack of a care system with expertise. The concept of the syncope unit has evolved as a response to better manage the application of guidelines.

In the Syncope Evaluation in the Emergency Department Study (SEEDS), patients were risk stratified for cardiovascular morbidity and mortality[36] and were divided into high-risk, intermediate-risk, and low-risk groups. Of the 263 patients who consented, 70 high-risk patients were hospitalized for inpatient management and 90 low-risk patients were discharged from the ED. Of 103 intermediate-risk patients, 51 were randomized to evaluation in the ED-based SMU and 52 to standard care.[36] Patients randomized to the SMU received continuous cardiac telemetry for up to 6 hours, orthostatic blood pressure (BP) monitoring and, if indicated, echocardiography, tilt-table testing, and electrophysiologic consultation. The probable diagnosis was established in 67% of patients randomized to the SMU group and in 10% of patients randomized to standard care (*P*<.001). Hospital admission was required for 43% and 98%, respectively. The SEEDS study showed that an ED-based SMU equipped with suitable resources and multidisciplinary teamwork improves diagnostic yield and decreases hospitalization without adversely affecting measured clinical outcomes.[37]

Syncope Management

An Italian study[31] compared 6 hospitals equipped with a syncope unit with 6 matched hospitals without such facilities and enrolled patients who were referred for urgent assessment of syncope. Although there was a reduction in number of tests performed, in particular echocardiograms and magnetic resonance imaging (MRI), there was no difference in the admission rates for patients

reviewed by the syncope unit, possibly because only 11% of potential participants were referred to the syncope unit. Hospitals with syncope units used recommendations by the European Society of Cardiology more effectively.[39] A UK study showed that the SMU reduced length of stay for patients admitted because of syncope and greatly increased elective outpatient activity compared with inpatient activity for syncope.[7]

Syncope Management: Outpatient

Another model of care is an outpatient secondary referral center,[38] which consists of a multidisciplinary grouping including cardiologists and specialist nurses with experience in arrhythmias, falls, and epilepsy. Evidence-based Web algorithms are incorporated in care pathways for the management of patients, with emphasis on differential diagnosis between syncope, epilepsy, and psychogenic episodes.

We have previously published our experience from a falls and syncope service (FASS) in the United Kingdom.[29] FASS has the capability of performing tilt testing, beat-to-beat BP monitoring, and ambulatory monitoring, as well as access to physiotherapy, occupational therapy, and specialist nursing skills. Data was prospectively studied at baseline for demographics, investigations, diagnoses, readmission rates, length of hospital stay, and assessments of gait and balance. After 1 year, a second audit of prospective patients was performed after guideline-based intervention with the introduction of Web-based algorithms. These teaching algorithms were visible in clinical areas as well as educational lectures, providing an outline for history taking, examination, and investigations, along with directions for inpatient versus outpatient management and subspecialty referrals to FASS. The total number of admissions with falls and syncope and rate of readmission within 30 days was reduced. Clinical investigations decreased, with fewer cardiological and neurologic investigations used. Thus, FASS showed evidence-based algorithms for syncope which advised for admission investigations and appropriate referral to FASS resulted in correct diagnosis, effective management, and reduced readmission rates and implemented good medical practices.

PROFESSIONAL SKILL MIX FOR THE SMU

It is probably not appropriate to be dogmatic regarding the training needs of personnel responsible for a dedicated syncope facility. These skills depend on the predetermined requirements of local professional bodies, the level of screening evaluation provided before referral, and the nature of the patient population typically encountered in each setting. Nonetheless, properly trained staff who are familiar with the validated and standardized risk stratification protocols are an important element of the SMU in order to make effective, efficient, and appropriate decisions for hospital admission and subsequent testing.

Staff responsible for the clinical management of the facility should be conversant with the various diagnostic and treatment guidelines for syncope and related disorders and guidelines on epilepsy.[6,39] A structured approach to the management of syncope also expedites clinical audit, patient information systems, service developments, and continuous professional training. We recommend that personnel involved in the initial assessment of patients with syncope should have relevant training in cardiology and components of geriatric medicine, neurology, and ENT. The common disorders that cause syncope or comorbidities associated with syncope drive the necessary training skills, namely hypotensive disorders, cardiac arrhythmias, Parkinson's disease and Parkinson's disease–like syndromes, autonomic neuropathies, diabetes, stroke and transient ischemic attack (TIA), epilepsy, falls, and ENT causes of dizziness. In addition, we emphasize that syncope is predominantly a cardiac or cardiovascular disorder, hence the emphasis on cardiology training (**Box 1**).

ROLE OF SYNCOPE UNIT
Initial Evaluation

During the syncope evaluation, the first goal is to establish a cause. This cause determines treatment, management, and risk of recurrent syncope, and thus achieves the second goal of risk stratification (**Fig. 1**).[6] A thorough history and physical examination can provide the diagnosis in approximately 50% of cases and is the most effective and efficient test at the bedside clinician's disposal.[40,41]

Although most of the diagnostic yield lies with the history, physical examination can also provide important information. Postural vital signs may suggest a diagnosis of orthostatic hypotension. BP measurements should be performed in the supine, sitting, and erect positions.[39] The cardiovascular examination focuses on identifying or excluding structural heart disease. Obstructive lesions such as aortic stenosis or hypertrophic obstructive cardiomyopathy can be identified with auscultation. Left or right ventricular dysfunction should also be evident from a careful precordial examination. The neurologic history and examination may reveal deficits that implicate other causes of transient loss of consciousness, such as seizures or conditions associated with autonomic dysfunction such as Parkinson's disease or Parkinson's disease–like syndromes. Gait and balance should also be assessed; impaired gait during hypotension makes loss of balance and falls more likely. A short cognitive test should be applied if impaired cognition is suspected (prevalent in 20% of patients >80 years old). Although amnesia for loss of consciousness is most common in older adults it also occurs in 20% of young adults with vasovagal syncope.[42] Carotid sinus massage is part of the standard physical examination in adults with syncope (usually >50 years old), and should only be performed with simultaneous phasic BP monitoring and continuous cardiac monitoring.[43] This information provides both diagnostic and risk stratification information.[41] A caveat to this is older patients with noncardiac syncope, for whom the diagnosis is frequently unclear after initial assessment.[44]

A 12-lead electrocardiogram (ECG) should be obtained in every patient with syncope. Although the diagnostic yield of a standard ECG may be as low as 5%,[45] its availability and low cost justify its routine use. The ECG may directly reveal the mechanism of syncope when arrhythmias are documented, or it may provide clues to underlying structural cardiac disorders that may predispose to syncope. An abnormal ECG is a consistent risk factor for an adverse prognosis across multiple studies, making it a crucial element of syncope evaluation.[46,47] Subtle ECG findings can be overlooked, which emphasizes the importance of a careful review of the baseline ECG and explicitly noting pertinent negatives. In particular, relying on automated interpretations and intervals is insufficient when evaluating a patient with syncope. Blood tests are frequently obtained in the initial evaluation of syncope, particularly among patients presenting to the ER. The yield of routine blood tests in the diagnosis of syncope is estimated to be between 2% and 3%. The main role of blood testing is to identify anemia or metabolic abnormalities. Cardiac biomarkers such as increased troponin and brain natriuretic peptide (BNP) have high specificity and low sensitivity for a cardiac cause.[48,49]

CARDIAC IMAGING

Echocardiography can play a central role in the risk stratification of syncope, but should be limited to patients in whom there is a suspicion of structural heart disease.[39] In a prospective study that used routine echocardiography in 155

Box 1
Domains that syncope specialists need to understand

Cardiology

  Disorders

    Neurally mediated syndromes (OH, VVS, CSS/CSH)

    Cardiac arrhythmias

    Hereditary cardiac disorders

    Ischemic cardiac disease

  Implantable cardiac devices (ie, cardiac pacing, defibrillators)

  Tests/technologies:

    Surface electrocardiogram

    Echocardiogram

    Ambulatory cardiac monitoring technology (Holter, external and implantable loops)

    Phasic BP monitoring

    Ambulatory BP

    Cardiac electrophysiology

    Coronary angiography

    Other cardiac imaging techniques

Neurology

  Disorders

    Epilepsy

    Parkinson's, multisystem atrophy, Lewy body dementia, pure autonomic failure

    Peripheral neuropathies

    Autonomic neuropathy

    Concussion

    Traumatic brain injury

    Stroke

  Tests/technologies

    Autonomic function tests

    Heart rate variability tests

    Neuroimaging

    Electroencephalography

Geriatric medicine

  Cognitive function assessment

  Comprehensive geriatric assessment

  Falls assessment and management

Psychiatry

  Mental health assessment

  Cognitive assessment

  Cognitive behavioural therapy

Pharmaceuticals

Abbreviations: CSH, carotid sinus hypersensitivity; CSS, carotid sinus syndrome; OH, orthostatic hypotension; VVS, vasovagal syncope.

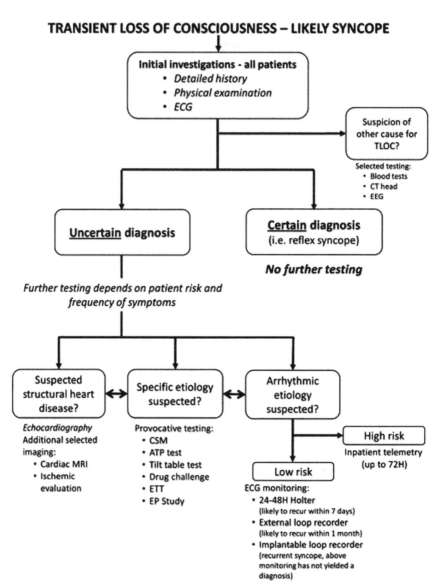

Fig. 1. Guidelines for risk stratification and diagnosis. Approach to the investigation of syncope. If an arrhythmic cause is suspected, high-risk features include those with (1) syncope while supine or on exertion, (2) palpitations with syncope, (3) a family history of sudden death, (4) nonsustained ventricular tachycardia, (5) severe conduction disease at baseline (ie, left bundle branch block or bifascicular block), and (6) ECG abnormalities suggesting an inherited arrhythmia syndrome (ie, long-QT or Brugada pattern). Additional high-risk clinical features that should prompt urgent initial investigations include severe structural heart disease or coronary artery disease. ATP, adenosine triphosphate; CSM, carotid sinus massage; CT, computed tomography; ECG, electrocardiogram; EEG, electroencephalogram; EP, electrophysiology; ETT, exercise treadmill test; TLOC, transient loss of consciousness. (*From* Krahn A, Andrade JG, Deyell MW. Selective appropriate diagnostic tools for evaluating the patient with syncope/collapse. Prog Cardiovasc Dis 2013;55(4):402–9; with permission.)

patients in whom a diagnosis was uncertain after initial evaluation,[50] 54% had normal echocardiograms; 31% had mild to moderate abnormalities that were irrelevant to the syncopal episode; and only 15% had relevant findings, including moderate to severe left ventricular (LV) dysfunction. The quantification of LV dysfunction by echocardiography is an important step in risk stratification and helps guide management (such as electrophysiologic testing). Only in certain circumstances (eg, valvular aortic stenosis) does echocardiography provide a likely cause. Other imaging modalities such as computed tomography (CT), MRI, radionuclide imaging, and cardiac catheterization have a limited role in the investigation of syncope and should only be used in selected cases. MRI is particularly useful in evaluating the right ventricle when there is a suspicion of arrhythmogenic right ventricular cardiomyopathy. Radionuclide imaging and cardiac catheterization are only of use when there is a strong suspicion of ischemia-induced ventricular arrhythmias as a cause for syncope. Most ventricular arrhythmias causing syncope are not related to ischemia.[6]

PROVOCATIVE TESTING

The goal of provocative testing is to either reproduce a syncopal episode or elicit an abnormal arrhythmic or physiologic response that strongly suggests the mechanism of syncope. The use of such tests (including carotid sinus massage, tilt-table testing, ATP test, and electrophysiology study) was recently reviewed in detail by Blanc.[43] Two useful and inexpensive tests, carotid sinus massage and active standing, are extensions of the physical examination. The remaining provocative tests require significant resources and/or are invasive and therefore should be used selectively. Exercise treadmill testing has a low yield (<1%) among unselected patients with syncope[51] but, in selected cases in which syncope occurs during or shortly after exercise,[52] yield is higher.[53]

There are a variety of other cardiac genetic disorders that predispose to exercise-induced tachyarrhythmias and include long QT syndrome, catecholaminergic polymorphic ventricular tachycardia (VT), arrhythmogenic right ventricular cardiomyopathy, and (rarely) exercise-induced anaphylaxis. Exercise testing may also provoke coronary ischemia with or without polymorphic VT or ventricular fibrillation in patients with coronary atherosclerosis or coronary anomalies. Some atrioventricular conduction abnormalities worsen with an increase in heart rate with exercise, and may be severe enough to provoke syncope. However, most patients with exercise-induced conduction abnormalities have an abnormal baseline ECG.[6,54]

HEAD-UP TILT TEST

Orthostatic tolerance (OT) refers to the ability to maintain cardiovascular stability when upright, against the hydrostatic effects of gravity, and hence to maintain cerebral perfusion and prevent syncope. Various techniques are available to assess OT and the effects of gravitational stress on the circulation, typically by reproducing a presyncopal event (near-fainting episode) in a controlled laboratory environment. The time

and/or degree of stress required to provoke this response provide the measure of OT. Any technique used to determine OT should enable distinction between patients with orthostatic intolerance (of various causes) and asymptomatic control subjects; be highly reproducible, enabling evaluation of therapeutic interventions; and avoid invasive procedures, which are known to impair OT.[55] Head-upright tilt testing (HUTT) was first described for the diagnosis of syncope in the late 1980s.[56] One of the main advantages of tilt testing is witnessed reproduction of symptoms in a controlled, monitored environment. Furthermore, it has some therapeutic benefit in that the frequency of syncopal events declines after tilt testing. Since its seminal description, it has been used to assess OT in patients with syncope of unknown cause, as well as in healthy subjects to study postural cardiovascular reflexes.[57–66] Tilting protocols comprise 3 categories: passive tilt, passive tilt accompanied by pharmacologic provocation (sublingual nitrate[63,65,68–70] or, less commonly, isoprenaline[66,67,70]), and passive tilt with combined lower body negative pressure. The main drawback of HUTT is its inability to invoke presyncope in all individuals undergoing the test, and corresponding low sensitivity. The main drawback of pharmacologic approaches are increases in sensitivity at the cost of unacceptable decreases in specificity. However, sensitivity and specificity are higher in older adults.[27,29,33,35,42,44]

ELECTROCARDIOGRAPHIC MONITORING

Electrocardiographic monitoring is indicated if there is a clinical suspicion of an arrhythmic cause of syncope. The best test for a diagnosis is symptom-rhythm correlation, which can only take place with simultaneous monitoring. Among patients older than 40 years with recurrent syncope and a normal initial evaluation and ECG, arrhythmias (including asystole) are identified as the likely cause in up to 50% of cases, although these arrhythmias most commonly have a reflex origin as in the cardioinhibitory component of neurally mediated syncope.[71,73]

Cardiac causes of syncope are more likely in older patients. The presence of some significant arrhythmias, defined as prolonged asystole, or high-grade second-degree atrioventricular (AV) block or third-degree AV block, rapid supraventricular tachycardias (SVT), or VT, when correlated with symptoms, is considered as diagnostic.[74–77]

In contrast, the absence of arrhythmia during monitoring while a syncopal episode occurs is also helpful and virtually excludes an arrhythmic cause. With the exception of some abnormalities, such as an asystolic pause of more than 3 seconds or an episode of SVT/VT, the interpretation of asymptomatic arrhythmias detected on continuous monitoring is controversial.[77,78]

Monitoring is indicated in patients with significant structural heart disease, baseline ECG abnormalities, palpitations at the time of syncope, absence of a prodrome with prompt recovery, or a strong family history of sudden death or arrhythmia.

INPATIENT TELEMETRY

In subjects deemed to be at high risk for an arrhythmic cause, the yield of up to 72 hours of inpatient monitoring is 16%.[79]

HOLTER MONITORING

Holter monitoring involves continuous ECG monitoring of typically 3 leads (or 12 leads) for a period of at least 24 hours. In several large studies only 4% of patients had symptoms during the monitoring period.[80,81]

The overall yield of detecting an arrhythmic cause for syncope is as low as 1% to 2% among unselected patients using Holter recordings in up to 15%.[80] However, Holter monitoring can exclude an arrhythmic cause when no rhythm abnormality is documented at the time of symptoms.[6,82]

EXTERNAL LOOP RECORDERS

External loop recorders have a memory loop that continuously records cardiac activity using a single-lead ECG rhythm strip. Examples include the King of Hearts monitor (CardioComm Solutions Inc), the Instromedix Inc device, and Mobile Cardiac Outpatient Telemetry (CardioNet), which can transmit data to a monitoring center when triggered automatically.[83,84] The overall yield for diagnosing an arrhythmia is 12% in patients with unexplained syncope, with an arrhythmia being excluded as a mechanism in a further 12%. However, compliance is a significant issue.[85]

A novel ambulatory monitor consisting of an adhesive patch containing both a solid-state recorder and single pair of electrodes is now available (Zio, iRhythm Technologies Inc, San Francisco, CA). It is capable of beat-to-beat recording for up to 14 days and can also be triggered by the patient. Its inherent advantages are its ease of use and patient compliance. Its role in the investigation of syncope is uncertain at present, although the diagnostic yield among patients with suspected arrhythmias (including syncope) discharged from the ER was 64% in a recent study.[86]

IMPLANTABLE LOOP RECORDERS

The implantable loop recorder is a device that, as with external loop recorders, records and deletes a single-lead ECG continuously, but is placed subcutaneously. Two devices are available: Reveal (Medtronic Inc) and Confirm (St Jude Medical Inc).[71–74]

The choice of monitoring device depends on the anticipated frequency of episodes based on history of frequency of events. Therefore, Holter monitoring is used in patients in whom syncope is expected to recur within a week. External loop recorders are used when syncope is expected to recur within 1 month. Implantable devices are used in patients with less frequent episodes but a strong suspicion of arrhythmia.

EXCLUSION OF OTHER CAUSES FOR TRANSIENT LOSS OF CONSCIOUSNESS

Metabolic disorders are typically easy to distinguish from syncope by history and directed laboratory testing. It can be difficult to distinguish between seizures and syncope, even after a careful history and physical examination. Routine neurologic investigation is indicated to investigate new focal neurologic signs or head trauma. The yield of the electroencephalogram (EEG) among undifferentiated patients with syncope is only 1.5%, which is similar to the background rate of epileptiform discharges in the general population.[87] Thus EEGs requested in the setting of syncope have a low yield.[88]

CT of the head or MRI are commonly performed (up to 50%) among patients presenting to the ER with syncope. However, its diagnostic yield is also extremely low. In the largest study evaluating the use of CT head among patients with transient loss of consciousness, only 5% had a cause determined, such as stroke or hemorrhage. All of these patients had focal neurologic findings or evidence of trauma.[89,90] Carotid Doppler ultrasound also need not be performed in patients with syncope. Carotid stenosis affects the anterior cerebral circulation and does not typically produce transient loss of consciousness.

Focal neurologic symptoms can occur during syncope in the presence of significant carotid artery stenosis.[91] Carotid Doppler studies are indicated in such circumstances. In a recent series from our group, almost 6% of patients who did not have carotid stenosis had focal neurology during syncope, and 6% of patients attending our ED with stroke or TIA had a history of presyncope or syncope associated with the event. In such instances a dual neurologic and cardiovascular approach is appropriate and important because an incorrect assumption that the diagnosis is TIA rather than syncope could result in overzealous treatment to further reduce BP and increase susceptibility to syncope.

SUMMARY

Syncope is common and costly, and presentation to acute hospital services is increasing. In general, the evaluation is haphazard and unstratified, and delivered by many specialties such as cardiology, neurology, geriatric, and emergency medicine. Syncope is predominantly the domain of cardiology or specialist syncope personnel. There is a wide variation in diagnostic tests and attributable diagnoses, coupled with variation in prevalence of unexplained syncope. A structured approach by an SMU results in reduced hospital admissions, better application of guideline recommendations, more accurate diagnosis, lower rates of unexplained events, and improved quality of life.

REFERENCES

1. Kenny RA, Bhangu J, King-Kallimanis BL. Epidemiology of syncope/collapse in younger and older Western patient populations. Prog Cardiovasc Dis 2013;55(4):357–63.
2. Ganzeboom KS, Mairuhu G, Reitsma JB, et al. Lifetime cumulative incidence of syncope in the general population: a study of 549 Dutch subjects aged 35-60 years. J Cardiovasc Electrophysiol 2006;17(11):1172–6.
3. Olde Nordkamp LR, van Dijk N, Ganzeboom KS, et al. Syncope prevalence in the ED compared to general practice and population: a strong selection process. Am J Emerg Med 2009;27(3): 271–9.
4. Landman J. Regret and elation following action and inaction: affective responses to positive versus negative outcomes. Pers Soc Psychol Bull 1987; 13(4):524–36.
5. Disertori M, Brignole M, Menozzi C, et al. Management of patients with syncope referred urgently to general hospitals. Europace 2003;5(3):283–91.
6. Krahn A, Andrade JG, Deyell MW. Selective appropriate diagnostic tools for evaluating the patient with syncope/collapse. Prog Cardiovasc Dis 2013;55(4): 402–9.
7. Kenny RA, O'Shea D, Walker HF. Impact of a dedicated syncope and falls facility for older adults on emergency beds. Age Ageing 2002;31(4):272–5.
8. Sun BC, Emond JA, Camargo CA. Direct medical costs of syncope-related hospitalizations in the United States. Am J Cardiol 2005;95(5):668–71.
9. Linzer M, Pontinen M, Gold DT, et al. Impairment of physical and psychosocial function in recurrent syncope. J Clin Epidemiol 1991;44(10): 1037–43.
10. van Dijk N, Sprangers MA, Boer KR, et al. Quality of life within one year following presentation after transient loss of consciousness. Am J Cardiol 2007; 100(4):672–6.
11. Ganzeboom KS, Colman N, Reitsma JB, et al. Prevalence and triggers of syncope in medical students. Am J Cardiol 2003;91(8):1006–8 A8.
12. Colman N, Nahm K, Ganzeboom KS, et al. Epidemiology of reflex syncope. Clin Auton Res 2004; 14(Suppl 1):9–17.
13. Calkins H, Byrne M, el-Atassi R, et al. The economic burden of unrecognized vasodepressor syncope. Am J Med 1993;95(5):473–9.
14. Ammirati F, Colaceci R, Cesario A, et al. Management of syncope: clinical and economic impact of a syncope unit. Europace 2008;10(4):471–6.
15. Jhanjee R, Can I, Benditt DG. Syncope. Dis Mon 2009;55(9):532–85.
16. Brignole M, Ungar A, Bartoletti A, et al. Standardized-care pathway vs. usual management of syncope patients presenting as emergencies at general hospitals. Europace 2006;8(8): 644–50.
17. Brignole M, Ungar A, Casagranda I, et al. Prospective multicentre systematic guideline-based management of patients referred to the syncope units of general hospitals. Europace 2010;12(1): 109–18.
18. Casini-Raggi V, Bandinelli G, Lagi A. Vasovagal syncope in emergency room patients: analysis of a metropolitan area registry. Neuroepidemiology 2002;21(6):287–91.
19. Del Greco M, Cozzio S, Scillieri M, et al. Diagnostic pathway of syncope and analysis of the impact of guidelines in a district general hospital. The ECSIT study (epidemiology and costs of syncope in Trento). Ital Heart J 2003;4(2):99–106.
20. Eagle KA, Black HR. The impact of diagnostic tests in evaluating patients with syncope. Yale J Biol Med 1983;56(1):1–8.
21. Farwell D, Sulke N. How do we diagnose syncope? J Cardiovasc Electrophysiol 2002;13 (Suppl 1):S9–13.
22. Farwell DJ, Freemantle N, Sulke AN. Use of implantable loop recorders in the diagnosis and management of syncope. Eur Heart J 2004; 25(14):1257–63.
23. Gordon TA, Moodie DS, Passalacqua M, et al. A retrospective analysis of the cost-effective workup of syncope in children. Cleve Clin J Med 1987;54(5):391–4.
24. Kapoor WN, Karpf M, Maher Y, et al. Syncope of unknown origin. The need for a more cost-effective

approach to its diagnosis evaluation. JAMA 1982; 247(19):2687–91.

25. Krahn AD, Klein GJ, Yee R, et al. Cost implications of testing strategy in patients with syncope: randomized assessment of syncope trial. J Am Coll Cardiol 2003;42(3):495–501.

26. Mendu ML, McAvay G, Lampert R, et al. Yield of diagnostic tests in evaluating syncopal episodes in older patients. Arch Intern Med 2009;169(14): 1299–305.

27. Nyman JA, Krahn AD, Bland PC, et al. The costs of recurrent syncope of unknown origin in elderly patients. Pacing Clin Electrophysiol 1999;22(9): 1386–94.

28. Schillinger M, Domanovits H, Mullner M, et al. Admission for syncope: evaluation, cost and prognosis. Wien Klin Wochenschr 2000;112(19): 835–41.

29. Parry SW, Frearson R, Steen N, et al. Evidence-based algorithms and the management of falls and syncope presenting to acute medical services. Clin Med 2008;8(2):157–62.

30. Sun BC, Emond JA, Camargo CA. Characteristics and admission patterns of patients presenting with syncope to U.S. emergency departments, 1992-2000. Acad Emerg Med 2004;11(10):1029–34.

31. Brignole M, Disertori M, Menozzi C, et al. Management of syncope referred urgently to general hospitals with and without syncope units. Europace 2003;5(3):293–8.

32. Blanc JJ, L'Her C, Touiza A, et al. Prospective evaluation and outcome of patients admitted for syncope over a 1 year period. Eur Heart J 2002; 23(10):815–20.

33. Kenny RA. Syncope in the elderly: diagnosis, evaluation, and treatment. J Cardiovasc Electrophysiol 2003;14(Suppl 9):S74–7.

34. Bartoletti A, Fabiani P, Adriani P, et al. Hospital admission of patients referred to the Emergency Department for syncope: a single-hospital prospective study based on the application of the European Society of Cardiology Guidelines on syncope. Eur Heart J 2006;27(1):83–8.

35. McCarthy F, McMahon CG, Geary U, et al. Management of syncope in the Emergency Department: a single hospital observational case series based on the application of European Society of Cardiology Guidelines. Europace 2009;11(2): 216–24.

36. Shen WK, Decker WW, Smars PA, et al. Syncope Evaluation in the Emergency Department Study (SEEDS): a multidisciplinary approach to syncope management. Circulation 2004;110(24):3636–45.

37. Shen WK, Traub SJ, Decker WW. Syncope management unit: evolution of the concept and practice implementation. Prog Cardiovasc Dis 2013; 55(4):382–9.

38. Petkar S, Bell W, Rice N, et al. Initial experience with a rapid access blackouts triage clinic. Clin Med 2011;11(1):11–6.

39. Moya A, Sutton R, Ammirati F, et al. Guidelines for the diagnosis and management of syncope (version 2009): the Task Force for the Diagnosis and Management of Syncope of the European Society of Cardiology (ESC). Eur Heart J 2009;30(21):2631–71.

40. Brignole M, Menozzi C, Bartoletti A, et al. A new management of syncope: prospective systematic guideline-based evaluation of patients referred urgently to general hospitals. Eur Heart J 2006; 27(1):76–82.

41. van Dijk N, Boer KR, Colman N, et al. High diagnostic yield and accuracy of history, physical examination, and ECG in patients with transient loss of consciousness in FAST: the Fainting Assessment study. J Cardiovasc Electrophysiol 2008;19(1):48–55.

42. O'Dwyer C, Bennett K, Langan Y. Amnesia for loss of consciousness is common in vasovagal syncope. Europace 2011;13(7):1040–5.

43. Blanc JJ. Clinical laboratory testing: what is the role of tilt-tablet testing, active standing test, carotid massage, electrophysiological testing and ATP test in the syncope evaluation? Prog Cardiovasc Dis 2013;55(4):418–24.

44. Parry SW, Kenny RA. Drop attacks in older adults: systematic assessment has a high diagnostic yield. J Am Geriatr Soc 2005;53(1):74–8.

45. Brignole M, Alboni P, Benditt DG, et al, The Task Force on Syncope, European Society of Cardiology. Guidelines on management (diagnosis and treatment) of syncope–update 2004. Eur Heart J 2004;25(22):2054–72.

46. Colivicchi F, Ammirati F, Melina D, et al. Development and prospective validation of a risk stratification system for patients with syncope in the emergency department: the OESIL risk score. Eur Heart J 2003;24(9):811–9.

47. Rose MS, Koshman ML, Ritchie D, et al. The development and preliminary validation of a scale measuring the impact of syncope on quality of life. Europace 2009;11(10):1369–74.

48. Hing R, Harris R. Relative utility of serum troponin and the OESIL score in syncope. Emerg Med Australas 2005;17(1):31–8.

49. Pfister R, Hagemeister J, Esser S, et al. NT-pro-BNP for diagnostic and prognostic evaluation in patients hospitalized for syncope. Int J Cardiol 2012;155(2):268–72.

50. Sarasin FP, Junod AF, Carballo D, et al. Role of echocardiography in the evaluation of syncope: a prospective study. Heart 2002;88(4):363–7.

51. Kapoor WN. Evaluation and outcome of patients with syncope. Medicine (Baltimore) 1990;69(3): 160–75.

52. Providencia R, Silva J, Mota P, et al. Transient loss of consciousness in young adults. Int J Cardiol 2011;152(1):139–43.

53. Doi A, Tsuchihashi K, Kyuma M, et al. Diagnostic implications of modified treadmill and head-up tilt tests in exercise-related syncope: comparative studies with situational and/or vasovagal syncope. Can J Cardiol 2002;18(9):960–6.

54. Woelfel AK, Simpson RJ, Gettes LS, et al. Exercise-induced distal atrioventricular block. J Am Coll Cardiol 1983;2(3):578–81.

55. Stevens PM. Cardiovascular dynamics during orthostasis and the influence of intravascular instrumentation. Am J Cardiol 1966;17(2):211–8.

56. Kenny RA, Ingram A, Bayliss J, et al. Head-up tilt: a useful test for investigating unexplained syncope. Lancet 1986;1(8494):1352–5.

57. Brignole M, Alboni P, Benditt D, et al. Guidelines on management (diagnosis and treatment) of syncope. Eur Heart J 2001;22(15):1256–306.

58. Brignole M, Alboni P, Benditt D, et al. Part 2. Diagnostic tests and treatment: summary of recommendations. Europace 2001;3(4):261–8.

59. Grubb BP, Temesy-Armos P, Hahn H, et al. Utility of upright tilt-table testing in the evaluation and management of syncope of unknown origin. Am J Med 1991;90(1):6–10.

60. Kapoor WN, Smith MA, Miller NL. Upright tilt testing in evaluating syncope: a comprehensive literature review. Am J Med 1994;97(1):78–88.

61. Benditt DG, Ferguson DW, Grubb BP, et al. Tilt table testing for assessing syncope. American College of Cardiology. J Am Coll Cardiol 1996;28(1):263–75.

62. Aerts AJ. Nitrate stimulated tilt testing: clinical considerations. Clin Auton Res 2003;13(6):403–5.

63. Athanasos P, Sydenham D, Latte J, et al. Vasodepressor syncope and the diagnostic accuracy of the head-up tilt test with sublingual glyceryl trinitrate. Clin Auton Res 2003;13(6):453–5.

64. Sheldon R. Evaluation of a single-stage isoproterenol-tilt table test in patients with syncope. J Am Coll Cardiol 1993;22(1):114–8.

65. Barron H, Fitzpatrick A, Goldschlager N. Head-up tilt testing: do we need to give an added push? Am J Med 1995;99(6):689–90.

66. Kapoor WN, Brant N. Evaluation of syncope by upright tilt testing with isoproterenol. A nonspecific test. Ann Intern Med 1992;116(5):358–63.

67. Janosik DL, Genovely H, Fredman C, et al. Discrepancy between head-up tilt test results utilizing different protocols in the same patient. Am Heart J 1992;123(2):538–41.

68. Wahbha MM, Morley CA, al-Shamma YM, et al. Cardiovascular reflex responses in patients with unexplained syncope. Clin Sci (Lond) 1989;77(5):547–53.

69. Del Rosso A, Bartoli P, Bartoletti A, et al. Shortened head-up tilt testing potentiated with sublingual nitroglycerin in patients with unexplained syncope. Am Heart J 1998;135(4):564–70.

70. Kurbaan AS, Franzen AC, Bowker TJ, et al. Usefulness of tilt test-induced patterns of heart rate and blood pressure using a two-stage protocol with glyceryl trinitrate provocation in patients with syncope of unknown origin. Am J Cardiol 1999;84(6):665–70.

71. Solano A, Menozzi C, Maggi R, et al. Incidence, diagnostic yield and safety of the implantable loop-recorder to detect the mechanism of syncope in patients with and without structural heart disease. Eur Heart J 2004;25(13):1116–9.

72. Brignole M, Sutton R, Menozzi C, et al. Early application of an implantable loop recorder allows effective specific therapy in patients with recurrent suspected neurally mediated syncope. Eur Heart J 2006;27(9):1085–92.

73. Pezawas T, Stix G, Kastner J, et al. Implantable loop recorder in unexplained syncope: classification, mechanism, transient loss of consciousness and role of major depressive disorder in patients with and without structural heart disease. Heart 2008;94(4):e17.

74. Ermis C, Zhu AX, Pham S, et al. Comparison of automatic and patient-activated arrhythmia recordings by implantable loop recorders in the evaluation of syncope. Am J Cardiol 2003;92(7):815–9.

75. Parry SW, Steen IN, Baptist M, et al. Amnesia for loss of consciousness in carotid sinus syndrome: implications for presentation with falls. J Am Coll Cardiol 2005;45(11):1840–3.

76. Davison J, Brady S, Kenny RA. 24-Hour ambulatory electrocardiographic monitoring is unhelpful in the investigation of older persons with recurrent falls. Age Ageing 2005;34(4):382–6.

77. Krahn AD, Klein GJ, Yee R, et al. Detection of asymptomatic arrhythmias in unexplained syncope. Am Heart J 2004;148(2):326–32.

78. Moya A, Brignole M, Sutton R, et al. Reproducibility of electrocardiographic findings in patients with suspected reflex neurally-mediated syncope. Am J Cardiol 2008;102(11):1518–23.

79. Croci F, Brignole M, Alboni P, et al. The application of a standardized strategy of evaluation in patients with syncope referred to three syncope units. Europace 2002;4(4):351–5.

80. Bass EB, Curtiss EI, Arena VC, et al. The duration of Holter monitoring in patients with syncope. Is 24 hours enough? Arch Intern Med 1990;150(5):1073–8.

81. Linzer M, Yang EH, Estes NA, et al. Diagnosing syncope. Part 2: unexplained syncope. Clinical Efficacy Assessment Project of the American

College of Physicians. Ann Intern Med 1997; 127(1):76–86.

82. Gibson TC, Heitzman MR. Diagnostic efficacy of 24-hour electrocardiographic monitoring for syncope. Am J Cardiol 1984;53(8):1013–7.

83. Rothman SA, Laughlin JC, Seltzer J, et al. The diagnosis of cardiac arrhythmias: a prospective multi-center randomized study comparing mobile cardiac outpatient telemetry versus standard loop event monitoring. J Cardiovasc Electrophysiol 2007;18(3):241–7.

84. Linzer M, Pritchett EL, Pontinen M, et al. Incremental diagnostic yield of loop electrocardiographic recorders in unexplained syncope. Am J Cardiol 1990;66(2):214–9.

85. Schuchert A, Maas R, Kretzschmar C, et al. Diagnostic yield of external electrocardiographic loop recorders in patients with recurrent syncope and negative tilt table test. Pacing Clin Electrophysiol 2003;26(9):1837–40.

86. Turakhia M, Hoang D, Zimetbaum P, et al. Clinical experience and diagnostic yield from a national registry of 14-day ambulatory ECG patch monitoring free. J Am Coll Cardiol 2012;59(13s1):E646.

87. Abubakr A, Wambacq I. The diagnostic value of EEGs in patients with syncope. Epilepsy Behav 2005;6(3):433–4.

88. McCarthy A, Neligan A, McNamara B. The role of the electroencephalogram as a tool for the investigation of syncope. Ir J Med Sci 2012;181(4):571–2.

89. Grossman SA, Fischer C, Bar JL, et al. The yield of head CT in syncope: a pilot study. Intern Emerg Med 2007;2(1):46–9.

90. O'Dwyer C, Hade D, Fan CW, et al. How well are the European Society of Cardiology (ESC) guidelines adhered to in patients with syncope? Ir Med J 2010;103(1):11–4.

91. Ryan D, Rice C, Harbison J, et al. Neurological events during vasovagal syncope. 2013. Submitted for publication.

Index

Note: Page numbers of article titles are in **boldface** type.

A

Adenosine
  in syncope and idiopathic AV block, 445–446
Adolescent(s)
  syncope in, **397–409**. *See also* Syncope, in children and adolescents
AECG monitoring. *See* Ambulatory electrocardiographic (AECG) monitoring
Ambulatory electrocardiographic (AECG) monitoring
  in syncope, **361–366**. *See also* Implantable loop recorders (ILRs)
American Heart Association (AHA)
  recommendations for driving with syncope, 470
ANS assessment. *See* Autonomic nervous system (ANS) assessment
Aortic stenosis
  syncope in children and adolescents due to, 401
Arrhythmia(s). *See also specific types, e.g.,* Bradyarrhythmia
  syncope due to, 389
    in children and adolescents, 401–402
Arrhythmogenic right ventricular cardiomyopathy (ARVC)
  in athletes
    as warning symptom of SCD, 426
ARVC. *See* Arrhythmogenic right ventricular cardiomyopathy (ARVC)
Atherosclerotic coronary disease
  in athletes
    as warning symptom of SCD, 426–427
Athlete(s)
  SCD in
    syncope as warning symptom of, **423–432**. *See also* Syncope, in athletes
  syncope in
    as warning symptom of SCD, **423–432**. *See also* Syncope, in athletes
Atrioventricular (AV) block
  idiopathic. *See* Idiopathic atrioventricular (AV) block
Autonomic nervous system (ANS) assessment
  in syncope evaluation
    function tests, 359
Autonomic syncope
  in children and adolescents, 398–400
    blood injury phobia, 400
    breath-holding spells, 400
    dysautonomic syncope, 399
    fainting lark, 400

  neurocardiogenic syncope, 398–399
  POTS, 399–400
AV block. *See* Atrioventricular (AV) block

B

Bifascicular block
  syncope and
    management of, 478
Blood injury phobia
  in children and adolescents, 400
Bradyarrhythmia
  EP study of, 369–373
Breath-holding spells
  in children and adolescents, 400
Brugada syndrome
  syncope and
    in children and adolescents, 402
    ECG of, 436–437

C

Canadian Cardiovascular Society (CCS) risk of harm formula
  syncope while driving–related, 467
Canadian Medical Association Driver's guide
  in determining medical fitness for driving with syncope, 469
Cardiac arrhythmias. *See also specific types, e.g.,* Bradyarrhythmia
  syncope due to, 389
Cardiac output (CO)
  low
    syncope and, 344
Cardiac pacing
  in syncope management, 477–478
Cardiac syncope
  in children and adolescents, 400–402
    causes of
      arrhythmias, 401–402
      obstructive, 400–401
      primary myocardiac dysfunction, 401
    management of, 478
Cardiogenic syncope
  in athletes
    as warning symptom of SCD, 424–429
Cardioneuroablation
  in syncope management in children and adolescents, 405

http://dx.doi.org/10.1016/S0733-8651(15)00055-7
0733-8651/15/$ – see front matter © 2015 Elsevier Inc. All rights reserved.